D0097964

Sports Rehabilitation and the Human Spirit

"The impeded stream is the one that sings."

— Wendell Berry

SPORTS REHABILITATION AND THE HUMAN SPIRIT

How the Landmark Program at the Lakeshore Foundation Rebuilds Bodies and Restores Lives

By Anita Smith with Randall Williams
Epilogue by Michael E. Stephens

NewSouth Books
Montgomery

NewSouth Books
105 S. Court Street
Montgomery, AL 36104

 Published in the United States by NewSouth Books, a division of NewSouth, Inc., Montgomery, Alabama.

Library of Congress Cataloging-in-Publication Data

Smith, Anita.
Sports rehabilitation and the human spirit : how the landmark program at the Lakeshore Foundation rebuilds bodies and restores lives /
by Anita Smith with Randall Williams ; epilogue by Michael E. Stephens.

p. ; cm.

ISBN 978-1-58838-295-5 — ISBN 1-58838-295-8 (hardcover)
ISBN 978-1-58838-296-2 — ISBN 1-58838-296-6 (paperback)

I. Williams, Randall, 1951- II. Title.
[DNLM: 1. Lakeshore Foundation. 2. Rehabilitation Centers—history. 3. Disabled Persons—psychology. 4. Disabled Persons—rehabilitation. 5. Sports Medicine—methods. WB 29]

617.1'027—dc23
2012050541

A limited deluxe hardcover edition was also produced.

All images courtesy the author
except page 255, top, by Matt Furman, photographer.

Design by Randall Williams

Printed in the United States of America
by Edwards Brothers Malloy

To all those who have served,
and will serve, at the Lakeshore Foundation;

And to all those who have been served by,
and will be served by, the Lakeshore Foundation;

All touched by a unique spirit.

CONTENTS

Introduction

The Spirit of Lakeshore

Anita Smith

Mike Stephens and I first came to know one another in the mid-1970s, when he had just been named executive director of Lakeshore Hospital and I was a medical reporter for the *Birmingham News.*

This was an exciting time for Lakeshore, early in its transition from a longtime tuberculosis sanatorium into a rehabilitation campus with facilities and programs to aid those with physical disabilities.

Through the years I wrote a lot about Lakeshore. Then, after I left the newspaper business to do other types of writing, I told Mike that if he ever decided to participate in a book about Lakeshore, I would love to work with him on it. Having seen so many lives enhanced, even transformed, on its campus, I thought of the Lakeshore Rehabilitation Complex as a magical place.

During the years when I was beginning my new career of writing books, the Lakeshore story was mushrooming in scope and impact. I was aware that Mike was at the helm of major mid-1980s initiatives that drove Lakeshore forward by leaps and bounds. Mike became the founder of the Lakeshore Foundation, which was given the mission of providing prototype sports, recreation, and fitness programs for those with physical disabilities. Mike also founded and led a multistate rehabilitation company, ReLife, Inc.—with Lakeshore Hospital as its flagship facility (there were many other ReLife facilities).

So it was that the time eventually came when Mike was ready for a book about Lakeshore. By then he was not involved in day-to-day operations of either a rehabilitation company or the Lakeshore campus. However, he was still very supportive of Lakeshore and still served on the Foundation's board of directors.

Mike told me that he knew the time had come to do a Lakeshore book when he observed a touching scene that brought home how the Lakeshore Foundation was helping physically disabled individuals assimilate into mainstream life and interact comfortably with the able-bodied. He told me: "There was this little boy in a wheelchair—around five years old. He was having the best time that day participating in events in the Foundation's fieldhouse. And alongside him was his able-bodied brother, a few years older, who also was participating and having fun. It was all so natural. Through Lakeshore's sports and recreation programs, the boy with a physical disability had found his comfort zone. And his able-bodied brother also felt at home. Anita, that's what it's all about—helping one person at a time, but also helping society to bridge gaps between the physically disabled and the able-bodied."

OLD HABITS ARE hard to break. The first 20 years of my writing career were spent as a newspaperwoman facing deadline after deadline.

By the time Mike and I started work on the Lakeshore book, I had been out of the newspaper business for another 20 years and had written several books. The books were nonfiction, heavy on research and interviews, and they tended to take a long time. But still there were occasions when I felt the sudden need to rush toward a deadline—just as I had done during my newspaper days—even if there wasn't one.

Mike and I had been working on the Lakeshore project for a few months. He was providing me with extensive background and was guiding me as I conducted initial interviews and research.

One afternoon after I had completed some interviews with individuals who had been helped by Lakeshore, I felt that deadline intensity, that it was time to start writing. I said so to Mike.

He was appalled. He knew that I had learned a lot about Lakeshore. However, he also knew that there was a lot—particularly relevant to the broader, developing Lakeshore story of recent years—that I *did not yet know.* Also, there was something else about my rushing that bothered Mike badly. He believed, rightfully so, that what I needed to understand were not just the *facts* of this Lakeshore story, but also *the feelings, the spirit.*

He was right.

Mike himself had incurred a severe physical disability while in his mid-twenties; by the time we started working on this book, he had been dealing with the aftermath for three and a half decades. Through his firsthand experience Mike had gained painful insights into the feelings, the hardships, the obstacles, the needs, and, oh yes, the *positive potential* of individuals with physical disabilities. Mike's insights had given him a special edge in guiding Lakeshore to lend life-changing helping hands to so many.

Since Mike had actually *lived* the story of one with a physical disability, and continued to live such a story, he knew that the stories of those I was interviewing were deep and complex—requiring my taking time, care, and reflection.

He said in no uncertain terms that I couldn't possibly understand enough yet to start writing. He said that I had to slow down and take the time to really *feel* the spirit of Lakeshore. He reminded me that we weren't on a newspaper deadline.

I realized that he was right again, for I had conducted just enough Lakeshore-related interviews to skim the surface and to tug at my soul just enough to know there was much more to learn and feel. If you're interviewing someone left paralyzed for life by an auto accident, or someone who has grave disabilities due to a birth defect, skimming the surface is *not* enough.

When I arrived home that evening, I shared the conversation with my husband, Jim Lunsford. I wasn't just seeking Jim's personal opinion; I also was seeking his professional opinion, for Jim had spent several years in the business of publishing and distributing books. Jim listened objectively, not like listening to the woman he loved, but like listening to an author. "Anita, Mike is right," Jim said. "This book project will greatly benefit from the meeting you and Mike had today."

I agreed. And now, several years down the road, I agree even more. This book took a long time to develop. But we kept working month after month and year after year, and I can now look back at that particular day as the beginning of my really getting to know the *spirit* of Lakeshore.

This book tells the stories of how individuals with physical disabilities have been helped, and continue to be helped, by two very different types of therapies. It tells about the more conventional rehabilitation therapies that have been provided at Lakeshore Hospital. And it tells about the incredible boosts to quality of life that the Lakeshore Foundation provides with sports, recreation, and fitness programs tailored for those with physical disabilities.

The internationally known Lakeshore Foundation and those served by it occupy the primary spotlight in this book. This is a foundation that is affiliated with the U.S. Olympics/Paralymics as an official training site. It is a foundation that is home base for far-reaching programs of sports, recreation, and fitness tailored for military personnel with physical disabilities, many of whom have been injured in combat in Iraq and Afghanistan.

But the book serves a purpose beyond Lakeshore and beyond Lakeshore's staff and client family, because the innovations and practices at Lakeshore draw from the steady advances that have been made in recent years in rehabilitation, recreation, sports, and fitness for the physically disabled. Mike Stephens and Lakeshore have been a leader in these advances, but they have also closely watched and learned from advances at other facililities. Thus this book will have usefulness and meaning to those similarly engaged in these programs at facilities around the world. Likewise, the stories of the remarkable individuals told in these pages will be inspiring to both the physically disabled and the able-bodied whoever and wherever they are, even if they have no direct connection to Lakeshore.

We haven't written a history book in the traditional sense. There are no references, footnotes, or appendices. Although the stories in the book are all true, we wanted the book to read more like a novel. That's only fitting, since the characters in this book have faced and dealt with obstacles that often seem beyond ordinary life.

The goal of this book is not just to let you see some of what has taken place and continues to take place at Lakeshore, but also to afford you a glimpse of the spirit that drives the process and the incredible successes. So many people I have interviewed for this book have commented on the Lakeshore spirit. Dr. Russ Fine, who at the time of his interview was director of the Injury Control Research Center at the University of Alabama at Birmingham (UAB), told me: "Lakeshore, I believe, became as much an *attitude* as a *place*."

In casting a spotlight on that driving spirit, on that "attitude," the book dwells not so much on *institutions* as it does on *people* whose lives have been transformed with the help of these institutions. Along the way are stories of some individuals whose courage and accomplishments have made my heart soar. I hope you have the same experience.

THE CONVERSATION WITH Mike Stephens that I have already mentioned was tense, but it was not out of character.

More than 30 years ago, when I was writing newspaper stories about Lakeshore in its early days as a rehabilitation campus, I had another tense discussion with him. I was trying to convince Mike that he should *tell his own story*—so the public could see why he felt so passionately about Lakeshore's mission, *and* so the public would want to join him in supporting that mission.

Mike is a very private person. It did not come naturally to him to bare his soul and talk publicly about his own physical disability and how his experience ultimately inspired him to help others. Still, Mike reluctantly came to the conclusion that he would tell his own story. He said that, after thinking about it, he could see how it could help Lakeshore if people could see *why* he felt so strongly that Lakeshore's mission was so vital. So I wrote a newspaper story about Mike's personal journey.

Then, when we started working on this Lakeshore book, I insisted that Mike tell his story in even more excruciating detail. I can tell you it was difficult, very emotionally painful, for him to relive those memories. But he did. As you will see, that's how this book begins—with Mike's story.

In my view, the entire book benefits from the fact that it was told through the eyes and guidance of Lakeshore Foundation founder Mike Stephens—not only his own story, but also how he has viewed the stories of many others who have been touched and helped by Lakeshore.

It might be understandable for someone to pick up this book and say, "Oh, this is great. This is a book meant to inspire individuals who have physical disabilities." Well, it is that. But we hope it is much more than that. We wanted this to be a book that can inspire people no matter what kinds of crises, obstacles, and/or losses they are facing.

In the process of researching and writing the book, what I learned from the individuals on these pages helped me to weather the single most devastating event that has ever occurred in my own life—the unexpected death of my husband Jim, in February 2008.

After Jim died, there were those who knew how close we were, who knew our love story, who in one way or another would say to me, "Anita, you are coping and going forward. Who is your therapist?" I could easily answer: "Lakeshore and its people and its *spirit* are my therapists—every day. If the people I have met at Lakeshore can go forward and cope, in many cases achieve at very high levels, after the ordeals they have endured, I can use them as my inspiration, indeed as my compass."

Part I

The Journey of Michael Stephens

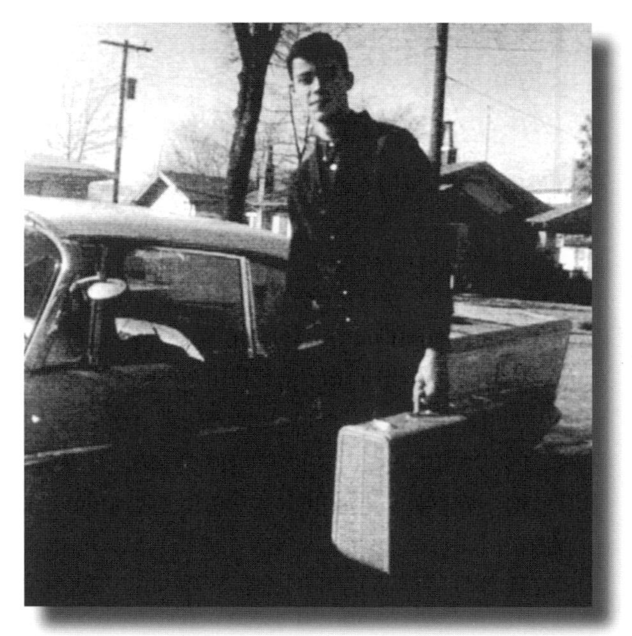

A young Mike Stephens before his injury, at the beginning of one part of his life journey.

1

Fateful Sunday

Mike and Susan Stephens had enjoyed a leisurely lunch on a Sunday afternoon in 1970 at the Cliff Terrace apartment of friends Larry and Linda Sinquefield in Birmingham, Alabama. The couples had eaten shish kebabs and sat around talking. They had planned a swim in the apartment complex pool, but time had gotten away. A salesman, Mike was starting a road trip the next morning and he had prep work to do before bedtime.

"Susan and I have to go, Larry," Mike said. "I need an early start tomorrow."

Fun-loving Larry protested, "Come on, let's at least jump in the pool and get wet."

Mike gave in and off they went. The wives continued visiting in the apartment.

Mike Stephens was an athletic and fit 26-year-old. He was a strong and experienced swimmer. When his legs flexed that afternoon on the concrete curbing of the Cliff Terrace pool and arched his body into the water, it was a dive like any of the thousands he had made before.

Maybe he slipped. Maybe the pool was shallower than he realized. At any rate, he dove so deeply that his head hit on the pool's hard bottom and bent so far forward that his chin touched his chest.

He never lost consciousness. But all his strength and swimming skill were now irrelevant. Somehow he kept air in his lungs. Miraculously, he floated to the surface. But all sensation and motion were gone from his body.

I can't move. My arms won't move. My legs won't move. I can't move my body.

He called out for his friend, who had just dived into the pool with him. "Larry, get me out of here. Something's wrong."

"Yeah, sure, Mike," Larry retorted.

Larry thinks I'm joking!

And why not? They were always joking around. Fear gripped Mike as he sank underwater, but again he floated to the surface.

"Larry, I'm serious. Get me out! I can't move!"

Puzzled but nevertheless responding, Larry pulled Mike to the side of the pool. "Just hold on," he encouraged. "Maybe the feeling will come back in a minute or so."

Mike tried to do as Larry said. But he couldn't.

"Larry, I can't hold myself up. And nothing is coming back. Something is really bad here. You've got to get me out of this pool."

Larry pulled him out. A small crowd of onlookers gathered near where Mike lay motionless beside the pool. Larry kept up his positive-spirited banter. "Mike, just lie there. Maybe you're just stunned. Maybe the feeling will all start coming back."

"I don't know, Larry. I heard something pop. And I don't know what it was."

Larry reached down to Mike's thigh and pinched him hard. Mike didn't even flinch.

For both Mike and Larry, the gravity of the situation was sinking in. Mike asked Larry to go tell Susan that he was in trouble and needed to go to a hospital.

An ambulance was summoned. Meanwhile, though he had not felt Larry's pinch, Mike began feeling almost unbearable arm and finger pain. Later he would learn that this was called "referral pain." On both sides of his body, searing pain ran down the backs of his arms into the pinkie and ring fingers on both hands.

Mike yearned for relief. "Larry, turn me on my stomach, and turn my head to the side. Maybe then I won't hurt so bad."

Suddenly, out of the gathering crowd, came a voice. "Don't do that. Don't turn him over. Leave him like he is. I'm a doctor. He has probably broken something in his back, and you could cause more damage by turning him."

Mike looked up at the stranger. "Thank you," he said simply.

The ambulance arrived and attendants rushed toward Mike with a stretcher. The doctor spoke up again. "Look, he needs to be placed on something stable, not like the stretcher you have. Go take a door off one of these apartments, and put him on that."

Within a few minutes, Mike was loaded onto an apartment door and was en route to the nearby UAB Medical Center.

The ambulance's wailing siren marked the end of one phase of Michael E. Stephens's life and the beginning of another. Unbeknownst to him or anyone else, it was also the beginning of a journey that eventually would offer hope and richer lives to many thousands of people with injuries or disabilities similar to the one Mike would now learn to live with.

2

Grim Reality

Mike was rushed to the busiest emergency room in Alabama, a level-one trauma center in the biggest hospital in the state—the University Hospital of the University of Alabama at Birmingham (UAB) Medical Center.

In those first few hours following his injury, Mike found his own circumstances and his surroundings to be terrifying. A gunshot victim was wheeled through the door. There were heart patients with chest pain. People were moaning, sobbing, screaming.

In the world outside his particular circle of hell, Mike's family had already contacted a neurosurgeon in a top Birmingham group. Yet in the emergency room where he lay, Mike didn't see much being done to help him. He had been x-rayed. Now he was lying on a hard gurney in a treatment room, feeling severe pain in his hands and down his back. Doctors and nurses occasionally glanced at him.

"I hurt like hell!" Mike complained. "I need something for pain."

"Yeah, I know you hurt," a doctor told Mike. "We would like to do something for you. But we can't give you anything right now. First we're just going to watch you."

"Watch me????"

"With the back injury you have, and where it is—up high, at the neck—we're concerned about your involuntary muscles, your heart and lungs," the physician replied. "We can't sedate you till we make sure they continue to function." He went on to explain that if Mike's lungs quit working, a tracheotomy would be performed so he could get air through a tube in his throat.

"What if my heart stops beating?"

The physician shook his head and walked out.

Mike saw the grim picture clearly. *I'm lying here paralyzed on this bed. And somebody just told me in effect that I need to listen for my every heartbeat*! Mike would say later that in a stroke of psychological genius the UAB doctor had put things in perspective, had let him know that he had bigger things to worry about than pain.

So Mike lay there in the UAB emergency room counting his heartbeats. His heart kept beating, and his lungs kept working.

Still, his situation was starkly grim.

Eventually neurosurgeon Dr. Griff Harsh III told Mike that x-rays confirmed he had broken his neck at the C-7 level—the seventh cervical vertebra. "Part of the vertebra has split off and is floating around like a razor blade," said Dr. Harsh. "We need to stabilize you."

Holes were drilled in Mike's skull and weighted Crutchfield tongs—resembling those used to move blocks of ice—were put in place to hold his neck straight and to reduce pressure in the injured area. Then he was placed horizontally on a Stryker frame—basically a board contraption with matting that rotates around the longitudinal axis. Every few hours hospital workers could turn him to prevent bedsores. Mike was tall and lanky. It was difficult to turn him without his feet getting caught up in the apparatus.

They're flipping me like a pig on a rotisserie!

Just like that, Mike had gone from being an adventurous, good-looking guy with the nice paycheck and the sharp suits that matched the flashy car, to total immobility and total dependence.

The gravity of Mike's situation was brought home even more graphically when he was transferred to a cramped semiprivate room on University Hospital's neurosurgery floor. One of his two roommates had crushing injuries to the frontal lobe of his brain as a result of having plowed his vehicle into the back of a pulpwood truck. The other was moaning in pain from the torment of traction to stretch his severely injured back.

ONE AFTER ANOTHER, those who loved Mike filed in to visit. Mostly, they could not handle the reality of what they saw, or Mike couldn't handle their reaction, or both.

Mike's parents were in near shock when they arrived and saw first-hand how badly their son was injured. Virginia Stephens was a strong-willed, action-oriented, stunningly beautiful woman whom Mike and his sisters had never referred to as "Mother" but, as others did, as "Gee Gee." In the initial minutes and hours after the accident, Mike had held onto his strength and presence of mind. Now, seeing his mother walk into his hospital room, he gave way to sobs that wracked his body.

I feel like I'm dissolving from a man into a little kid. I wish there was something Gee Gee could do to help me!

But that day Gee Gee Stephens could do nothing to change her son's circumstances. She reached for her first cigarette in 90 days.

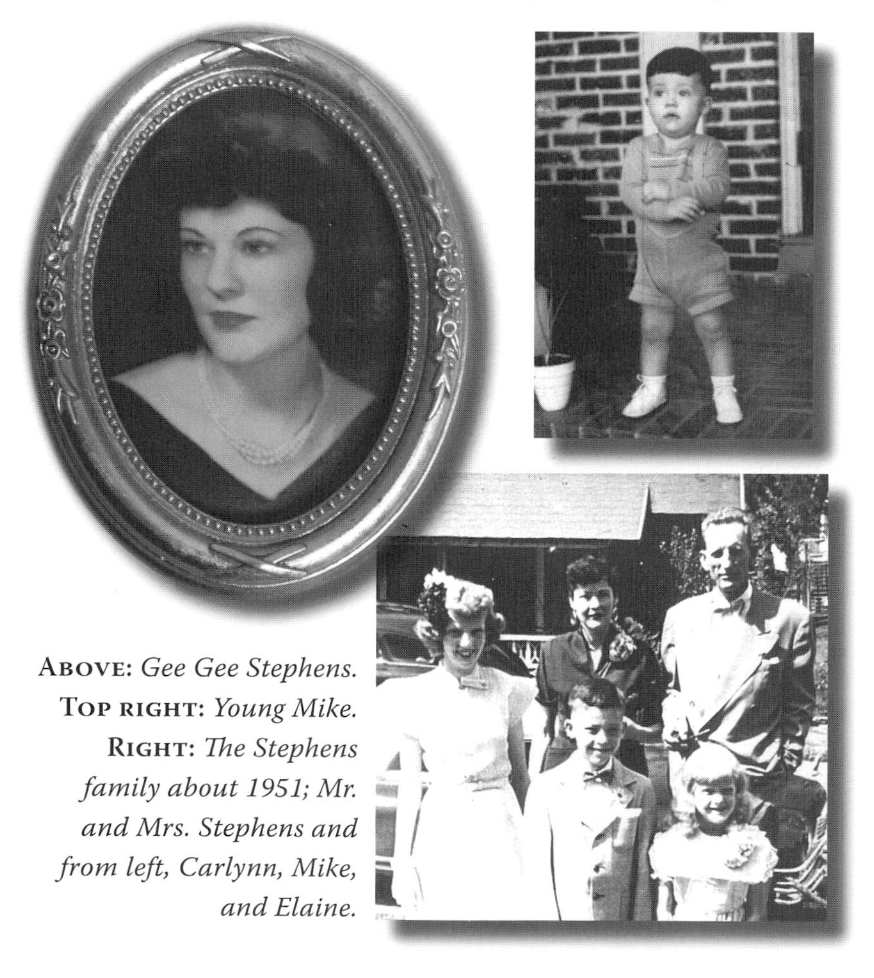

ABOVE: *Gee Gee Stephens.* **TOP RIGHT:** *Young Mike.* **RIGHT:** *The Stephens family about 1951; Mr. and Mrs. Stephens and from left, Carlynn, Mike, and Elaine.*

Then there was the stoic coping of Mike's wife, Susan. A federal probation officer, Susan was accustomed to confronting crisis with firmness. During his first dismal night in the hospital, Mike asked her to place a magazine on the floor where he could see it when orderlies turned him on the Stryker frame to face downward. Not long after Susan placed the magazine on the floor inches below Mike, she saw a tear drop onto the magazine.

"Crying is not going to do you any good," she said matter-of-factly.

"Well, okay," said Mike, as he managed to stop his tears, at least temporarily.

Some of Mike's macho male friends were so anguished they couldn't even speak to him. One, a former Auburn University football player, saw Mike being wheeled off the hospital elevator and into his room. As this big, strong young man gazed at Mike with the Crutchfield tongs in his skull and his body strapped into the Stryker frame, his face became a mask of shock and horror. He awkwardly mumbled a few words of support, bent down and kissed Mike tenderly, and fled.

Another friend was standing at the bedside when Mike woke the next morning. This muscle-bound guy—6'4" and 250 pounds—had played pro football. And he had known Mike as also athletic, fit, agile. Now he looked down at a helpless and motionless form suspended in a strange hospital apparatus. When Mike awakened and saw his friend standing at the foot of his bed, he said, "Well, hey, Charlie, how are you doing?" Big, hulking Charlie couldn't handle it. Tears started flowing down his cheeks, and soon he made his exit.

IN THE DAYS and weeks that followed, Mike played a dark waiting game for movement to return to his body. But the movement was not returning, and every passing day increased the odds of permanent paralysis from the chest down.

During this period, Mike felt the only way to get through the visits from friends and family was to put up the appearance of being in good spirits. He started timing his pain pills for 15 minutes before visiting hours. The pills numbed his brain just enough that he could put up a decent front for visitors and maybe in the process he could even give himself a false sense of security. He also tried some liquid spirits.

They're pouring all this awful cranberry juice down me to keep my urinary tract flushed. Hell, I'm going to ask the Doc to give me some beer instead!

Mike's doctor wrote a prescription for two bottles of beer a day. Soon Mike's friends were bringing in cases of beer, and friends and off-duty hospital workers were stopping by to have a beer with Mike and offer him some words of support.

Mike's party plan took the edge off his harsh reality for only a short time. Then he plunged into a deep depression. His physical condition also went downhill. He spiked a fever of 106 degrees, and the hospital staff began packing him in ice to get the temperature under control.

Playing the jolly host to a steady stream of visitors was no longer possible. A "No Visitors" sign went up. Mike was realizing that he had to build within himself the strength to cope rather than trying to draw strength from other people.

By this time, Mike had been moved from the Stryker frame into in a CircOlectric bed that allowed him to be turned somewhat like on a Ferris wheel. Mike was spending his time in a vacant world. The main events of the day came when he was turned one way or another in his Ferris wheel bed.

I'm lying here looking at the ceiling for six hours and counting the holes in the ceiling. Then I look at the floor for six hours. My world has been reduced to a very small screen.

EXCEPT FOR CLOSE family and a few carefully chosen friends, the main exception to Mike's "No Visitors" sign was his minister.

Mike had been exposed to considerable religious teaching from birth on into adulthood. In fact, his maternal grandfather was a Methodist minister and Mike was brought up in the Methodist Church. As a young adult, he joined the First Christian Church in Birmingham, attended services often, and gave generously to the church. But in later years he would reflect that until his 1970 accident and its aftermath, he had never been deeply spiritual. He would say that he had spent most of his time focusing on the superficial, looking out for himself, and having a good time.

As Mike lay paralyzed in Birmingham's University Hospital, people reached out to him with prayer. In fact, an entire day of prayer was designated for him as a result of a Catholic family friend taking Mike's mother, a lifelong Methodist, to a Birmingham convent to pray.

At this convent, it was unusual for worshipers to encounter the nuns who lived and worked there; usually the nuns were in the background, going about their daily chores and prayers. However, as fate would have it, as Gee Gee Stephens and her friend were praying, there suddenly appeared before them the most famous nun at this widely known convent, Mother Angelica, familiar nationally to millions of television viewers as the founder/leader of the high-profile Birmingham-based Eternal Word Television Network.

Herself a victim of a spinal injury years ago, Mother Angelica sat with Mike's mom and shared memories of her own accident, a fall while she was using an electric machine to scrub a soapy floor. The nun hiked up her dress enough for Gee Gee to see the residual effects. "See. I'm still in braces. I can relate to some of what your son is going through," said Mother Angelica, who had undergone surgery and was hospitalized for a lengthy period after her accident. "It's very important to me that we try to help your Michael."

Mother Angelica promised that she would designate a round-the-clock day of prayer for Michael Stephens. On that day, nuns in the convent would pray for Mike when they paused for prayer times that were interspersed with their chores and periods of rest and sleep. "This means that not only am I myself going to pray for your Michael," Sister Angelica told Gee Gee Stephens. "I'm going to have all the sisters I know—my fellow nuns—to pray for him as well."

Mike received a little card in the mail telling him of the date Mother Angelica had selected for the special day of prayer for him at the convent. Hour after hour that day, as Mike lay there in the hospital, he was keenly aware of those prayers. He thought about the contrast in the hell-raising life he had been living and how all these good, spiritual people now were praying for him—a young man they had never even met. Mike had plenty of time to think about the life he had been living prior to his recent accident.

Some of his guilt-ridden thoughts turned to a particular night when he and Larry Sinquefield had been out kicking up their heels until 4 o'clock in the morning. When Mike returned home there was a message that he should call his mother immediately, and he learned that while he had been having a good time, a person very important to his life and dear to his heart had died—his paternal grandmother. She had broken a hip and had been in the hospital. Mike knew he should have been more attentive about visiting her. He felt he should have been with her the night she died.

She loved me, and she was always there for me. But there at the end of her life, I was not there for her.

Then, one night after his accident, as he lay paralyzed and asleep in the hospital, Mike had a dream—maybe a vision. He felt the spirit of his grandmother come to him in this dream.

In my dream, I feel the presence of a woman floating toward me. Out of the corner of my eye, I catch a glimpse of beautiful white hair. She touches me. I feel a spiritual comfort, a sense of peace. Although she never speaks, in my heart I know that I am receiving a message from my grandmother.

From that night forward, Mike experienced a lifting of the heavy guilt he had felt for not being with his grandmother at the end of her life.

DURING THIS PERIOD, Mike was beginning to look inside himself, embarking on what for him was an unprecedented process of soul-searching.

His pastor was visiting one day when Mike was having especially bothersome pain because his limp body had slumped into a contorted position in the CircOlectric bed. Mike told the pastor that he was going to call for orderlies to adjust his position.

The pastor felt that he needed to leave. Mike protested, but when the orderlies arrived the minister did leave. As the door closed behind him, Mike was overcome with feelings of rejection and abandonment—because the minister was leaving without saying a prayer. To Mike, it seemed like the closing of a door on his desperate need to find inspiration and strength outside himself.

I want my minister to pray for me—to talk to God and negotiate my getting well. Now he has left without saying a prayer, and I'm doomed to be paralyzed the rest of my life.

The incident reinforced for Mike his need to find inspiration and strength inside himself.

The minister had barely left Mike's room that day when the orderlies approached his bed and pulled his body up and readjusted him. As they did, Mike felt a sensation down his back—a little snap of rapid-fire feeling, the first time since Mike was injured that he had felt a sensation in his back.

The next morning, he could wiggle a big toe just a little. Soon he could move the next toe. Then he could move five toes. Then he could move his foot. Small sensations began traveling up one side of his body and down the other side. He felt a twinge of movement in one arm.

Mike was excited. He told his neurosurgeon, "Look, I'm getting some return, I'm moving my toes."

Dr. Griff Harsh didn't want Mike to get his hopes up and then have them crushed. He had been a neurosurgeon a long time. He had seen body sensations and little movements occur with paralyzed patients when it turned out to mean little or nothing in terms of their increased mobility. Dr. Harsh cautioned Mike not to get too excited about what could be just muscle spasms. But he said he would have Mike moved to UAB's nearby Spain Rehabilitation Center to "get as much activity going as will be possible for you."

He also warned, "Frankly, Mike, I must tell you that, based on the severity of your injury and the length of time of since your paralysis, it is my opinion that you are not likely to ever walk again."

3

Bucking the Rehab System

Mike would later recall his arrival at Spain rehab hospital as "my introduction to hell." There he confronted the possibility that his neurosurgeon might well be correct, that he might spend the rest of his life paralyzed and in a wheelchair.

He would not, could not, buy into that prognosis. In the Spain cafeteria, he turned his back on other patients: *It bothers me too bad even to look at them. I can't become a part of their world.*

Spain was and is a top-flight rehabilitation center in the heart of the vast UAB medical complex. The doctor's orders for Mike's care called for therapy aimed at getting him as independent as possible in three months—independent while still in a wheelchair.

"Don't expect to walk again," a therapist told him. "We're just going to try to get as much activity out of you as we can."

Other patients, or "clients," had their own grim stories of how they had lost their ability to walk or talk or hear or see. Some were like Mike—recently disabled by accidents or by medical problems such as strokes. Others were patients who returned again and again for recurrent problems, sometimes decubitus ulcers resulting from skin breakdown, sometimes for another round of therapy to build on their limited body strength.

Mike's first attempt at physical therapy was a dismal failure. Therapists put him on a mat, put a belt around him, lifted him up, and said, "Try to hold yourself on your hands and knees." He collapsed into a heap. After ten failed attempts, he heard someone say, "He's had enough." He was placed in his wheelchair and returned to his room.

I'm never going to be able to do anything.

Like many rehab centers, Spain was a tough environment. Staff members believed that to teach any degree of independence to individuals with severe disabilities, they had to be especially strict. Some felt they had to be especially blunt as well, reminding patients of the reality of their circumstances. In Mike's eyes, no one was tougher than the "Drill Sergeant," a female staffer who worked the 11–7 shift and woke patients every morning and hollered at them to get dressed. She hollered a lot, and sometimes she called them "DDs"—"dead dicks."

That woman doesn't have a heart about anything—calling us DDs because we're paralyzed. Well, I'm going to show her one day!

Mike's roommate was Nelson Wedgeworth, a repeat Spain patient due to recurrent problems, who was paralyzed from being shot in the back during a drive-by shooting. Nelson was streetwise and savvy from life in rough black neighborhoods. He also was a bitter, defiant man who made fun of anything spiritual and who refused to participate in some of Spain's programs. In group therapy, Nelson refused to say a word. He thought the whole process was just plain stupid. Nelson also thought it was stupid for Mike to carry around a little red bag with a piece of so-called blessed cloth in it. He would point to the bag holding the cloth and make snide statements.

A defiant streak was something Nelson had in common with his roommate. However, Mike's defiance was soon driving him to push himself rather than to sit on the sidelines. After a few days at Spain, Mike decided he very much did want to participate in some of the center's programs; he just wanted to pick them.

Mike first progress came in rebuilding his strength.

As he became stronger, all he wanted to do was to build up his body by working out, including with weights. He began pulling every trick he could think of to free himself from his assigned periods in psychotherapy and occupational therapy so he could get to the gymnasium and do more physical therapy.

Some of the physical therapists told him he was overdoing it. "Your back is not going to hold up. Your legs are too weak to support this," a Spain physical therapy administrator warned. "You're going to mess up your back." The rebellious Mike kept lifting weights. He pushed his body, and then he pushed some more. (Years later, the warnings from those Spain physical therapists would stick in his mind when he suffered chronic lower back problems.)

Then Mike got a yearning to do something else. One day he asked his physical therapist, Marilyn Bennett, "Don't y'all have a pool there in the back?" She said yes. Mike said he'd like to get into the pool. Marilyn thought that was a good idea, and she began helping Mike with simple pool exercises, like tossing large lightweight beach-type balls while the water buoyancy stabilized Mike's weakened body. For Mike, who always had an open appreciation for beautiful women, there was a bonus with these water exercises—physical therapist Marilyn was striking in the yellow two-piece bathing suit she wore to the water-therapy sessions.

Some two and a half weeks later Marilyn threw a beach ball to Mike. The ball ended up in the shallow end of the pool. Mike maneuvered into the shallow water and picked up the ball. Marilyn was stunned; she would never have expected this from someone with Mike's level of injury. "Mike! Look at you! You're standing in 18 inches of water. If you can do that, you can walk on our parallel bars!!"

So it was that they stopped the pool exercises and Mike graduated to the parallel bars. It was a monumental breakthrough and Mike was ecstatic—except for one thing: *I'll sure miss seeing that yellow bathing suit.*

Mike became as focused on the parallel bars as he had been with the weight lifting. He pushed, and he pushed, and he pushed some more. There came the day when—in one day—Mike moved from parallel bars to a walker, to a pair of four-pronged canes, to two regular canes, then down to one cane.

Mike was feeling increasing sensation, strength, and movement in his lower body. He began "walking" the halls of Spain—a form of walking in which Mike would drag therapist Marilyn down the halls, with her fingers locked into the belt loops of Mike's jeans. That walking was far from normal, but he was beginning with great effort to move his body from one place to another.

With no idea that Mike had begun to walk, the tough night-duty Drill Sergeant entered his room one morning, doing her standard screaming routine. She was yelling for him to get up so she could transfer him to his wheelchair, which was across the room. To her amazement, Mike got up from his bed, limped the few steps to his chair, and sat down. When he looked up, this seemingly callous woman was sobbing.

"What the hell is wrong with you?" Mike demanded.

She continued to sob. "You don't know how long I've waited to see one of you boys do this. You just don't know how long I've waited. It means so much."

Before long the Drill Sergeant was transferred to a different job in another unit. Mike believed he understood why. *Now that her soft spot has shown through, she can't be as tough as she was. She's had to move on.*

Mike wanted to move on, too. Now that he was relearning to walk, he was like the stubborn two-year-old—learning how to maneuver on his own, and wanting to do everything for himself, with as little support as possible.

Finally he pushed his therapist too far. They had a heated argument when Marilyn tried teaching Mike to climb stairs using a cane. Steps are treacherous for someone whose legs are weak, as his still were. She demonstrated how to grip the handrail and how to position his cane. He retorted that he wasn't going to use a cane. She replied that that was too risky. He insisted.

Marilyn had had enough of Mike pushing, pushing, putting himself at risk and defying her guidance. Her temper flared. "Well, Mike, if you think you know so much, why don't you just pack up your things and leave Spain and do your own rehab!"

Always defiant, Mike would not back down. She got him situated in his wheelchair and returned him to his room.

Mike knew he had crossed the line and that if Marilyn recommended he be "expelled" from Spain that it was likely to happen. He had completed six weeks of a scheduled 12-week program. The prospect of prematurely being on his own scared him but he was not going to admit it.

It came as no surprise to Mike that he soon had a visit from Dr. Cecil Nepomuceno, a rehabilitation medicine specialist who was overseeing Mike's care. Much-loved and much-respected, "Dr. Nepo" was known as both an excellent physician and a gentleman.

"We can't have you treating our therapists the way you just treated Marilyn," Dr. Nepo told Mike. "She's responsible for you."

Mike said he understood that but was simply enthusiastic about his progress and wanted to keep going.

A deal was struck. Mike would apologize to Marilyn, and he would stay one more week. He did both, meaning that he completed seven weeks of Spain's rehab program.

LEAVING SPAIN ALSO meant leaving behind Nelson Wedgeworth, Mike's bitter, sarcastic roommate who showed up for group therapy sessions in body only—never saying anything, never participating. As mentioned, Nelson had also ridiculed an object that had become important to Mike, a little red bag containing a piece of cloth.

The cloth had come to Mike from his aunt, his mother's sister who lived in Boston. The donor, a friend of the aunt who had heard of the nephew's accident, simply said, "Send this cloth to your nephew."

According to legend, the Virgin Mary had appeared on a hill and handed a woman a blessed cloth, saying, "Divide this cloth among the sad and crying in the world, for them to shed their tears upon."

Mike's aunt believed, and she sent the cloth to Mike's mother. Mike's mother also believed, and she made a little red bag to hold the cloth, with a sewn-on loop to hold the bag on his arm. Wherever Mike went, so went the little red bag with the special cloth. When he lay in bed, the little red bag was at his elbow.

At the beginning, Mike didn't necessarily believe, but he wasn't taking any chances. *Maybe it will help—the piece of cloth in this little red bag. I'll keep it with me.*

When it came time for Mike to leave Spain, he went through the group therapy ritual for departing patients. Spain saw few patients like Mike, who walked again against all odds, so there were quite a few questions.

But finally the other patients had asked their questions, wished him well, and said their goodbyes. The social worker who was leading the session was bringing the meeting to a close when Nelson raised his hand. The social worker was taken aback, as was everyone else in the room.

"Yes, Nelson?" she asked softly.

Nelson pointed. "Mike, that little red bag you've got there . . ."

"Yeah, Nelson?" said Mike, expecting another wisecrack about the bag and the cloth it held.

"I was wondering, Mike, if I could have a little piece of that cloth."

Nelson Wedgeworth had just expressed how badly he wanted to move and walk again, as was true with every other paralyzed patient in the room.

4

Walking, Against All Odds

As Mike was discharged from Spain Rehabilitation Center, the defiance and stubborn determination that had driven him were very much alive, as his wife Susan quickly saw. She drove into the center's discharge area in Mike's beloved 1969 green Grand Prix, expecting to have Mike placed in the passenger seat and to drive him home.

"I'm driving!" Mike greeted her.

"Are you sure?" she said.

"Yeah," said Mike, climbing with great difficulty into the driver's seat. He cranked his car. It took all the strength he could muster to move his weakened foot from the gas pedal to the brake and back again. *I won't tell Susan that I might or might not be able to hit this brake quick enough!*

On that day when Mike was discharged from Spain, he was aware that his and Susan's perspectives were far apart—punctuation to an increasingly strained marriage (that would eventually lead to divorce). Mike Stephens guided the Grand Prix slowly out of the driveway of UAB's Spain Rehabilitation Center, headed for a new life that was filled with daunting uncertainty.

I'm not the same person I was before I was injured. I can see how people who suffer devastating injuries have to grapple with painful feelings of losing their independence. My focus right now is on believing I can get better, and on taking whatever steps I have to take to make myself get better.

Later in his life, Mike would be told many times that the main thing that enabled him to walk following his injury was his determination. Some experts would say that by all odds Mike's spinal injury had been too severe to permit him to walk, but that he had defied the odds by pushing himself to almost superhuman limits. When he left Spain five weeks earlier than scheduled, he stepped up his pursuit of building up his ability to walk.

His first challenge was his own home, in a hilly Birmingham community appropriately named Bluff Park. There were steps and a steep embankment in front of the house. With his pitifully weak legs, Mike knew his best bet was to enter through the basement. Even there, he faced a set of 12 steps, and he had to crawl up them to the living area.

His legs were so limp when he first got home that they were dragging. At Spain, he had been aided in his walking by some kind of support, either rehabilitation equipment or a person, or both. Now, when he first got home and was on his own, sometimes he had to crawl from room to room.

Mike knew he had to strengthen his legs and he knew that in his defiant frame of mind he would have to do it himself. His stubborn, verbally abrasive reaction to a therapist who was trying to prevent him from hurting himself had in effect gotten him kicked out of Spain rehab center. Now that he was out on his own, he was a little scared, but he was still determined.

Okay, Big Mouth. Now you need to design and carry out your own rehabilitation program to pick up where Spain left off. You've got to practice walking—practice, practice, practice!

MIKE KNEW WHERE to find a tough training course. One day not long after he got home, he limped painfully to his car and drove himself to downtown Birmingham. In the heart of Birmingham's retail and business district, he knew he could find lots of sidewalks and tall buildings with lots of steps.

Day after day Mike drove to downtown Birmingham, where he walked and then walked some more. He limped severely, feeling persistent pain, constantly aware he was precariously unsteady, moving very slowly at first, gradually picking up a bit of steam. Out of breath but still pushing, he walked the sidewalks. Struggling to make the muscles in his legs bend and move, he climbed hundreds of stairs.

A key component in Mike's downtown training course was the 16-story Brown-Marx Building, with retail space on the ground level and business offices on the higher floors. He started with walking up and down six flights, again and again. He stumbled on the stairs. Sometimes he fell. Gradually he moved up to eight flights, then ten.

On the city sidewalks, despite using a cane, Mike still stumped his toes, occasionally fell against a building, and, on a bad day, crumpled to his knees. In a downtown area crowded with people, he never knew what obstacle he might encounter—a dropped item, a slippery candy wrapper, a spilled soft drink, or just the usual cracked or broken concrete.

Mike was human. Embarrassment engulfed him when he stumbled or fell with people watching him. He knew he had to get past that. *If I fall, I've just got to get back up and keep going.*

When he reached a particularly difficult curb or flight of stairs, he could feel his desire to succeed waging battle against fears that he might fail. *I've got two choices here—flight or fight. Right after I was injured, I chose flight from the reality of what had happened to me. Then at Spain I started changing to fight. Now I've got to keep fighting.*

He knew the choice to fight fit the personality of the Mike Stephens who had existed before the accident—the brash, I'll-do-it-my-way and to-hell-with-the-rules young man, the same kind of guy who had resurfaced at Spain.

Mike now felt surges of adrenaline that seemed to be generated by a powerful well of anger. It wasn't like conventional anger toward a person. It wasn't even like anger toward his situation. It was more like a grinding urge to forge ahead, no matter what was in front of him.

For a change of pace from walking in bustling downtown Birmingham, Mike started driving over to a nearby quaint suburban shopping center. There he practiced walking around several blocks of appealing one-story and two-story buildings containing fashionable shops and a mix of eateries.

One day, Mike decided to take a lunch break inside a popular hot-dog stand. Exhausted from a long session of walking, he sat down at a

Pac-Man machine and put in his quarter. He sat quietly and played the then-popular arcade game just long enough to catch his breath. Then he decided to get in the growing line to place orders. As he rose from his seat at the Pac-Man machine, he found out the hard way that he had overdone the walking. He stumbled forward a couple of steps and realized to his horror that his legs were totally numb. His legs simply could not support him. He fell hard in a twisted heap.

No one offered to help. No one asked, "What's wrong?" or "Are you hurt?" or "Can I help you get up?" In fact, a couple of customers stepped around him as they hurried to claim their places in line, while Mike still lay sprawled on the floor.

Grittily, he pushed against the floor with his hands and grappled his way to his feet. Then he left without ordering a hot dog.

That was a lonely moment. But the next day he was back on the streets walking.

5

At a Career Crossroads

Mike was a natural salesman. Prior to his accident, he was doing well in his job with publishing giant Prentice Hall, selling reference materials called "loose-leaf legal services" to attorneys, accountants, physicians, hospital administrators, and other professionals who needed to keep current with the latest regulations in their various fields. He was on the road more than he was home, and on his business trips he lugged large, heavy binders of samples—each tailored to a particular subject area.

After Mike was injured, the physical toll of the travel and the lifting of the samples was an obvious problem. Rehabilitation medicine specialist Dr. Cecil Nepomuceno warned, "Mike, you're going to have to get a desk job." Typically, Mike resisted. *Since my injury, the folks at Prentice Hall have been real good to me; and I've been doing pretty well at keeping in contact with my clients by phone.*

He gave the old sales job a try, but it didn't take long to realize that Dr. Nepo was right. Mike had to take mental inventory of the facts. *All this driving and lugging these big binders around is hell. The physical part is sapping so much of my strength that there's not enough energy left to interact with my clients.* Mike had to admit to himself that he couldn't produce for Prentice Hall the way he did before.

Another problem was that even before the accident he had become bored with the job. He liked Prentice Hall, but he no longer loved the job, and now it was too taxing for his body. Further, he realized that he had eventually gotten bored with every job he'd had.

He needed a career change, and at this critical juncture of his life he arrived at a clearer professional goal than he had felt so far in his 28 years. He decided that he wanted to become a hospital administrator.

No doubt the weeks he had spent as a hospital patient contributed to the decision. However, Mike's first seeds of interest in hospital management were planted prior to his injury—by having hospital administrators among his Prentice Hall clients. Their work interested him. He noticed that none of his clients faced more diverse or more interesting challenges than did hospital administrators. They needed to know about laws governing issues and situations ranging from personnel to building codes, construction bids, safety, taxes . . . and the most precious commodity known to our society—human life. *Now, if I could become a hospital administrator, wouldn't that be some interesting career! I bet I'd never get bored with that job!*

So Mike quit his job at Prentice Hall and prepared to return to college for the education he would need to become a successful hospital administrator.

Returning to college was a big step. Mike needed an undergraduate and a master's degree, and to date he had two years of college and no degree. That would be a challenge. During the on-and-off stints of his time as a college student, Mike Stephens had cut a hell-raising path of academic disaster and bad-boy behavior at the University of Montevallo, a small state-supported liberal arts college located 30 miles south of Birmingham in Shelby County. Its rich history dates to 1896 when it was founded as Alabama College, a Methodist-affiliated girls' school. It eventually was taken over by the state and went co-ed; the present name was adopted in 1969.

THE PRE-ACCIDENT AND post-accident periods of Mike's enrollment at Montevallo were a study in contrasts.

He was as natural a student as he was a salesman. Mike was fortunate in being able to quickly absorb and retain large amounts of information—when motivated. But in his first stint at Montevallo, Mike was mostly focused on having a good time. He had an eye for good-looking women. He liked to stay out late and party. He enjoyed playing practical jokes and getting into mischief with the guys he hung out with.

Later Mike would label this his "creative behavior" period.

After one prank that unintentionally destroyed a Coke machine, he was hauled before the dorm's disciplinary council. Fortunately for him, he was well-liked by his fellow students and was fined only a dollar.

Mike and his friends especially liked to play pranks on campus "nerds." They blindfolded one young man and drove him to the woods, tied him to a tree, and left him. But the victim was smarter than they were and was able to describe the pranksters and their car make and model by sounds. Armed with this information, administrators traced the prank back to Mike and cohorts.

On the academic side, Mike was constantly in trouble. Not bothering to study, he made such poor grades that he was placed on academic probation. Then Mike got caught giving a fellow student the answers to a test in one of his classes. This time he was sent to "trial" before the Student Court, resulting in a recommendation of two semesters of probation.

The university dean overseeing the review was the same dean who had overseen the case in which Mike and his friends had played the prank on the blindfolded student. The dean confronted Mike and announced to him that his track record was catching up with him and that this time he was going to be kicked out of school for a year. Then the dean added, "Mike, you have such strong abilities. You could be an outstanding person, if you just had the right attitude."

Even strong-spirited Mike believed that it would do no good to argue with the angry dean. Convinced that he would soon be officially kicked out of school, Mike left the University of Montevallo and went job hunting.

FOR A TIME, he sold shoes in a small specialty shoe store. Then he worked in a killer job on an assembly line in a bakery. For eight-hour shifts as a "pan-shagger," he stood in the same spot pulling miniature cakes from 24-pound, blazing-hot molds and transferring them to a conveyor belt. If he let his tired arms drop, he would be burned by the steaming-hot surfaces.

Weary of the bakery, Mike applied for a job at a machine shop. A key factor in Mike's not getting this job was that the owner, who interviewed him, didn't know what to make of Mike—since Mike, trying to be truthful, confessed that he had been expelled from Montevallo for bad behavior. But when the man called the university, he was told that Mike hadn't been expelled. The machine shop owner didn't hire Mike, but, when he mentioned his confusion, Mike realized the dean had outfoxed him. The dean had thought Mike should be kicked out, and he convinced Mike that he would be, but then after Mike left on his own, the dean never took the academic steps to formally expel him.

Ironically, in later years Mike would come to respect and greatly admire that dean, his old nemesis, as someone whose high standards and strict actions helped shape his life for the better.

Mike returned briefly to the University of Montevallo. He stayed long enough to earn a few more college credits, then he withdrew again. Along the way, he married Susan Walker, a fellow student he had met at Montevallo. He was then 21, married, with a good job. And he was fit and healthy.

In his early 20s, Mike left college behind and began focusing on a sales career. He sought to build a stable career in which he could make financial headway, rather than just going from one undesirable job to another. For three years he did a good job selling life insurance for Metropolitan Life. Then he moved on to a different sales position with Prentice Hall, where he did extraordinarily well for three years selling loose-leaf legal services.

When Mike returned in 1970 to the Montevallo campus for a third time, several months after his severe spinal cord injury, the university was much the same, but he certainly was not. Mike was not only changed physically, but he was a totally different type of college student. This was, in fact, his first serious entry into the University of Montevallo. For the first time, Mike had plans that connected his studies with a specific career goal. He now wanted to become a hospital administrator. To do that, he had to have two college degrees. His goal was to earn his bachelor's degree at Montevallo and then pursue graduate studies at another university that offered a healthcare administration curriculum.

Mike knew he had to bear down this time. And he had not been back on campus very long before Professor Sara Morgan put him to the test in her business law course. She had known him in his earlier bad-boy student days; he had failed one of her courses. Dr. Morgan had a maternal streak and a track record for taking a special interest in students with a history of academic and/or behavior problems. When she encountered these formerly low-achieving students after they returned to school, she zeroed in. She wanted them to succeed; so she challenged them.

Thus, when she looked out into her classroom and saw Mike—now a 28-year-old and the oldest student in the room—Dr. Morgan bore down on him. Her trademark style was to call on students to explain cases of precedent—prior judicial decisions that usually governed how courts would rule on current and future cases. If she called on a student and the student didn't know the answer, often she would say "Wrong!" without looking up. In Mike's class, she began calling on various students and each time one got something wrong, she in turn would call on Mike. "Mr. Stephens, you tell them," she would say.

Mike still had not become accustomed to studying, and often when Dr. Morgan called on him he didn't know the answer either. He would ad-lib something, but he knew his responses were nowhere near correct, and he knew that Dr. Morgan knew. Yet she continued to call on him. Day after day, she would say, "Mr. Stephens, you tell them."

I'm just making this stuff up. And it isn't working. Dr. Morgan is just going to keep calling on me. I had better start studying.

So Mike started studying—not just for Dr. Morgan's class but for all his classes. Before long, the same Mike Stephens who had been on academic probation, and who had behaved so badly he thought he had been kicked out, made the Dean's List. Then he made the Dean's List the next semester. And the next. And the next.

Two years after he returned to Montevallo, Mike was inducted into a honorary academic fraternity. Mike's grades were so high his last two years that they overcame the poor grades from his "bad-boy" years.

At the 1973 University of Montevallo graduation ceremonies, honor student Mike Stephens was among those who walked across the stage to receive their diplomas. He walked with a severe limp, but he walked. In the audience to watch him receive his bachelor's degree in business administration were his proud parents, Henry Ed and Gee Gee Stephens. There had been many times when his parents had reason to wonder if they ever would see the day when their only son would be graduating from college.

Mike himself had wondered. *I remember when I first went off to college, my dad said, "Son, I want you to have a good time. But at least bring home decent passing grades." Well, at the beginning I was bringing home D's and F's. Even though I was living what at the time I thought was a fun life, it was in many ways also a tough life—always in trouble with somebody, hearing my parents gripe, hearing the university administrators gripe, trying to get out of jams—something always biting me in the ass. All in all, it turned out to be easier to make good grades than it was to make bad ones.*

He didn't know it yet, but he had just completed the last "easy" thing he would do for a long time.

6

Surprising Paths

On the surface, it seemed so simple, maybe even easy. Mike Stephens had decided to become a hospital administrator. Now he was on track to pursue that goal.

With his bachelor's degree in hand, he was ready to enter a master's program in healthcare administration. Conveniently, the University of Alabama at Birmingham (UAB) had such a program on the same campus where Mike had been hospitalized and undergone rehabilitation following his accident.

UAB's graduate program in healthcare administration was relatively new, and by all reports it was very good—in fact, it ranked among the top 10 programs of its type in the nation. However, it was not that easy to get into the UAB program. There were 25 openings for the next class, and 150 qualified applicants, most of whom had not fooled around for their first two undergraduate years and thus had better grade point averages than Mike's.

My chances don't look too good. And I want this real bad. What am I going to do?

As it turned out, there wasn't much he could do except submit his application. Then life took a strange twist. While Mike had been learning how to become a serious student during his third try at college, he had also been carrying out his first experiment in entrepreneurism. He was acting as his own project manager in building an upscale four-unit apartment building in the Birmingham suburb of Hoover. This was an apartment building he would own, lease to tenants, and manage. It was the first of Mike's many entrepreneurial ventures.

On a Sunday afternoon, Mike showed one of the units in his new building to a woman named Dawn. She didn't rent the apartment, but in making small talk during the showing Mike learned that she worked at UAB. He mentioned that he wanted to become a hospital administrator and was trying to get into the UAB graduate program.

That was it. Mike knew Dawn only from that casual conversation, but afterwards he would always associate her name with the dawn of an exciting new era in his professional life.

What Mike didn't know on that Sunday afternoon was that Dawn apparently had seen in him some qualities UAB was looking for in its carefully selected healthcare administration graduate students. She had reason to be familiar with these qualities, for she worked in the office of the director of UAB's healthcare administration program. She told the director about Mike Stephens and suggested he take a close look at Mike's application.

Mike was accepted into the program. He was now on the path to fulfilling his dream, thanks to a surprise encounter with someone who had operated quietly behind the scenes to open a door for him.

IN GRADUATE SCHOOL, Mike worked hard and made good grades. He also had some luck when it came to the on-the-job training part of the program. He was selected for the residency he wanted—at Baptist Medical Centers (BMC), a large and rapidly expanding multi-hospital system headquartered in Birmingham.

His residency at BMC corporate headquarters would be under the preceptorship of one of the nation's best-known and most progressive healthcare administrators, BMC's president and CEO, L. R. "Rush" Jordan.

Learning hospital administration firsthand from Rush Jordan! Man, this is great!

Mike's career possibilities looked bright at that point. As his residency got underway, the BMC training experience proved every bit as exciting and enlightening as he thought it would be. He was spending a lot of time with Rush Jordan—not only at BMC's corporate offices, but also accompanying Jordan to meetings such as with the Alabama Hospital Association and to sessions with attorneys in Washington,

D.C. Mike also interacted with other BMC leaders and spent time in corporate finance. For a short period he was assigned to work with executive Dick Lind, who was heading BMC's management-contract planning for an old Birmingham-based tuberculosis hospital to be converted into a rehabilitation complex—a campus that would bear the name of Lakeshore.

Mike was soaking up every minute, learning more than he ever thought he could in such a short time. He would be involved with BMC for a year. Just think what he could learn in a year!

THEN, SIX MONTHS into his residency, the bottom suddenly fell out of Mike's world.

Rush Jordan and his team got into an irresolvable confrontation with powerful members of BMC's governing board and medical staff. The result was one of the greatest shakeups to date in the rapidly growing U.S. healthcare industry. Within a matter of hours, whole careers collapsed. Mike Stephens looked in disbelief at the professional carnage.

After more than a decade of leading Baptist Medical Centers to greatness, Rush Jordan has resigned under pressure! And that's just the tip of the iceberg—14 top administrators have also resigned in support of Jordan. This is not the same hospital system I came to. Who the hell is in charge here?????

One of the answers to Mike's question about who was in charge would prove to be a stunning shock. In the wake of the exodus of BMC administrators, the BMC board improbably turned over the tremendous responsibility of running the Montclair hospital to a pair of inexperienced master's-degree-candidate residents, one of whom was Mike Stephens himself. During this difficult interim period, he and fellow resident Pat McDonald were tapped as "co-administrators" of Baptist Medical Center Montclair.

Even before the shock wore off, Mike realized that the interim position could be an awesome opportunity—one that matched his specific ambition to become an administrator in an acute-care general hospital like BMC-Montclair. As Mike and Pat got down to the business of overseeing the day-to-day Montclair operations, Mike was scared and excited all at the same time.

He was not quite 31 years old. He was thrust unexpectedly into a difficult leadership role that demanded fast-paced decision-making, problem-solving, and crisis-management—experiences that helped toughen and prepare him for the career that lay ahead.

Mike and Pat held things together at BMC Montclair until the cavalry arrived in the form of more seasoned administrators. After Texas hospital executive Emmett R. Johnson—a leader who was much the opposite of Rush Jordan—was recruited as BMC's president/CEO, Mike watched as Johnson planted the seeds of his own administration. While Jordan had been a visionary, flamboyant, high-energy, risk-taking innovator with the approach of a private-enterprise entrepreneur, Johnson was an even-keeled, quietly competent, easygoing man who brought a calming balance to BMC's very troubled environment.

However, although Mike learned from Emmett Johnson and his "steady-the-ship" and "get-things-in-order" style, Mike never felt the connection with Johnson that he had felt with Jordan. Mike's own personality was more like that of the forge-ahead-and-take-a-risk Jordan.

Too, from the time Johnson stepped onto the plush carpet of his BMC office, he had his hands full putting Humpty Dumpty together again. Johnson was aware of and appreciative of how young Mike Stephens had stepped up to the plate during the turbulent weeks following Jordan's sudden departure, but Johnson didn't have time to interact much with or to really get to know Mike. For his part, Mike realized it wasn't necessary that he and Johnson have a close relationship for the recent developments at BMC to pay off for his career.

AMIDST ALL THIS change within the Baptist Medical Centers system, Mike was watching for professional opportunity for his near future. BMC had recruited a new CEO, but the majority of those other 14 administrative vacancies were not filled. In light of his unexpected recent experience as an interim Montclair administrator, Mike felt sure he could be hired for one of those BMC positions when his residency was finished—which would be soon.

So it came as no surprise when one day Mike was summoned into the office of BMC leader Emmett R. Johnson. He quickly got to the point: "Mike, your residency is coming to an end. You've done a great job with us here. And I'm sure you've thought about what you want to do. What do you want, Mike?"

"Mr. Johnson, I want a career in an acute-care hospital," Mike replied. "I really have enjoyed my experience at Baptist Medical Center Montclair. I would like an administrative position at Montclair."

Johnson took that in, repeated that Mike had done a good job under difficult circumstances, and conceded that he deserved to have what he wanted. But then Johnson went off on a tangent.

"As you know, Mike, several months ago Baptist Medical Centers entered into a management contract to plan and operate a new rehabilitation hospital—the Lakeshore Hospital. Mike, considering your background, we think you will be a good fit to become the new executive director at Lakeshore."

It was an offer, of course, even if it wasn't close to what Mike had expected or wanted.

Mike had spent part of his residency at Lakeshore with a BMC administrator, so he had insight into what the hospital was all about. True, the Lakeshore project was billed as a "new" rehabilitation hospital. But the only thing new about it was the rehab part. This was a "new" rehab hospital housed on an aging campus tucked away in a remote wooded location in the Birmingham suburb of Homewood.

The campus had operated as a tuberculosis sanatorium for decades. The complex included some distinctive old stone buildings that dated to the 1920s and to the Works Progress Administration of the Great Depression, and some newer brick structures. While the old stone buildings were quaintly distinctive and attractive, none of the existing structures seemed fit for use as any kind of hospital, rehabilitation or otherwise.

Mike knew that converting that old TB-care campus into the

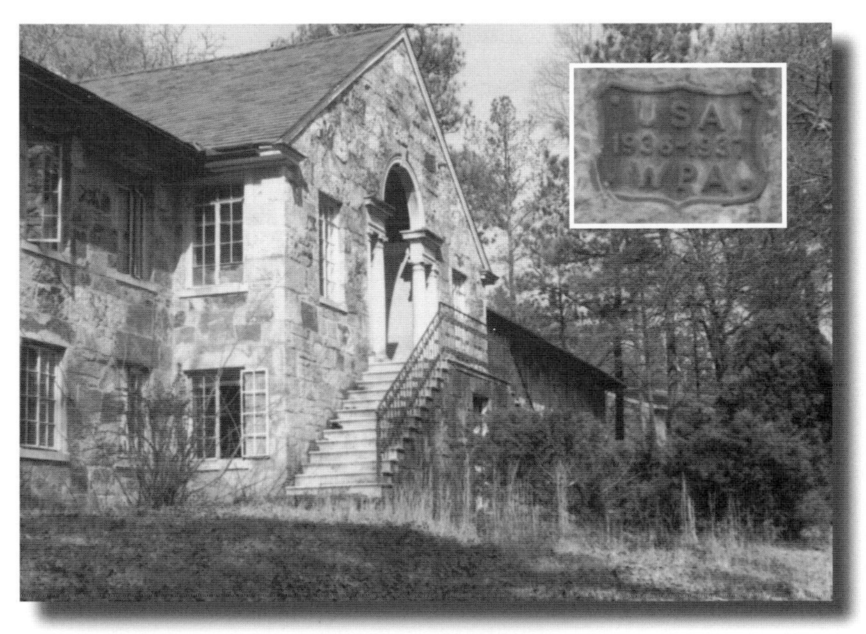

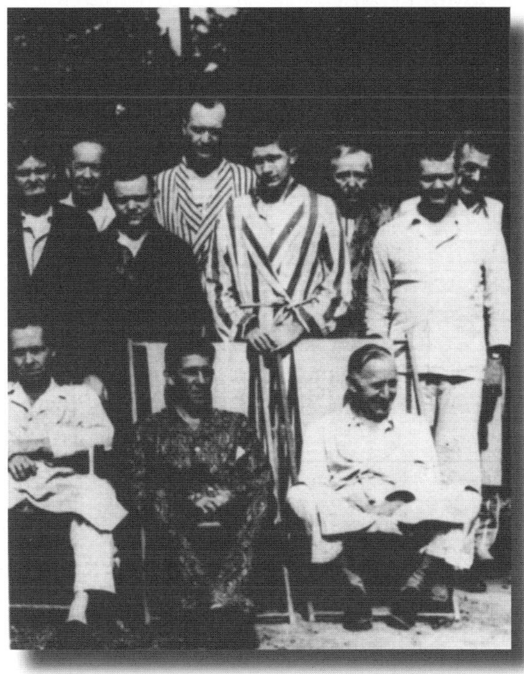

Lakeshore Hospital operated from stone buildings on a remote, wooded campus; for years, the facility had served tuberculosis patients. Inset into top photo shows a bronze plaque on one of the buildings denoting its Works Progress Administration-era status.

Lakeshore rehab hospital had gotten off to a slow start and had a long way to go to meet expectations of Dr. John Miller III, the UAB rehabilitation leader who had been the leading advocate for the concept. Miller dreamed that Lakeshore could become a joint effort of the community and the state of Alabama, and with UAB's help grow into a modern version of the famous Stoke Mandeville rehab Mecca in England.

Further, some in positions of responsibility at BMC seemed to hold an uncomfortable attitude toward Lakeshore Hospital. Mike had gotten the impression that a number of current BMC leaders didn't know what to do with Lakeshore and were questioning why BMC had ever entered into a contract to manage it—particularly in light of BMC's full plate managing its own recent change and turmoil.

And, very significant to Mike, he had overheard talk that one of the first two BMC administrators dispatched to Lakeshore had been an unhappy camper in those buildings out in the woods.

They've already had one guy who couldn't wait to get out of being executive director at Lakeshore. And now they want to send me.

PUTTING IT CHARITABLY, Mike's gut feelings about the Lakeshore position were less than enthusiastic. Professionally, he was more interested in acute care than rehabilitation. Personally, he was the guy who caused such a ruckus as a patient at Spain Rehabilitation Center that he essentially got kicked out of the program before he'd finished his treatment.

Another nuance involved the suspicion that Johnson had offered the job because he had a stereotyped image of Mike.

I still don't walk very well. I can get around without using a wheelchair but only with a lot of effort. Emmett Johnson hasn't really gotten to know me. So when he looks at me, he sees a guy who has a bad limp. To him it makes sense: find a guy who limps and send him to run the rehab hospital.

Mike knew better than to burn his bridges by insulting BMC President/CEO Emmett Johnson with an outright rejection. So he decided to ask for a starting salary higher than he could imagine Johnson approving, and he asked for some perks.

Johnson didn't blink an eye. He said fine to all.

So Mike ventured a bit further.

He said he would take the job at Lakeshore Hospital if Johnson would make a deal: "I will make you a commitment that I will go to Lakeshore for two years and I will do all I can for Lakeshore. But after those two years, Mr. Johnson, I want you to get me out of there. I'm asking you to commit that at the end of two years, you will appoint me to what I really want—a good administrative position in one of BMC's acute-care hospitals."

Again, Emmett Johnson agreed.

So it was, with great doubts and reservations, that Mike Stephens began his stint as Lakeshore Hospital's executive director —with "acting" before his title until he could finish up his thesis and earn his master's degree. He intended to stay two years. Yet, more than 30 years later, with more twists and turns than he can recite, he would still be actively involved with the remote, wooded campus that he helped build into a world-renowned rehabilitation hospital and paralympic sports training facility.

Decades later he would look back and say, "I sincerely believe I was led to Lakeshore Hospital by a divine spirit." By then he could look around with pride and even awe at what had been accomplished.

Yet there would be many times, particularly during the early years, when Michael E. Stephens encountered challenges and obstacles beyond his imagination. There would be times when he wondered if he was being followed around in those buildings out in the woods not by a divine spirit but by the devil himself.

Part II

Lakeshore and Michael Stephens Intersect

7

From TB Sanatorium to Rehabilitation Complex

The development in 1946 of an antibiotic treatment for tuberculosis set the stage for the gradual decline of the Jefferson Tuberculosis Sanatorium. By the 1970s, the sturdy stone buildings erected by President Franklin D. Roosevelt's Works Progress Administration were underutilized and suffering from neglect. Several potential uses for the facility were nominated, but planners eventually agreed it should be used for the rehabilitation of physical disabilities.

If any one person's vision stood out in converting the sanatorium campus into the Lakeshore Rehabilitation Complex, it was that of John M. Miller III, M.D. The Alabama-born Miller was a powerhouse at the University of Alabama at Birmingham. He served as chairman of UAB's Department of Rehabilitation Medicine and also as director of both Spain Rehabilitation Center and UAB's Rehabilitation Research and Training Center.

In a March 1982 interview with *Birmingham Magazine*, Mike Stephens would describe Lakeshore as "a comprehensive approach to rehabilitation, the utopian dream of Dr. John Miller."

Beginning about mid-1972, Miller served as president of the medical staff during the transition from Jefferson Tuberculosis Sanatorium to Lakeshore Rehabilitation Complex. He supported the developing Lakeshore programs by loaning and sharing physicians and other experts from UAB's Spain Rehabilitation Center.

Perhaps most importantly, Miller had a strong hand in developing the master plan for Lakeshore's newly emerging mission in rehabilitation. Those who knew Miller noted that some of his ideas were inspired by approaches that had been taken in providing services to patients with spinal cord injuries at Stoke Mandeville, where the Paralympic Games were founded in 1948.

Believing that Lakeshore should help those with physical disabilities beyond the acute-care phase, Miller wanted Lakeshore to rehabilitate individuals for reintegration into the community.

He advocated a plan that called for the campus to have both a hospital component and a vocational rehabilitation training component—with state and federal vocational rehabilitation funds contributing to a funding base.

He strongly believed Lakeshore's service should include "transitional living"—offering a place on the Lakeshore campus where those with physical disabilities could progress from treatment-and-training to life in the outside world—and "residential living"—a cluster of long-term housing units designed for individuals with physical disabilities and located on the Lakeshore campus.

Dr. Miller also had ideas about coordinating the services offered by UAB's Spain Rehabilitation Center with those offered by Lakeshore. His concept was that Spain could take care of those with physical disabilities in the early days of their therapy—soon after an injury or illness occurred—and that Lakeshore could offer long-term resources to further the rehabilitation Spain had begun. In addition to Miller, others at Spain—including Dr. Don Patrick and Dick Lind, who helped chart the Lakeshore master plan—had supported that continuum of services.

By early 1974, discussions about Lakeshore referred to two types of facilities on its campus. There was "Lakeshore Hospital," which received its first rehab patients in November 1973. And there was "Lakeshore Rehabilitation Facility," which began providing services to rehab clients in July 1974. The former addressed healthcare needs. The latter offered vocational rehabilitation services—job retraining and job placement.

It was indeed a partnership. In time, the two components became known as the Lakeshore Rehabilitation Complex.

Although idea after idea came forth from Dr. Miller, unfortunately the full scope of his vision for Lakeshore would never be known. He

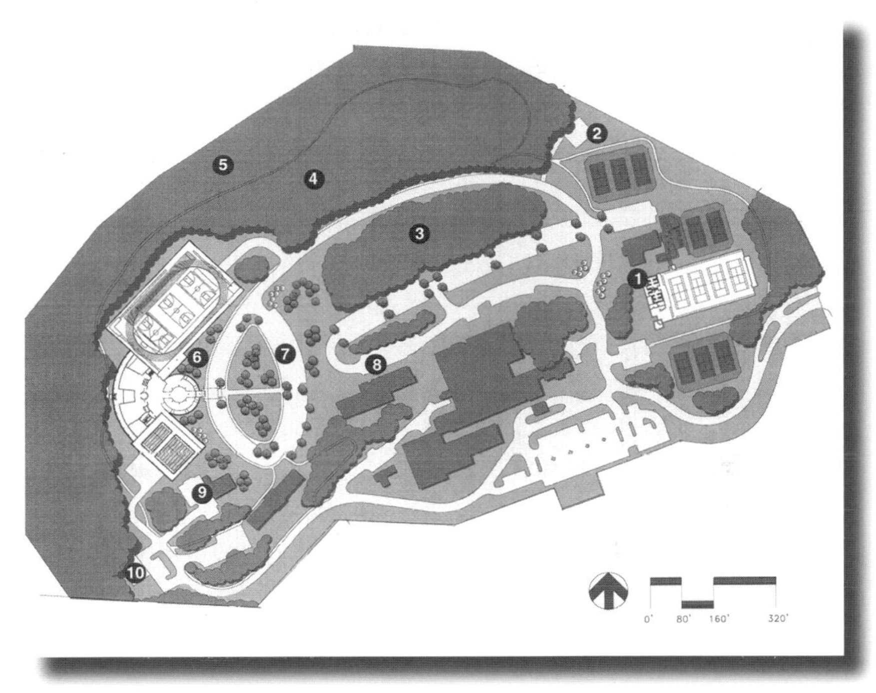

Eventually the Lakeshore Foundation would craft an expanded master plan with special-purpose buildings for sports and fitness, but the campus's original structures, shown in gray above, encompassed Lakeshore Hospital and Lakeshore Rehabilitation Facility.
Below: *A 1974 aerial view of the campus.*

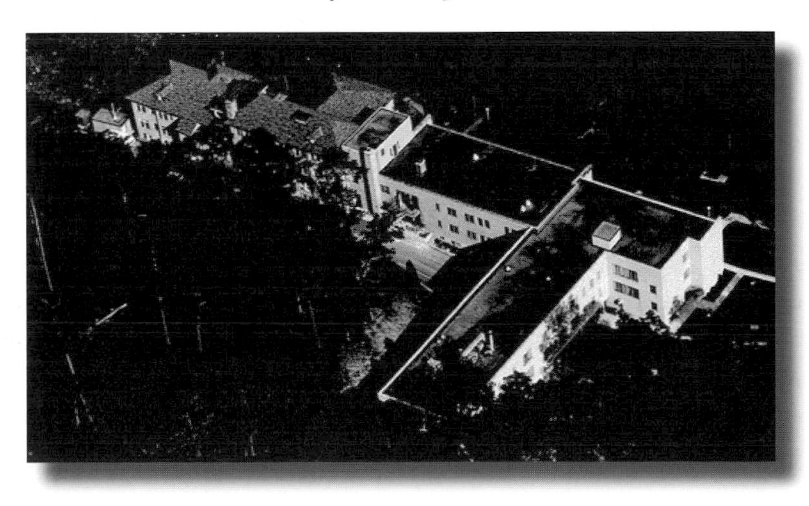

was stricken with a viral heart infection and, following an extended illness, died February 29, 1976. He was 44.

IN THE EARLY years on the Lakeshore rehab campus, Lakeshore Hospital and Lakeshore Rehabilitation Facility were closely paired. Located in adjacent buildings, the two entities aimed to work seamlessly in the different services they delivered to those with physical disabilities.

Lakeshore Hospital came to the aid of patients with healthcare needs by using the skills of physicians, nurses, and physical and occupational therapists.

Lakeshore Rehabilitation Facility made available the counselors, testing experts, teachers, and other staff to provide adult education, driver education, and testing, retraining, and placement for new jobs. Some of its first jobs programs offered training for switchboard receptionists, computer programmers, and microfilm technicians.

Lakeshore's initial patient-client emphasis was on individuals with disabilities related to spinal cord injuries, amputations of limbs, orthopedic disorders, and cerebral vascular accidents. Gradually, that list expanded to cerebral palsy, multiple sclerosis, muscular dystrophy, arthritis, sight problems, and other disabilities.

When Lakeshore Hospital officially opened as a rehab facility in November 1973, the initial patients were transfers from UAB's Spain Rehabilitation Center. The close ties between Spain and Lakeshore would continue, but the 1972–73 master plan also included strategies to identify other individuals who needed Lakeshore's services.

Early plans projected patient referrals from physicians in the community, Spain Rehabilitation Center, and Alabama's statewide vocational rehabilitation program. For example, a Spring 1975 Lakeshore report to state vocational rehabilitation staff noted that Spain's Dr. Cecil Nepomuceno was screening and examining patients for admission to Lakeshore Hospital. (This was the same "Dr. Nepo" who had been Mike Stephens's rehabilitation physician following his swimming accident.)

ON THE VOCATIONAL rehab side, two of Lakeshore's key early players were Drs. Donald Patrick and George M. Hudson.

In March 1974, Patrick (a Ph.D.) was named director of the Lakeshore Rehabilitation Facility. Patrick was not new to the Lakeshore campus. In 1973, he had been loaned to Lakeshore by UAB to direct a three-month federally funded study to decide the future use of the TB sanatorium collection of buildings. This was the study that led to Lakeshore's having a multi-disability rehabilitation mission. Patrick's appointment was another reflection of the close ties that existed between Lakeshore and UAB while the rehab campus was being planned and birthed. Patrick initially was to be a part-time director of the Lakeshore Rehabilitation Facility; he would also continue part-time in his post as associate project director of UAB's Rehabilitation Research and Training Center.

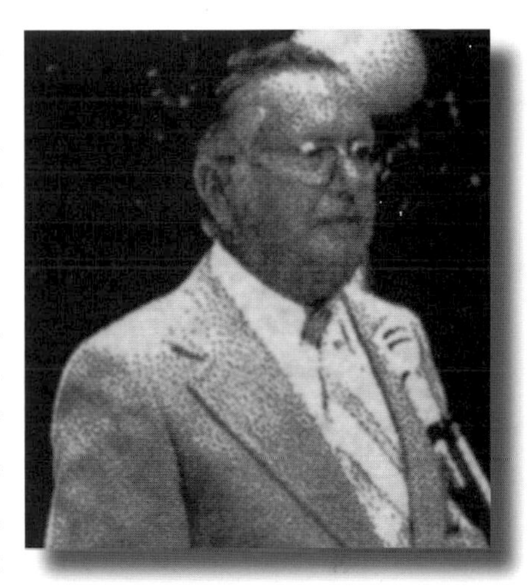

Dr. George Hudson.

From the beginning of Patrick's work at Lakeshore, he worked closely with the state official who directed Alabama's Division of Vocational Rehabilitation and Crippled Children's Service, Dr. George M. Hudson, and with Hudson's assistant, Bill Cowen, who was instrumental in writing grants and driving initiatives forward. Hudson's division was then under the Alabama State Department of Education. In later years, a separate rehabilitation department would be established at the state level—the Alabama Department of Rehabilitation Services.

Meanwhile, on the Lakeshore Hospital side, a search was underway for a visionary leader. The task of finding such an administrator was in the hands of Baptist Medical Centers (BMC), which had a management contract with the Lakeshore board of directors.

In August 1972, during the conversion of the Lakeshore campus from TB sanatorium—TB patients were still in the facility—to rehab complex, BMC had placed Lakeshore Hospital under an administrator who ended up staying for only five months. Then for the next year and a half, BMC put the hospital's administrative reins in the hands of a BMC official whose main focus was to conduct long-range campus planning, not to entrench himself as a day-to-day rehab hospital administrator.

By 1975, BMC President Emmett Johnson recognized the need to recruit a Lakeshore Hospital administrator with multiple strengths—the ability to organize and put in place crucial operating systems, the leadership skills to get routine operations on an even keel, the vision to plan ahead for success, and the determination to convert those plans into reality.

As Johnson consulted with other BMC officials about the ideal person to fill the Lakeshore Hospital's executive director position, his eye kept coming back to a young hospital administration resident who had performed admirably in the leadership vacuum left after the exodus of 15 top BMC executives in 1974: Michael E. Stephens. He was only 31 and he was inexperienced. But Johnson could see that the young graduate student was determined, smart, and a born salesman and natural leader. Also, he had personal experience as a rehab patient.

As related earlier, Johnson offered Mike the job, and Mike, with grave reservations—and with Johnson's commitment that in two years he could trade the Lakeshore post for one in an acute-care hospital—accepted.

MIKE STEPHENS BECAME Lakeshore's acting executive director just a few months before Dr. John Miller's death. He was already familiar with the anatomy of the rehab hospital he would head due to the time he had spent on the Lakeshore campus during his master's degree residency. He well understood the key ingredients of the Lakeshore vision—operating a rehabilitation hospital and a vocational rehabilitation facility on the same campus.

Mike also had enough information about the Lakeshore project to know that rough sailing likely lay ahead. He knew that a long list of concerns was headed by financial needs, physical-plant issues, and society's tendency to discriminate against those with physical disabilities.

"There would be so many times when I would wonder about the full extent of Dr. Miller's ideas for Lakeshore—ideas that would have emerged gradually and been modified as Lakeshore developed," Mike said. "As we went forward and Lakeshore would take this turn or that turn, I would sometimes wonder, 'Now, what would Dr. Miller have thought about this?' "

Mike knew the comprehensive rehab campus concept was new in the Birmingham area and, for that matter, new around the state. Some strong selling would have to be done. Mike knew it would be an uphill battle to sell the Lakeshore concept to physicians, patients, and families, and also to leaders in various communities who could help reshape negative societal attitudes toward those with physical disabilities.

He was painfully aware that Lakeshore Hospital had inherited decades-old buildings that were not designed for their current use. And Mike could see no capital funds in sight to deal with that. Perhaps even more pressing was the day-to-day cash-flow need of a struggling new rehab hospital that was trying to get its feet on the ground. Mike did not have to look deeply into the Lakeshore Hospital crystal ball to see looming obstacles.

As it turned out, a far-reaching piece of federal legislation passed two years before Mike took his new job would make all the difference.

Under the Rehabilitation Act of 1973, additional grants became available to the states for retraining individuals with disabilities. The new law also barred firms doing business with the federal government from employment discrimination against the disabled.

In a December 1975 article by Dr. Donald Patrick, he referred to the Act as "the recent shot heard 'round the rehab world.' " His article appeared in *Viewpoint*, published jointly by two of UAB's rehabilitation entities—Spain Rehabilitation Center and the Rehabilitation Research and Training Center.

In his article, Dr. Patrick said the new legislation opened the doors for significantly expanded employment of individuals with physical disabilities. He said that "with the increased emphasis on services to the severely disabled," the Lakeshore concepts "appear to be ideas whose time has come."

There could be no doubt that without the injection of federal and state vocational rehabilitation funding the Lakeshore dream could not have been birthed and sustained.

At the beginning of Lakeshore's life in 1973–74, vocational rehabilitation monies even subsidized patient care. As Lakeshore Hospital received its first patients on Tuesday, November 6, 1973, its leaders said that all of the first hospital patients would be clients of the state's vocational rehabilitation program and that funds from that program would pay the bills.

This arrangement was intended to be, and proved to be, short-term. When Lakeshore Hospital opened, application had been made for the hospital to receive reimbursement for Medicare and Medicaid patients. Applications also had been made for the hospital to work with Blue Cross-Blue Shield and other insurance companies. In April 1974, Lakeshore began admitting its first Medicare/Medicaid-sponsored patients. And private insurance approval would follow.

However, it would be a slow, painful process to get the patient population to a financially viable level. Dr. Patrick wrote that the first three months of Lakeshore's existence "were very trying ones financially."

Those deep Lakeshore money woes would last far beyond three months.

8

A Reluctant Arrival Takes Charge

Mike Stephens was far from enthusiastic when he arrived at Lakeshore Hospital in 1975. *Well, I'm here—even though I have come fighting it the whole way.* He reported for duty with the official title of "Acting Executive Director." The "acting" part would be removed a month later when Mike received his master's degree in hospital administration from the University of Alabama at Birmingham (UAB).

A July 28, 1975, article in the *Birmingham Post-Herald* officially announced that Michael E. Stephens had been selected as Lakeshore's new executive director. The article also reported that Richard A. "Dick" Lind, who had preceded Mike in Lakeshore's top administrative slot, had on July 1 begun his new job in Florida—as assistant director of the Halifax Hospital and Medical Center in Daytona Beach.

The irony was not lost on Mike. *Dick Lind is going forward in a career that I want, and that I intend to have in a couple of years—a career with a general acute-care hospital, not a struggling rehab facility.*

Mike already knew the campus from his brief stint there as a resident. But at that point Dick Lind had been in charge at Lakeshore Hospital. Now, Mike was looking at problems through a new perspective.

What Mike saw was a beautiful, serene wooded setting accented by two stone buildings that were the original structures on campus, intermingled with more recently built brick structures. Altogether the campus looked like a picture postcard—that is, if one were on a rustic vacation at a remote lodge.

Lakeshore's isolated location was intentional. In decades gone by, it was common for TB patients to be cared for in secluded settings away from the general population to prevent the spread of the highly contagious *Mycobacterium tuberculosis*.

Pervading what was now the Lakeshore rehabilitation campus was an air of both seclusion and yesteryear. The remote, historic feel was fed not only by the wooded location, but also by the antiquated appearance of the TB sanatorium's original stone buildings. The resulting effect struck some as suitable for a murder mystery movie set on an isolated British estate. No wonder the Jefferson Tuberculosis Sanatorium had become the subject of tall tales and folklore. "Once a security guard went to check out a concern in the original 1920s stone building and reported, 'I believe that something strange is going on there. Maybe there is a ghost,' " Mike recalls. "Needless to say, I had a lot to think about as I was getting settled in at Lakeshore. I was going to work at a place where folks actually thought ghosts were running around."

As the young executive took inventory, his mind was racing. He could hear the echoing voices of some of his fellow UAB healthcare administration graduate students, who had warned him of possible consequences of "taking a job out there in that remote rehab place. You could be throwing away your whole career!"

IT WOULD TAKE a whale of a renovation job to transform the older buildings into an acceptable 1970s hospital facility. Even Lakeshore's more recent structures posed a major challenge; they were designed with narrow passageways for ambulatory TB patients, and now they had to accommodate rehab patients, most of whom were in wheelchairs.

By the time Mike arrived on the scene, only minimum renovations had been completed. Few beds were open to receive patients at Lakeshore, and, since the patient census was pitifully small, most of those available beds were not occupied.

As Lakeshore had been transitioning from a TB sanatorium to a rehabilitation center, some of the cleanup had been hurried, spotty, and makeshift. In one big 1950s building, enough cleanup had been done to create an area on the first floor that could accommodate rehab patients. However, the second floor of that building looked like a huge cluttered attic. Outdated TB sanatorium furnishings and pieces of equipment clustered in disorganized and dusty disarray. Mike liked order. What he saw on that floor was the definition of disorder.

This is how bad it was:

One night a patient in a wheelchair, a patient at Lakeshore for rehab due to a brain injury, accidentally pushed the wrong elevator button and ended up alone on that darkened, cluttered floor. "No harm came to the patient," said Mike. "But it's not surprising that he was so confused by the mess he saw that he thought he had arrived in some kind of 'Twilight Zone.' " The patient found a phone at the abandoned nurses' station on the deserted floor and called the police and told them he was at Lakeshore Hospital and that "everyone else is gone. Something has happened—don't know what. Maybe a bomb went off or something. It's all a big mess!"

Mike was the first to agree that it indeed was a big mess.

There was also an appalling roach infestation on the campus. These and similar problems gave Mike reason to worry about state hospital inspections, and they raised his concerns about the challenges of marketing to bring in new patients.

Man, look at the dark, dingy halls in these buildings! Who's going to want to refer a patient, or come as a patient, to this decrepit old place?

Yes, operating a hospital in these outdated facilities was going to be a challenge. Generating a cash flow was going to be a challenge. Attracting patients was going to be a challenge. Everything was going to be a challenge.

AROUND THAT TIME, Mike Stephens met George Traugh, Lakeshore's new medical director. Traugh was smart, colorful, and would prove pivotal in Lakeshore's early history. Very knowledgeable in rehabilitation medicine, Dr. Traugh was a "physiatrist," a physician who specialized in physical medicine. He was effective, innovative, progressive, and caring and committed toward his patients. Like several other key professionals

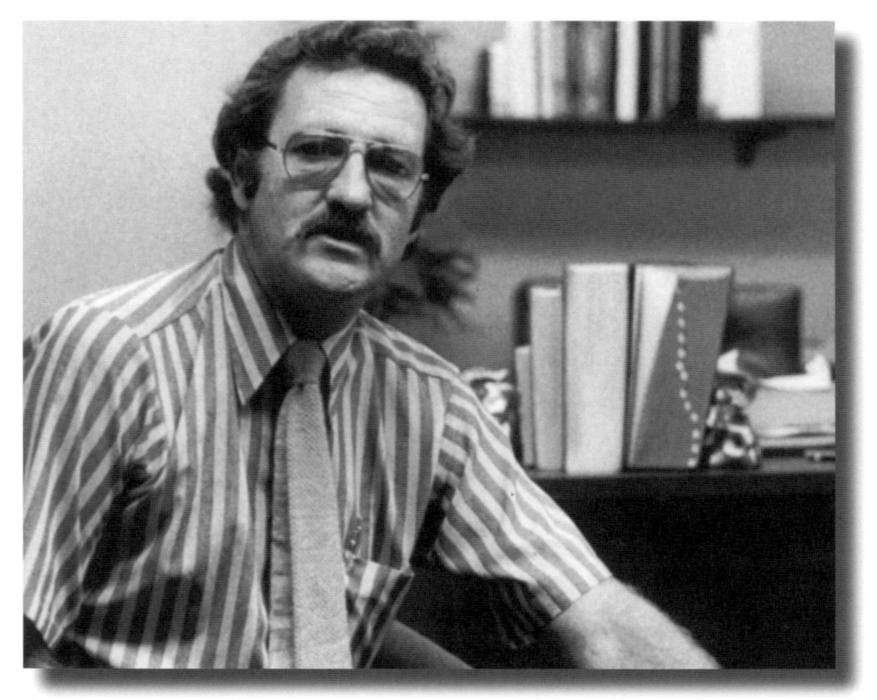

Dr. George Traugh.

in the early days of Lakeshore, Traugh came from UAB and had treated patients at UAB's Spain Rehabilitation Center.

Traugh was also well known nationally because he had been in the media spotlight as the physician who guided the rehabilitation of Alabama Governor George C. Wallace after the governor was paralyzed by a would-be assassin's bullets on May 15, 1972.

George Traugh was not only strong and effective, but also flamboyant and independent. He said exactly what he thought, proudly wore his cowboy boots to work, was unpredictable, obviously enjoyed being difficult at times, and was so far from mainstream that some would describe him as eccentric. All-in-all, he was a man who marched to his own drummer.

But then, some of those same descriptions could describe independent-minded Mike Stephens—minus the cowboy boots.

On the day they first met, the two were being escorted on separate tours of the Lakeshore campus in preparation for assuming their new jobs. Partway through their respective tours, their paths crossed. They said hello, agreed they needed to talk later, and went on.

As the tours came to an end later that day, their paths again crossed and Traugh said, "Well, now is the time to talk."

Mike suggested his office, but George had other ideas. "No, let's get into my truck," replied the doctor.

Mike was bemused as he climbed into Dr. Traugh's truck. As befitted its interesting owner, the 1950s-era orange pickup had its own distinctive style. The truck bellowed smoke as Dr. Traugh drove it to Ireland's, a nearby popular bar and restaurant.

They sat in the bar for a long time that day, talking and drinking. As hospital administrators and physicians are prone to do, they approached a variety of subjects from differing points of views. They talked about Lakeshore's potential and they talked about Lakeshore's problems. They batted possible approaches and solutions back and forth. Neither was short on opinions nor shy about voicing them.

At the end, George looked at Mike and said, "I wanted to see what you are all about. I like you."

That day marked the beginning of a good working relationship and friendship between Lakeshore's new executive director and new medical director. Each felt the pulls, needs, and constraints that were common for those in their respective positions. Both wanted good patient care. As a hospital administrator, Mike had to strive toward that end with budget realities always at the forefront of his mind. As a physician, George tended to push budget concerns toward the back of his mind.

An example of their constructive interaction came early in their days at Lakeshore when Dr. Traugh felt a strong need for an intercom system.

"Mike, I'm all over Lakeshore Hospital—from one end of that place to the other. There could be someone who really needs me and can't get in touch with me," the doctor told the young administrator. "I need a paging system—a public-address system."

Mike answered, "I would like to get a paging system for you. You're covering a lot of patients, and I believe you need an intercom system. But Lakeshore can't afford it."

Then Mike began to explain how George could help Lakeshore Hospital with its finances and in the process "earn" his paging system—by bringing in a steady stream of patients to Lakeshore.

"Listen, this is a two-way street," said Mike. "You maintain a census of 20 patients for 30 days, and I'll see to it that you get a paging system."

Now it was Dr. Traugh's turn to be bemused. He respected strength, candor, and innovative approaches. From young administrator Mike Stephens, he had just gotten all three.

Dr. Traugh responded to Mike's challenge. He worked hard at bringing in patients to Lakeshore. Soon he was up to the goals Mike had outlined. As promised, he got his paging system.

Mike would later recall that incident as the official launch of getting in a baseline of patients for Lakeshore Hospital. Working together, Stephens and Traugh would lead the way for many good things to take place on the Lakeshore rehab campus.

AS DIFFICULT AS budgets are in an administrator's job, personnel issues can be even more of a headache, as Mike learned in a hurry on a Monday morning when he had been in his Lakeshore position for only a month.

Because he had been appointed to the Lakeshore job by Baptist Medical Centers, Mike made it a point to stay in close touch with BMC administration. On this particular Monday morning, he stopped by to visit with administrators at BMC Princeton in west Birmingham. He had barely walked through the door when an administrator friend fired at him: "Well, Mike, what are you going to do about all this mess?"

The "mess," which Mike had not yet heard about, was airing in radio news bulletins about a fatal domestic dispute. A husband had fatally shot his wife after she confronted him about an affair he was having. The wife had also called the other woman's husband to tell him about the affair, and that distraught man then shot himself and was now in the hospital (he survived).

The mess was Mike's mess because the cheating husband, now an accused wife-killer, was Lakeshore's director of maintenance and housekeeping. And the "other woman" was also a Lakeshore employee, an attendant in the transitional living unit.

There was more. This was 1975, barely a decade after the civil rights protests and KKK bombings and other violence that had roiled Birmingham in the 1960s. And the male Lakeshore employee was black while the female employee was white.

As soon as Mike heard the news that Monday morning, he knew he had to place the sordid situation high on his growing list of priorities, even though he felt his full attention needed to be on Lakeshore's core problems of patient census, money, and buildings. *We have enough problems to deal with around Lakeshore without all this kind of crap. I should be telling myself, "Mike, you'd better get out of here. The place is falling apart."*

Instead, he hunkered down, living and breathing Lakeshore night and day as he dealt with both the litany of Lakeshore core problems and the nightmare of a personnel crisis.

I know that I'm not leaving, not yet. I'm going to hang in there, give Lakeshore the two years I promised to Emmett Johnson, and during those two years really work at making something out of this place.

AS HE SETTLED into the work at Lakeshore, Mike sometimes reflected on the facility's roots in tuberculosis treatment and how he had gleaned his first childhood impressions of the disease. Those impressions had come from a lady named Maudie, from Maudie's daughter, and from Mike's mother, Virginia "Gee Gee" Stephens.

This was Mike's story:

"I remember that, when I was a child, a lady named Maudie lived across the street from us. Everybody loved Maudie.

"Maudie had a daughter that I had not known. The daughter had been away from home for months, and then she returned home. When she returned, she came with her mother to visit at our house. The daughter had known my mother, and it was important to her

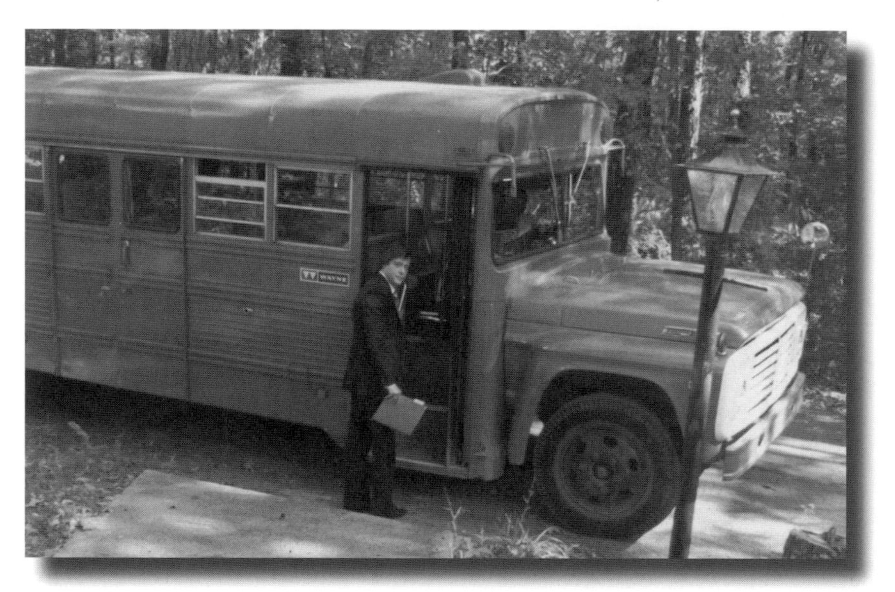

It might not have looked like much, but Mike Stephens was proud of this much-used school bus donated by an arm of the state vocational rehabilitation services. It was the first major piece of equipment Lakeshore received during its critical period of trying to find funding for needed expansion of programs. The bus was used to take clients into the community to reduce their isolation.

to be able to again visit with Gee Gee Stephens.

"When she came to our home for that visit, she had just been discharged from a tuberculosis sanatorium. As most people in that day and time were, my mother was terrified of tuberculosis—I mean really terrified. When Maudie and her daughter came to our home, my mother would not allow my two sisters and me to be around the daughter.

"My mother was very gracious to Maudie and her daughter. Consistent with her custom when visitors came, she served them coffee and cake. But after they left, she boiled the dishes to destroy any germs. Her fear was so typical of the deep fear of tuberculosis that existed in those days."

Gradually as his Lakeshore tenure proceeded, Mike began to see interesting parallels between the two societies of patients who had come to be served on the same campus—first the tuberculosis patients, and then those with physical disabilities.

"With TB, the approach of isolating patients for treatment had continued for decade after decade. Then both the treatment and the image surrounding TB changed. Gradually TB patients were treated within the community, integrated into the community, and accepted by the community. Instead of being isolated for treatment in sanatoria, TB patients were mainstreamed to receive the healthcare they needed in acute-care general hospitals. With the improvement of pharmacological agents for treating TB, more and more TB care was carried out on an outpatient basis—with patients taking anti-TB drugs, undergoing periodic checkups in outpatient clinics, and living at home during treatment. As people became more accustomed to TB patients being treated in non-isolated environments, the stigma of tuberculosis gradually diminished and over time was virtually eradicated.

"Little did I realize when I was assigned to Lakeshore in 1975 that to help place those with physical disabilities back in society, I was embarking on a mission that also meant we had to attack significant impediments related to social stigma and isolation."

Mike saw that in some ways, many of those with physical disabilities were as isolated from their communities as TB patients had been.

"There were customs in play that seemed bent on isolating people in wheelchairs from other segments of society. In both cases, part of the isolation that had to be combated was related to stigma. I found it both ironic and touching that these two societies of patients, who on the surface seemed so different, would have so much in common in that both groups—the tuberculosis patients and individuals dealing with physical disabilities—would be isolated to receive services on the same campus in Homewood, Alabama."

In the isolation of that serene, beautiful wooded acreage in Homewood, obstacles would be confronted and tremendous progress would be made via a comprehensive approach to rehabilitation. As time went by, many a person with physical disabilities would see his or her life dramatically changed for the better on this campus that had come to be known as Lakeshore.

However, before steady and significant progress would begin to show its face at Lakeshore, Mike Stephens would see the struggles of some pioneer rehabilitation patients in Lakeshore's "early days"—struggling patients whose experiences would forever be seared into his mind and heart.

9

Of Sandwiches and Senators

Mike Stephens may have been a reluctant rehab hospital administrator, but he was effective. One reason why is that he was empathetic with the patients. Johnny Bolt's sandwich is a good example. Empathy can only take an administrator so far, however, and another reason Stephens was effective is that he was determined. Some might say stubborn. His filibustering of a U.S. senator is a good example of that. The sandwich led indirectly to the senator, and the senator led directly to $1.7 million in critically needed funding to replace a condemned hospital building and make other expansions.

This is how it happened.

Johnny Bolt was a young Lakeshore patient paralyzed from the waist down by a gunshot wound. He was from the town of Jasper in rural Walker County, about 50 miles northwest of Birmingham. He was not yet 21 when he was shot one night while trespassing. Johnny was not exactly a master criminal—he had been stealing watermelons—and Mike liked him: "He was so genuine you couldn't help but like that kid. Johnny just had this big ole country-boy way about himself."

Johnny was at Lakeshore specifically for treatment of a decubitus ulcer—a pressure sore, or bedsore, which is a common problem for paralyzed persons who have impaired circulation and immobility. The body's weight presses vulnerable tissue against a bed or wheelchair and an ulcer develops. Improperly cared for, such an ulcer can spread and lead to infection in surrounding muscle, tendon, and bone, and ultimately can cause death. Treatment is tedious, involving constant cleaning, medicating, and sometimes surgically cutting away decayed tissue.

Meanwhile, Johnny spent much of his time lying on a bed or a gurney with his behind stuck up in the air, which was his situation when Stephens encountered him one evening on an elevator in Lakeshore's main hospital building, a decrepit stone structure built in the 1920s.

Stephens had been Lakeshore's executive director for less than six months. One of his early acts was to impose a strict no-food-in-patient-rooms rule. He hadn't wanted to. He knew intimately the simple pleasure of having a snack handy when a craving hit during the lonely hours of rehabilitation. But—and there's no way to sugar-coat this—Lakeshore was crawling with roaches. "Those damn roaches were all over those buildings. The situation was just horrible," Stephens remembers.

He and Johnny were alone in the elevator. Johnny was face-down on a gurney that he could self-propel, and he had a pillow that he could rest on. They exchanged hellos. "Right off the bat I became suspicious," said Stephens. "So I said, 'Johnny, what have you got under that pillow?' "

"Awww, Mr. Mike . . .," said Johnny, knowing he was busted. He lifted the pillow—revealing a sandwich he meant to eat later in his room.

"Johnny, you know the rules. You can't take that sandwich to your room. Take it back to the cafeteria."

Johnny did.

IN JOHNNY'S PRESENCE, Stephens maintained a kind, firm, and composed demeanor. He didn't show Johnny how he really felt, but the incident got to him emotionally. Johnny was devastated, and so was Mike, and it was no passing feeling. "I knew what that sandwich meant to Johnny. I had been there in his situation. To me, Johnny became a heartbreaking example of how at that time we had such lousy facilities that we couldn't even permit a slight pleasure in life for our patients who already had suffered and lost so much."

Like Johnny, Mike had been a young man who one day went from being strong and able-bodied to being paralyzed. Like Johnny, Mike had been a patient in a rehabilitation hospital.

Mike knew the things that were important to a patient in Johnny's situation. "Once you're hurt your world becomes so small, so narrow.

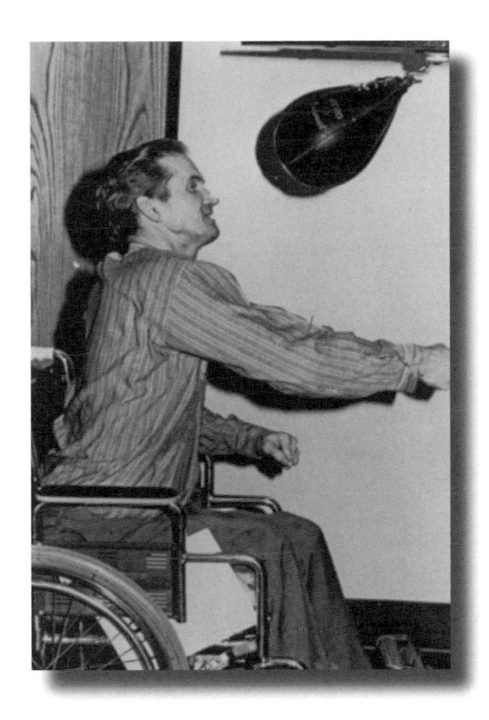

Johnny Bolt, working out on the speed bag.

It's a big victory just to be able to make your way into a closet and get your clothes. When you have a severe physical disability, to the point you can't even move parts of your body anymore, and are learning how to live with that, little things take on a whole level of increased importance. It can be very, very special to take something from the cafeteria back to your room so you can look forward to having that snack at night."

As in many rehab hospitals, Lakeshore patients were not even allowed to have televisions in their rooms because watching TV encourages inactivity. Rehab is about physical activity so patients can gain strength and as much mobility as possible. Rehab patients are pushed so hard day after day that their challenges can be compared to army boot camp, Stephens says. He recalls even today how he looked forward to the slightest diversion when he was a patient at UAB's Spain Rehabilitation Center.

"During the day, I was busy in the various therapy sessions. Then, at 5 p.m., most of Spain's staff left for the day, and I went back to my room, where there was nothing for me to do. So there I was, paralyzed, sitting in my wheelchair or lying in my bed. It was boring, a terrible existence. I recall times when the one thing I had to look forward to at night was food I had brought back to my room from Spain's cafeteria. I knew I could eat that treat at 10 P.M., and that was something I could look forward to.

"Oh yeah, I knew how Johnny Bolt felt."

ROACH INFESTATION OF its buildings was only a part of Lakeshore's dismal picture in 1975. The bottom line was that the Lakeshore campus was ill-suited to function as a rehabilitation hospital. Subpar old stone buildings were mixed in among newer brick structures that had not been designed or built to accommodate rehab patients; the combination was a looming disaster. Of particular concern to Stephens was the oldest building on campus, a 1920s stone structure that was not up to current codes, but which housed Lakeshore Hospital's crucial ancillary services of pharmacy, laboratory, radiology, and dietary. Limited renovation funds had not been able to solve the problems and Stephens knew that Lakeshore was headed for a showdown with hospital inspectors about building-related issues. It was just a matter of time—a short time, as it turned out.

About a year after Johnny Bolt had to be denied his sandwich, inspectors from the Alabama Department of Public Health (ADPH) condemned the building. Stephens recalled the moment: "I mean, those inspectors came on Lakeshore's campus and took a good look at that building and said, 'You've just got to tear this building down and move these services somewhere else.' "

This was a rare and drastic step by ADPH, but it was one that was devastating for an Alabama hospital because the inspectors determined whether a hospital retained its license to operate.

The condemnation could not have come at a more pivotal time. On the one hand progress was being made, while on the other hand an ongoing money crisis was playing out.

On the progress side, Lakeshore Hospital was gaining a real foothold in helping individuals with challenging physical disabilities; Lakeshore had started some great work that needed to continue. Stephens and the staff and board felt it would be a tragedy if Lakeshore were forced to close.

On the money woes side, the hospital had a mounting cash flow problem because it didn't yet have enough patients and because there were ongoing problems in getting insurance companies to reimburse adequately for care of patients in a rehabilitation setting.

"At the time, Lakeshore Hospital was $140,000 in the hole, and there were no funds to draw from. In short, we were out of money. During this period there was one occasion when the board chairman countersigned a loan in order for the hospital to meet payroll," Stephens recalled.

He knew that to save Lakeshore Hospital, something drastic had to be done.

In his desperate search for lifelines, Stephens noticed wording in the nation's Medicare law that was more than a bit interesting. "There was this Medicare provision that if you could procure a federal grant to build something, and you got it built, then there was an allowable cost under Medicare reimbursement to depreciate it—that is, you could get reimbursement for depreciation of the building."

That Medicare provision struck him as possibly addressing two big Lakeshore problems: the need for a building to replace the one that had just been condemned and the need for cash flow. *This could be the answer. Get this federal grant here. And then charge them over here. Get us a building and a cash flow. This could save us!!*

So Mr. Stephens went to Washington.

The timing could have been better. It was early 1977 and the nation had just gotten a new president whose eyes were focused on keeping a tight, tight rein on federal dollars. One of the economic policies that new President Jimmy Carter had just put in place was a controversial budget-control technique he had used in modified form as governor of Georgia. The technique was called "zero-based budgeting," and it had federal officials and members of Congress shaking their heads in frustration.

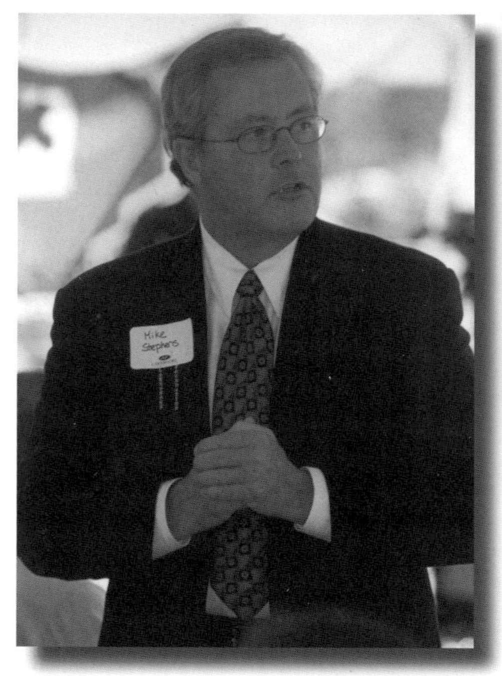

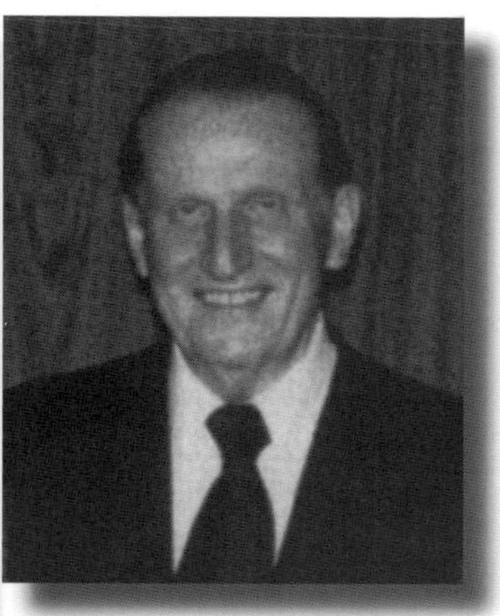

A determined Mike Stephens sought aid from Alabama's congressional delegation, and got it from Senator James B. Allen Jr.

Before Carter, Washington had been accustomed to incremental planning based on modifying previous budgets. In that traditional approach, last year's budget was used as a baseline and then adjusted for inflation and additions or cuts. Under Carter, federal agencies and departments would start at zero for each budget period and have to justify every expense.

The powers-that-be in Congress were suddenly very skittish about lending their support to extra expenditures.

On the other hand, Stephens knew that he had no choice about the timing. He had to go to Washington to seek help, and he had to go right then.

Stephens also knew whose key support he must have—that of James B. "Jim" Allen, the powerful second-term junior U.S. senator from Alabama. During his eight years in the Senate, Allen already had amassed an impressive record. His effectiveness was due in part to his prior political experience, including eight years in the Alabama legislature and two terms as Alabama's lieutenant governor.

Stephens had done his homework and felt that he likely could count on the support of other key members of Alabama's congressional delegation, including Alabama's longtime senior senator, John J. Sparkman. It was Senator Allen that Stephens had to convince.

He knew he faced a tough selling job on Allen, for Allen had become known as one of the most conservative Democrats in the Senate. In this period of zero-based budgeting, he expected Allen would be even more frugal-minded than usual toward new projects.

But Stephens was a salesman. Prior to his injury and prior to coming to Lakeshore, his first career had been as a successful salesman of insurance and then in the legal publications business. He was about to need all that experience and more.

IN WASHINGTON, STEPHENS made his calls at the offices of members of Alabama's congressional delegation. As expected, things went pretty well until he reached Allen's office and was stonewalled by a staff member.

Stephens recalled that long, long day. "A staffer came out into the reception area and asked me to explain what I needed. After I did, he began giving me all this stuff about 'Well, we can't give you any support for this Lakeshore project this year. Senator Allen will try to put it into the budget for you next year.' "

That would be too late; Lakeshore had to have concrete plans now for a building replacement plan that ADPH inspectors would accept. So Mike challenged the staffer.

"Well, now this is not meant as any disrespect to you. But I've got to hear this from Senator Allen himself. I represent a certain population of people in the Birmingham area, including a board of directors that has some members who are supporters of the senator. I just don't feel comfortable returning to Birmingham without having talked to Senator Allen himself."

The staff member was accustomed to people pushing him to see the senator. He held firm. Mike held just as firm, saying, "That's fine. I'll just sit right here and wait until he can see me."

As the hours ticked by, Mike sat and waited all afternoon.

Finally, at 5:30 P.M., he was called in to see Allen. Mike rose from his seat and made what seemed a long, long walk into the senator's office.

Well, I'm getting what I asked for. I'm getting in to see Allen. But now I'm scared to death. I've never even met this guy. But here goes.

Once into Senator Allen's office, a different kind of feeling began to come over him. He no longer felt afraid. Instead, he felt determined—very determined.

Mike's conversation with the senator was like Part I and Part II. Part I was a repeat of what Allen's staff member had told Mike several hours earlier: wait till next year.

"I just can't support federal funding for this project this year," said Allen. "But don't worry. Next year I'm going to put it in the budget. And the year after that you'll get it."

Mike didn't hesitate. "Senator, Lakeshore Hospital can't wait. Lakeshore Hospital can't survive that long!"

So Mike and Allen entered into Part II of their conversation—the part where it became obvious that Allen more and more understood both the urgency of the situation and the merits of saving Lakeshore Hospital.

Salesmanship, determination, and commitment came through.

In the following weeks, U.S. Senator Jim Allen took on Lakeshore as a personal project. He explained the multi-disability center to his colleagues in the Senate. He explained that the hospital had an immediate need for construction funds.

"You would have thought he was Gregory Peck in the courtroom in *To Kill a Mockingbird*," Mike said. "He spoke on behalf of Lakeshore like the truly eloquent Southern politician that he was."

An appropriation of almost $900,000 for the Lakeshore project was included in the Senate version of the Labor-Health, Education and Welfare Appropriations Bill. In the House of Representatives, that appropriation was also supported.

But the battle wasn't over. Within days of a vote on the appropriations bill, the Lakeshore funding was removed by powers-that-be in the Senate.

Once again, Alabama's junior senator went to bat for Lakeshore, directly challenging a colleague who was the most powerful member of the Senate when it came to appropriations: Warren G. Magnuson, longtime powerhouse Democratic senator from the state of Washington. Magnuson was chairman of the largest committee in the U.S. Senate, the committee that held sweeping jurisdiction over all discretionary spending legislation in the Senate—the U.S. Senate Committee on Appropriations.

The Congressional Record reflects that on June 29, 1977, at the 11th hour before a final vote, and when the funds seemed lost and Lakeshore's doom thus sealed, Allen asked Magnuson this simple question on the floor of Congress: "I understand that the House-passed version of the Labor-HEW Appropriations Bill contains $900,000 for the Lakeshore Hospital in Birmingham, Alabama. I would like to ask Senator Magnuson to explain the Senate Appropriation Committee's rationale for apparently deleting funds for this excellent, multi-disability facility."

Magnuson replied that the decision had been to save federal dollars and that "the committee's action was not based on the merits of the specific Lakeshore Hospital . . ."

But Allen by this time was as determined and as effective a salesman as Stephens had been with him. The Lakeshore grant was restored to the appropriations bills. When the dust settled, Lakeshore got $810,000 in federal funds, to be matched with $889,000 in state funds. That total, plus what little Lakeshore itself could muster, made a funding package. Consistent with the coalition of partnerships that supported Lakeshore, the state funds came from what was then known as the Division of Rehabilitation and Crippled Children in the State Department of Education—with the approval of that division's director, Dr. George Hudson, as well as the support of Alabama Governor George C. Wallace and State Superintendent of Education Dr. Wayne Teague.

"**We were able** to move all our ancillary services into a new building," said Mike. "And we didn't tear down the historic building that had been condemned for hospital use. Instead, we converted the old stone building into an administrative building. Too, just as planned, the depreciation on our new building helped us with cash flow that began to turn us around financially."

Lakeshore thus got what it had to have—plus some bonuses. The core structure would be called a "social center" and would house ancillary services that had been located in the condemned building, and more. This spacious building would provide space for a much-needed new kitchen, laboratories, x-ray, and pharmacy. The new facility would double the space for physical and occupational therapy and would create new recreational space, a speech therapy area, and a workspace for fitting Lakeshore patients with tailor-made artificial limbs and braces.

As "bonuses" in this construction package, Lakeshore would have enough funds to build a new Lakeshore entrance and a new transitional living facility—a dormitory-like center where individuals with physical disabilities could live while they were in Lakeshore evaluation, rehabilitation, or workshop activities; it also was a center that would help individuals transition from life on the Lakeshore campus to life in the outside world. (Transitional living had been the topic of the thesis written by Michael Stephens when he obtained his master's degree in healthcare administration from UAB.)

On many future occasions Stephens would say that Lakeshore was grateful to all members of the Alabama congressional delegation who helped procure crucial funding for the new building. They included U.S. Representatives John H. Buchanan, Jack Edwards, and Tom Bevill, and U. S. Senators John J. Sparkman and James B. Allen Jr.

But he also emphasized that if not for the pivotal leadership by Senator Allen, the vital construction project would never have become a reality, and there likely would have been no more Lakeshore.

"Lakeshore owed a tremendous debt of gratitude to Senator Allen. He helped save Lakeshore Hospital," Stephens said.

Less than a year later, on June 1, 1978, U.S. Senator Jim Allen died in Gulf Shores, Alabama, of a sudden heart attack. He was 65.

10

'Don't Mess with My People'

The two years that Mike Stephens had promised he would stay at Lakeshore were coming to a close. In exchange for spending two years at Lakeshore, Mike had extracted a commitment from Baptist Medical Centers' President Emmett Johnson that he would help find Mike a hospital administration position in a general acute-care hospital.

As it turned out, Mike never asked Johnson to come through on that deal. During those two years at Lakeshore, something had happened. "Call it a feeling. Call it a spirit," said Mike. "It wasn't something that happened suddenly. But, at the end of two years, I no longer wanted to leave. I felt I had been led to Lakeshore for a purpose. I was where I wanted to be."

The spirit that drove Mike bubbled up from his ever-deepening connection with the people on whose behalf he worked every day. He had seen firsthand the needs of those with physical disabilities—at Lakeshore, at Spain Rehabilitation Center, and out in the community. He had felt those needs. In some cases, he had lived those needs personally.

"I just felt that these people needed a voice," said Mike. "Actually, they needed many voices. But at least I could be one voice."

Mike was fueled by the increasing numbers of successes that Lakeshore was having in helping many individuals who had physical disabilities. He wanted more successes. Time and again, newspaper headlines were recording those successes. In the mid-to-late-1970s, Lakeshore was getting an increasing amount of favorable news media and community attention.

As the roots of the two Lakeshore entities dug deeper and deeper into the rehabilitation community, more success stories began to emerge. At Lakeshore Hospital, patients were finding help with their medical problems. At Lakeshore Rehabilitation Facility, individuals with various types of disabilities were going through counseling and retraining to enable them to build good lives despite their disabilities.

But Mike knew that deep down he was driven even more by the failures than by the successes. He was driven by the gaps that still needed to be filled at Lakeshore and out in the community. Too often, the larger society was still not ready to embrace disabled individuals—not ready, not equipped, and not willing to be helpful and accepting.

As one spotlight after another was shining on society's deficits in this area, Mike was both sad and angry.

ONE CASE THAT would forever haunt Mike Stephens was that of Millie Ragland. She was a young single mother who came to Lakeshore a few months after giving birth in a Birmingham acute-care hospital.

What should have been a joyous day was marred by tragedy. Soon after Millie went into labor, she was given saddle block anesthesia. "Saddle block" is a common term for anesthetics injected with a fine needle into the spine, thus numbing the abdomen, lower back, and legs.

Millions of women around the world have undergone the saddle block procedure during childbirth with no lasting side effects. Millie Ragland was in that unfortunate small percentage who have damaging complications. Millie was permanently paralyzed from the waist down.

Her life was in a shambles. Alone, and unable to work, she was unable to support herself and her baby. On top of that, she was depressed—unable to relate to and accept her baby because she associated the infant with the paralysis that had ravaged her life. Social workers realized that even if Millie could accept her baby emotionally, she couldn't take care of her baby financially. So Millie's little girl was taken from her.

It gets worse.

Millie developed decubitus ulcers and one of her paralyzed legs became severely infected and had to be amputated.

She spent an initial period at Spain Rehabilitation Center and was then referred for additional services to Lakeshore.

So Millie came to Lakeshore. She would be served on both sides of the campus. She would receive medical care at Lakeshore Hospital and would become one of the first residents in the hospital's transitional living unit. Also, she would receive job counseling and retraining at Lakeshore Rehabilitation Facility.

Mike and the Lakeshore Hospital staff felt that it was vital to have specified goals for each patient. When Millie Ragland was transferred from Spain to Lakeshore, Mike asked, "What will be the Lakeshore objective with Millie? What are we shooting for? How will we know that Millie has been rehabilitated—that we have really helped her?"

Mike consulted with Dr. Cecil Nepomuceno, the physician at Spain who had been working with Millie.

Nepomuceno responded: "Well, if you can get Millie to accept her baby, that would be a good objective. If Lakeshore can provide services to Millie that help her to accept and take care of her baby, then her Lakeshore rehabilitation can be deemed a success."

That sounded reasonable to Mike. "That's a good goal for Millie," he said. "We'll work toward that."

As the Lakeshore staff pulled together to help Millie, one of the services they provided was to get her fitted with an artificial leg.

Lakeshore Medical Director Dr. George Traugh took the lead in working with prosthetics specialists and with Millie on this project.

Traugh had a way with patients. He had an infectious sense of humor, and it happened that, before her tragedy, Millie loved to laugh. As Traugh worked with Millie, soon she was laughing again. When she laughed, her beauty showed through. Millie Ragland was a strikingly beautiful girl; some said she looked an awful lot like superstar singer Diana Ross. At Lakeshore, flashes of Millie's old personality began to sparkle, and those at Lakeshore saw not only her exterior beauty but her inner beauty as well.

When it came time to design her new leg, Millie asked, "So what are you all going to do here, Dr. Traugh?"

"Well, Millie, to make a replacement for your leg, we're going to take a mold of your good leg and use it as a pattern," Traugh explained. "Once the prosthetics folks here make the mold, they will reverse it, so you'll have a left leg and a right leg that match."

Millie threw back her head and laughed: "Oh, no you don't! I don't want another leg that looks like the one I have. The leg I have left is too skinny; it's just plain ugly! Now, it wasn't that way before I became paralyzed. But with the paralysis and all, my leg is all shrunk up. Since I need this new leg, I want it to be a curvy, beautiful leg. I want you to find the prettiest woman you can find with the best-looking legs around, and make me a leg just like hers!"

Millie had fun with that. But, even though she was laughing, she was serious. Traugh and the prosthetics experts listened. Millie got her sexy new leg—and she was pleased.

ON THE VOCATIONAL rehabilitation side of Lakeshore, staffers focused their attention on retraining Millie for work she could do from a wheelchair and on finding her a clerical job.

Although more jobs gradually were opening up for those with physical disabilities, it was a slow process. Jobs still were hard to find. Often disabled persons had to settle for jobs beneath their abilities.

That was the case with Millie. Vocational rehabilitation job placement counselors found her a job sorting checks at a downtown Birmingham bank. Unfortunately, it was a second shift job; she wouldn't get off work until 10 P.M.

But Millie was glad to be working. She was glad to be able to pay her own bills. Further, she wanted her baby back and was delighted when the little girl came home. So it was that Millie and baby settled down in a tiny apartment. Millie had someone who could care for her daughter while she worked.

Millie had a life back. She was enjoying a taste of happiness, family life, and independence that she had thought would never again be possible.

The goal that had been set for Millie's rehabilitation had been met. Millie Ragland was ready to get out in society and make her own way.

Sadly, society was not ready for Millie Ragland.

To this day, Mike Stephens can't tell the end of Millie's story without his voice cracking.

"Every night when Millie got off work in downtown Birmingham, she had to call a taxi to take her to her apartment. But then the taxi drivers got tired of dealing with her. Millie was in a wheelchair. The taxi driver would have to help Millie get into the taxi, fold up her wheelchair and put it in the trunk of the taxi, then get the wheelchair out when they arrived at her apartment and help Millie out of the taxi and back into the wheelchair. The long and short of it is that the taxi drivers stopped responding to Millie's calls. There were days when she couldn't get to work and nights when she was left stranded in downtown Birmingham after she got off work. Millie was without transportation," Mike recalls.

The predictable happened. Since Millie had no transportation, she lost her job at the bank. And since she no longer had a job, she couldn't take care of her baby. Welfare workers came and took her daughter again.

"Millie had developed such a love for that baby," said Mike.

Losing her baby was the final straw for Millie Ragland. One day she got her hands on a shotgun and killed herself.

Although Millie's life had ended, the messages embedded in her story remained much alive. Mike said he was determined that her story would be told again and again, about the importance of society accepting individuals who were dealing with physical disabilities.

At the YWCA of Central Alabama, located in downtown Birmingham, Mike donated funds to support a child development center. And, within that childcare center, a preschool classroom was named in memory of Millie C. Ragland, who had so loved her own child.

As the years went by, Mike had many occasions to write messages about rehabilitation in articles, booklets, and brochures. Sometimes in writing these messages he would attach the by-line of Millie Ragland, or he would insert quotes attributed to Millie.

"Millie had inspired the quotes; and I felt in that sense they really were her quotes," said Mike. "I wanted to keep Millie's name front and center to keep reminding myself how society had failed her. I took that failure personally, and it was horrible. I felt that we had failed Millie, that I personally had failed Millie. That failure helped drive my advocacy for individuals who had physical disabilities. I wanted the Millie Ragland legacy to be that she also inspired some corrections in society, to make progress in accepting and embracing individuals with physical disabilities. I just never want Millie Ragland to be forgotten."

Mike said he could never get over cases like those of Johnny Bolt and Millie Ragland that pointed out the inadequacies in rehabilitation services and in societal acceptance of those with disabilities. "I knew we had to do more to help the Johnnys and the Millies; and we had to provide that help at the time when the help was really needed in someone's life. Because waiting till tomorrow to extend that help could be too late. For my part, all this meant my staying at Lakeshore, staying in the fight on behalf of people who needed support."

MIKE WAS DRIVEN, too, by memories of those with whom he had shared his own rehabilitation experience at Spain Rehabilitation Center. On more than one occasion, he would hear about a new chapter, often a disturbing chapter, in the lives of some of his fellow Spain "alumni."

Two who especially dug a hole into Mike's consciousness were Nelson Wedgeworth and Charles Green.

Nelson and Charles, both with extensive paralysis, had felt a surge of hope when they saw Mike start walking while at Spain. "Being around someone who becomes a walker can affect other rehab patients in a variety of ways—with their own belief systems, their hopes for their own futures, their motivations to reach for higher goals," Mike said. "That's what happened after I started walking at Spain. Other rehab patients around me got fired up."

Even though Nelson was Mike's roommate at Spain, Mike never learned a lot about him at the time. Nelson kept his thoughts and details about his life very private.

But Mike knew that Nelson was a product of the streets. He knew that long before Nelson became paralyzed from the waist down in a shooting incident, Nelson was living a difficult life on the streets of Birmingham.

For most of the time Mike had known Nelson at Spain, Nelson had been a cynical, embittered man who refused to be forthcoming and cooperative with his fellow patients, with his therapists, with anybody. Nelson, as we saw earlier, was the patient who made fun of the prayer cloth Mike's aunt had sent him and that Mike carried everywhere he went at Spain. Then, as Mike was leaving Spain, Nelson shocked everyone by publicly asking Mike for a little piece of the cloth.

Mike had been touched by Nelson and he tried to keep up with him. Nelson did complete his rehabilitation at Spain, but then he returned to the streets. One day he overdosed and died on one of those streets.

Charles Green's story tugged equally deeply on Mike.

Before an injury that left him paralyzed from the chest down, Charles had been a promising young racing mechanic on the NASCAR circuit.

When Mike met him at Spain Rehabilitation Center, it had been several years since Charles's injury. He was what some in the rehab world called a "retread"—one of those injured people who continued to have complications and to return for additional treatment.

As Nelson had, Charles began thinking hopeful new thoughts about his own situation after Mike became a "walker" at Spain.

He became inspired and worked hard on his rehabilitation and began making plans to seek a racing job he could do despite his paralysis, something like dispensing parts from one of the big rigs parked near the pit area at the track.

Mike remembered vividly the weekend before his own discharge from Spain.

"There was a race at the Talladega Superspeedway this particular weekend. And Charles asked for a weekend pass from his inpatient treatment at Spain to go to the track. He wanted to talk to a crew chief who had supervised him back when he was a mechanic."

The day Charles returned to the race track was very hot. He sat in his wheelchair in the sun waiting to see the crew chief.

"As he waited in the blazing sun, Charles was getting into bad trouble with the heat. He had a problem that quadriplegics tend to have—he had lost his ability to sweat. Since he couldn't sweat, the heat was trapped inside his body and his internal temperature soared," Mike said.

Charles passed out and had to be rushed back to Spain. He remained in bed the next week receiving IV fluids.

When Mike next heard from Charles it was several years later when Charles was admitted to Lakeshore Hospital, where Mike was by then executive director.

Charles's medical situation was gut-wrenching.

"He had developed pressure sores—decubitus ulcers—that needed emergency care," said Mike, "and he had gotten into this shape because he had been living out of his car! The sores were bad and had become infested with maggots."

AS MIKE SERVED as executive director of the developing rehabilitation hospital at Lakeshore, he had questions regarding the Nelsons and Charleses of the world.

A person is injured, and somehow he gets medical care. Then somehow he has access to rehabilitation. But then what? Thousands of dollars and many man hours are invested in his medical care and his rehabilitation. But then, when they consider him 'rehabbed,' he's put out on his own in the same terrible environment from where he came. So who's out there in that environment to help him then? What's out there for him? What's next in his life?

To Mike, those questions and the voids they represented had to be translated into new programs, into new forms of outreach.

Charles was one of those individuals with a severe disability who wanted to do something constructive. He wanted to get back in society and to be productive . . . But there was no one out there to help him make it happen—in my view a real sad commentary on the weak state of our vocational rehabilitation and other rehab programs when Charles needed those programs so badly. There have to be some better ways. We have to find some better ways.

As Mike Stephens became an advocate for those served by Lakeshore, he didn't overtly use the fact that he himself had once been paralyzed and that he still walked with effort and with a limp. However, those who knew Mike knew his history.

"I believe that, as I made my case repeatedly on behalf of those with physical disabilities, it did become a factor that some folks ultimately realized that I had been down some of the same paths—that I had been severely injured, that I had been paralyzed, that I had been through rehabilitation," said Mike. "I felt this come into play many times when I was arguing with various individuals, with representatives of various institutions and agencies, about how to approach something on behalf of those with physical disabilities. Sometimes I felt it was like a light bulb went on and they were willing to listen to my point of view. It was like, 'Well, Mike actually is the only one at the table here who has been through what we're talking about. Maybe he does know more about this than we do.' "

Mike said his biggest advantage in this regard was the drive he felt to be an advocate for these people he understood and who needed help so badly.

I feel a kinship to the people I represent and to their needs. This understanding is kind of like holding a trump card that makes me feel stronger, that makes me know that I know what I know about certain things and that I have to fight for them. I have this feeling that comes over me like "Don't mess with my people."

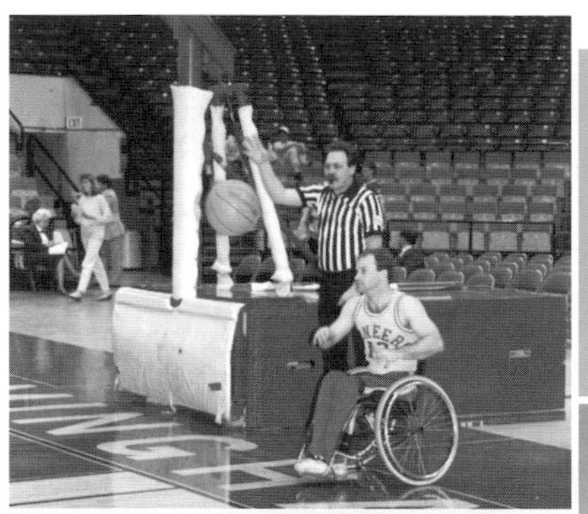

A progression of Lakeshore basketball, clockwise from top left: Joe Ray inbounds on a borrowed court; one of the first teams in the new Wallace Center;

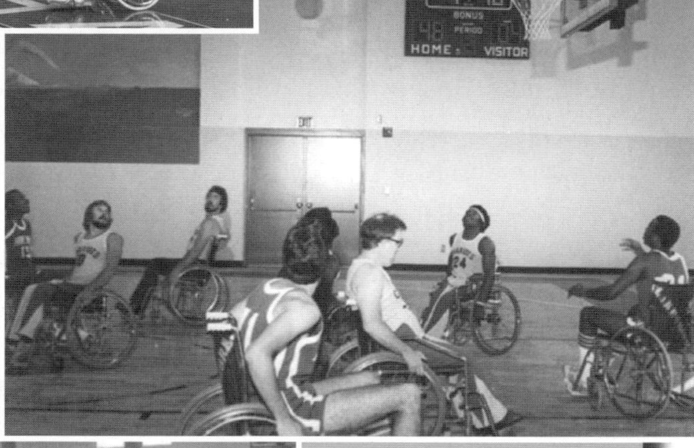

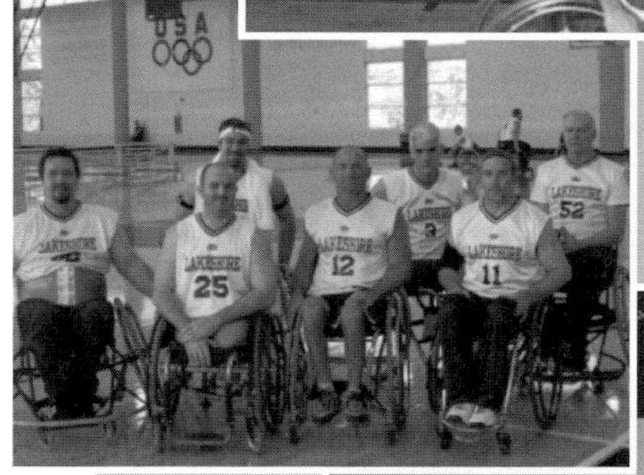

the '86 national champs; some of the same guys in the new fieldhouse.

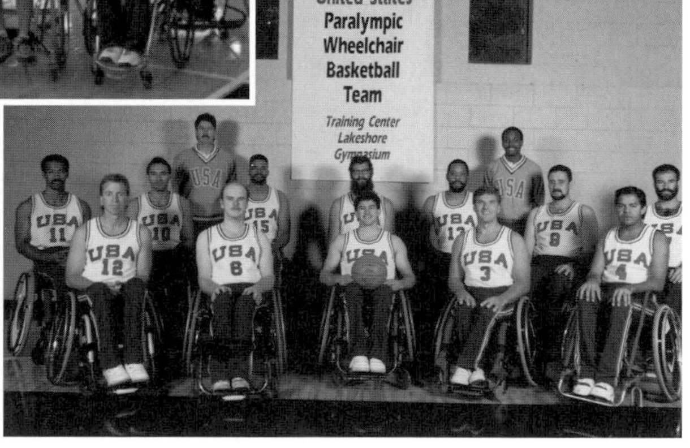

11

The Power of Sports and Recreation

Prior to being injured, Mike had been very athletic. After his rehab, he learned about and started playing some wheelchair basketball. He liked it. He looked around and saw others with physical disabilities who, like himself, were letting off steam and having fun.

Sure, they were in wheelchairs. But the ball was the same. The court was the same. The exhilaration of racing down the court, dribbling, passing, finding the open man, blocking out, shooting, and scoring was the same. Sweating, throwing the occasional elbow—it was basketball. It was good.

When he started playing in the early 1970s, wheelchair basketball—in Birmingham at least—was in its infancy. Getting together enough people to play was a challenge. Finding a gym to play in was a bigger challenge. The obstacles foreshadowed those that athletes with physical disabilities would face in the coming years as they pioneered other wheelchair sports.

But the opportunities were coming. You could feel it.

Before long Mike was both playing and coaching. In 1974, local recreation specialist Mary Lou Humphrey founded a wheelchair basketball team called the Birmingham Chariots, later known as the Birmingham Pioneers and then the Birmingham Storm.

Mike got involved.

The Chariots struggled at every turn, recalled player-coach Howell Whitson in a March 15, 1982, interview in the *Birmingham News*.

UAB Coach Bill Truss helped out on his own time in the beginning, but had to drop out due to commitments at UAB.

For a time, UAB let the Chariots use Bell Gymnasium. But, as UAB's enrollment grew and the university became more involved in athletics and intramural sports, there was no room for the Chariots. For brief periods the Chariots variously used a recreation center in the north Jefferson County municipality of Gardendale, the gym at Ramsay High School on Birmingham's Southside, and a community center in the west Jefferson County community of Ensley.

"We were always having to beg for a place to practice and play," said early Chariots player Jim Wooten. "Few buildings were wheelchair accessible at the time. We had one situation in which we had to go up steps to get to where we were practicing. Somehow all of us guys had to get ourselves and our heavy wheelchairs up those steps. It was tough."

Nor were the wheelchair athletes always welcomed by the able-bodied who used the same gyms.

"At the Ensley Community Center, we were assigned very specific hours on specific days," said Wooten. "Since we had the gym only for an hour to an hour and a half, it was important that we get to start on time. But it didn't always work out. We would arrive to play at the time we had been told. And sometimes we couldn't get these able-bodied guys off the court because they still were playing, and they didn't want us there anyhow. We would be waiting for them to finish and they would be calling us 'gimps' and 'crips.' They would say things like, 'Well, here comes this bunch of crips, trying to run us off our court!' We had some real interesting conversations with those guys."

WOOTEN WAS A tough guy, a competitor. He would tell you that wheelchair basketball saved his life.

At Meek High School in the little northwestern Alabama town of Arley, Jim lettered in football, basketball, and baseball. In his two favorite sports, football and basketball, he was the team captain. He also loved to fish and hunt.

Howard College (later Samford University) wanted to give him an athletic scholarship. If he could add a few pounds to his lanky 6'2"

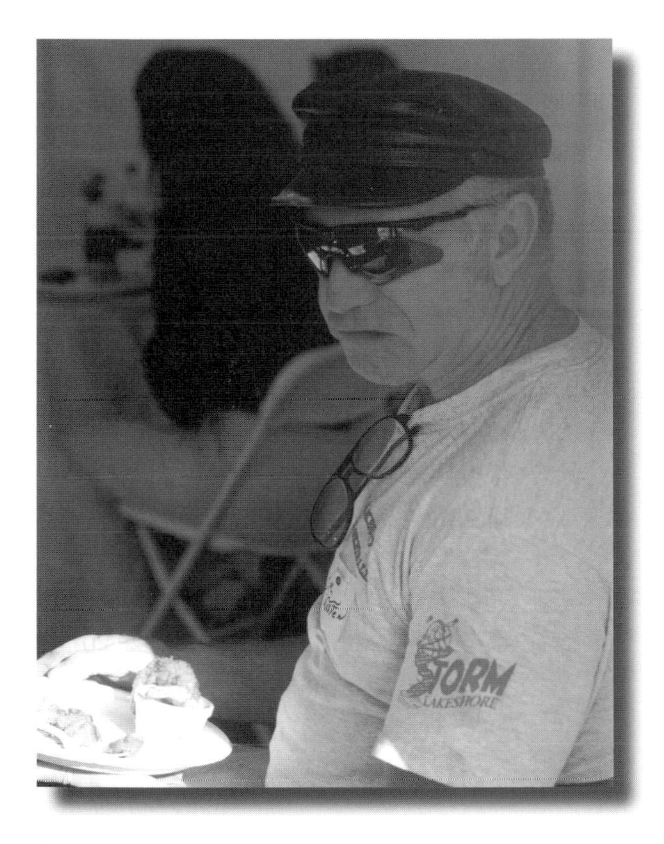

Jim "Danger" Wooten.

frame, he would play football. If he stayed at the same weight, he would play basketball.

Those dreams ended November 12, 1961. Eighteen-year-old Jim was driving just outside of Arley; the road had recently been paved and he hit gravel and lost control. The accident left him with a broken back and paralyzed legs.

After his hospitalization and rehabilitation, Jim returned home. Sports had been his main interest, and his talent was to have been his ticket to college. Back in Arley, Jim felt disconnected, bored, bitter, depressed. He floundered for a decade.

"I saw nothing for a person with my disability to do there, nothing for someone in a wheelchair," said Jim. "Oh, I did a little fishing and hunting. As far as working, I was just piddling, doing a little work on cars and some welding. I had a chip on my shoulder most of the time.

I got off into alcohol and I don't know how deep that would have gone if I had not run into something I liked a lot better."

The something better was wheelchair basketball.

Not long after the Chariots were founded, Jim badly burned his heel while welding and went into Birmingham for treatment. He ran into Howell Whitson, who looked the still strongly built Wooten up and down and asked him how he would like to play some wheelchair basketball.

Jim had never heard of wheelchair basketball, but Whitson talked him into at least coming to watch a game.

He was more than a little excited about what he saw. He recalled being amazed that the game was so fast, that it was so high-scoring, that the players obviously were using both mental and physical skill.

He was hooked. "After seeing that first game, I started playing wheelchair basketball; and after that you could not have run me out of it," Jim said.

Jim was very serious about wheelchair basketball. Though already in his early 30s when he started playing the game, his toughness and skill would make him an internationally recognized wheelchair sports athlete. His competitiveness also earned him the nickname "Danger."

Mike Stephens was one of his coaches on the Chariots. "Jimmy 'Danger' Wooten was something else!" recalled Mike. "When I first met him he had long sideburns and an attitude and demeanor that matched his nickname. But he was a talented player—focused, committed, skilled, and tough."

Jim was the kind of player that Mike liked to coach, because Mike himself was a tough, driven competitor. Jim played to win, and Mike coached to win.

They got along fine. They won a lot of games.

Today, Mike still laughs about one they didn't win. That day, on the opposing team was a giant of a wheelchair basketball player.

"This guy was a single amputee, missing one leg," said Mike. "If he was standing he would have been around 6'5"; he probably weighed

275 to 285 pounds, and he was solid. He would wheel by like lightning, his teammates would throw him the basketball, and he was so tall and so strong that he would just hold the ball up above his head so that nobody on our team could block him. The guy was scoring against us right and left."

During a Chariots time-out, Mike called on Danger.

"Wooten, go out there and intimidate that guy!" ordered Coach Mike. "You can't let this guy keep doing this. Intimidate him!"

"Yes sir!" Jim replied. After all, intimidation was Danger's specialty.

Mike recalled: "Wooten went out there, and I saw him put his elbow right into the middle of this big guy's chest. I mean it sounded like a tree cracked! But it didn't faze him."

The big guy just kept hitting his baskets, building his team's lead.

Mike called another time-out and motioned for Jim. "Wooten, I thought I told you to intimidate him," said Mike.

"Well, Coach, when I hit him in the chest with my elbow, he just looked down at me and said kind of quiet-like, 'You don't want to do that anymore.' " Pause. "And, to be honest, Coach, I don't."

The Chariots lost that day, but for Mike Stephens and Jim Wooten, no game was a total loss when they were having an opportunity to be involved in a wheelchair sport they both loved.

AFTER HE BECAME executive director of Lakeshore Hospital, Mike was determined to get the Lakeshore campus involved in sports and recreation. Having personally seen and tasted the magic of wheelchair basketball, he wanted to learn all he could about other wheelchair sports and forms of recreation for those with physical disabilities.

The more Mike learned about wheelchair sports and recreation, the more he could see why wheelchair sports were taking hold around the world.

Mike saw their value in terms of ongoing physical and mental therapy. He saw their value as an outlet for pent-up energy and as a means toward achievement, self-confidence, and recognition. He saw their value as a social outlet. And he saw their value as a reentry into society for many—as a reintroduction to believing in oneself, to being competitive, to focusing on what can be accomplished instead of what cannot be done.

"I had experienced the range of emotions when some accident or illness leaves you with a physical disability and changes your life so drastically," said Mike. "And if you think beyond that to people who have had physical disabilities since birth, they have gone their whole lives being limited by these challenges."

Mike knew how difficult it could be for a person with a physical disability once he or she was discharged from a hospital or rehabilitation center out into the real world. "For some people, going home after rehab to a purposeless existence can be a big hit from which they never recover. At that point, having access to wheelchair sports can mean everything. After I had a little exposure to sports and recreation programs for people with physical disabilities, it didn't take me long to become a believer in the power and potential of such programs—when they are done well, and when they reach the people who need them."

In fact, Lakeshore's original master plan called for building a dedicated sports and recreation center. But in the early years, even though Lakeshore staff encouraged patients and clients to become involved in sports and recreation, available recreation facilities on the campus were limited, and there were no facilities expressly designed for wheelchair sports.

Mike set out to change this.

He was convinced of the urgency because sports and recreation were so consistent with Lakeshore's mission to reintegrate into society those who had physical disabilities. Beyond that, Mike felt that Lakeshore's beautiful and spacious wooded setting made it an ideal location for what could be a model recreation center.

He realized that for Lakeshore to have a truly functional sports and recreation home for those with physical disabilities, the facility had to have at least three elements: a gymnasium, a swimming pool, and space for recreational activities such as table tennis and chess and for parties and other social gatherings.

When Mike was desperate for money to finance a replacement for Lakeshore's condemned ancillary services building, he sought and got the key support of U.S. Senator Jim Allen. Now, to fulfill the vision of a sports and recreation facility at Lakeshore, he knew that this project, too, would need powerful political support.

The high-profile elected official who, above all others, could understand the need for such a project—and who had the clout to secure funding—was George C. Wallace.

Mike already knew Alabama's governor. The two shared common ground.

Both had gone through devastating life-changing experiences that had dealt them lasting physical disability. Mike's diving accident occurred in 1970, and in 1972 Wallace was paralyzed from the waist down by bullets fired by a would-be assassin.

Soon after it happened, George Wallace had learned of Mike's accident from Mike's relatives who lived just around the corner from Wallace's personal residence in Montgomery. This was the house that was to have been the retirement home for Wallace and his wife, Lurleen. When Wallace was told of 26-year-old Mike Stephens's grave injuries, he conveyed his concern through his neighbors who were Mike's relatives.

Wallace was not then the governor. However, he was running for the office, against Governor Albert Brewer, who was elected as lieutenant governor in 1966 and was serving out the unexpired term of Lurleen B. Wallace, who in 1968 had died of cancer after serving as the state's first woman governor for not quite 16 months.

After George Wallace was returned to the governor's office in 1970 and became paralyzed a year and a half later—at age 52—it was Mike's turn to express his concern; when Wallace was shot, he sustained a spinal cord bruise that was similar to Mike's injury from the diving accident.

Mike and Wallace had other things in common.

Following their injuries, both had received services at Spain Rehabilitation Center. And both had close ties with Dr. George Traugh. Based at UAB at the time Wallace was injured, Traugh became the governor's physician. Three years later, Traugh became medical director at Lakeshore and Mike's close friend and associate.

Wallace was already familiar with Lakeshore and its mission and he and Mike had already met. On August 28, 1976, Mike was among those hosting the official dedication of and the first public open house for the Lakeshore Hospital and Lakeshore Rehabilitation Facility. Governor Wallace was among those speaking at the dedication ceremonies and touring the Lakeshore complex.

And Wallace had already lent his support to the expansion of Lakeshore—including state matching funds for construction of the new ancillary services building on the Lakeshore campus. (Although Lakeshore Hospital itself was a private entity, the hospital could receive some state support due to its relationships with Alabama's vocational rehabilitation program and with UAB, a state university.)

Mike had every reason to believe that of all politicians, George Wallace could understand Lakeshore's need for a sports and recreation center. He knew about Lakeshore's services and reputation. And, not least, he had a love for and a record in sports.

Short in stature but solidly built, Wallace had been an outstanding youth and high school athlete, winning Alabama Golden Gloves boxing championships in 1936 and 1937.

Through the years, Wallace had kept himself physically fit. After he was paralyzed, he understood the importance of exercise in an ongoing rehabilitation regimen. When he returned to Montgomery following his hospitalization and rehab, he had a mini-workout center installed in his bedroom in the Governor's Mansion.

Even so, Mike knew the governor was inundated with requests to support many projects. He also knew that Wallace's calendar was full. It was difficult to get an audience with him and even perhaps more difficult to get an audience in a setting where Wallace could focus his full attention on one subject without interruptions. This was especially true in the bustling Governor's Office in the Capitol, where there was a constant buzz of activity and distraction.

If and when Mike made a pitch to Wallace, the timing would have to be right.

Ironically, Mike's opportunity came when he was asked to approach Wallace for funding for a different project, a state research-oriented urology laboratory that was planned for Spain Rehabilitation Center. The lab was the idea of UAB rehabilitation medicine leader Dr. Samuel Stover, and the lab's mission would be to conduct badly needed research on urinary tract infections that were an ongoing and potentially fatal threat to paralyzed individuals.

"Those at UAB who asked me to make the pitch to the governor did so because they were aware that Wallace and I shared common ground. They felt he and I could communicate well about the need for this urinary tract infections research," Mike said.

Of course Mike agreed to help.

At the same time, he knew he would make two pitches to Wallace if he got the chance—one about the state urology lab at UAB, and a second pitch about the sports and recreation center for Lakeshore.

"I didn't tell anyone else that I had that in mind. I didn't tell Dr. Sam Stover at UAB. I didn't tell Dr. Don Patrick at the Lakeshore Rehabilitation Facility. And I didn't tell Dr. George Hudson in the Alabama Vocational Rehabilitation Service office." After the dust had settled, all three of these powerful men would support the far-reaching results triggered by Mike's meeting with Wallace.

By the time Mike went to Montgomery to have the meeting, Wallace was nearing the completion of his third gubernatorial term. He would serve a fourth term in 1983–87; between George and his late wife, Lurleen, a Wallace was in Alabama's highest elected office for almost 18 years. It was clearly the most powerful gubernatorial reign in the state's colorful political history.

As it turned out, Mike's meeting with Wallace was not scheduled to take place in the Capitol. Instead, the meeting was in the Governor's Mansion, in Wallace's bedroom office. Since Wallace's injury, he had used this upstairs room in the mansion not only as his bedroom and workout center but also as a second office.

Mike had learned from others that Wallace had a personal triage system for evaluating requests that came to him in his bedroom office. The system worked like this:

A proposal for something Wallace didn't believe in was simply tossed on the floor. One that involved something Wallace thought was a good idea but which he was going to let his staff push forward went on a stack to his left. A proposal that Wallace strongly believed in and that he thought needed his personal pushing went on his right. The latter were his pet projects.

When Mike went in to meet with Wallace, he pitched the UAB project—the state urology lab projected for location in UAB's Spain Rehabilitation Center.

Since his late wife's battle against cancer and since the onset of his own battle with spinal cord injury and paralysis, Wallace had become a stronger and stronger supporter of health-related causes. As someone who was paralyzed and personally at high risk for urinary tract infections, Wallace readily understood the need for a UAB lab to conduct research in that area.

Mike finished his verbal presentation and watched as Wallace placed to his left the written proposal Mike had given him containing information on the state urology lab. Later, UAB did receive state funding for the urology lab and it became a reality at Spain Rehabilitation Center.

Then Mike took a breath and launched into his second pitch, seeking Wallace's support of state funding for the construction of a sports and recreation center at Lakeshore.

Mike spoke to the governor straight from his heart, as one injured man to another, as one athlete to another.

"Governor, you've been an athlete. You were a boxer," said Mike. "You know the feeling of pushing yourself as an athlete, to the point you are just dead tired. Don't you remember how good that felt? And don't you also remember how pushing yourself physically relieved anxiety?"

Wallace listened. And Mike went on.

"You also know what it's like to get hurt—like you and I got hurt—and you know what it's like to be limited in being able to push yourself physically. I don't have to tell you, Governor, how frustrating it is to the many people who have physical disabilities who, because of their disabilities, also have lost their physical outlets. And I don't have to tell you what it could mean to people with physical disabilities if we could provide them with such a place here in Alabama."

Mike described the dream of building a first-class recreation center at Lakeshore where the disabled could release pent-up emotion, anxiety, and energy . . . "a place where they can get tired, and a place where they can enjoy wheelchair sports and recreation and have fun and achieve . . . Can you help us with that, by supporting state funding that will enable us to build this new sports and recreation center?"

When Mike finished, Wallace was polite but somewhat subdued. He said nothing one way or another to voice his reaction to the Lakeshore pitch Mike had just made. He neither said he would commit nor that he wouldn't commit.

Mike was disappointed and also surprised. He had fully expected the Lakeshore request to strike a responsive note with Wallace.

Mike sensed that he had stayed as long as he should and that the meeting with Wallace was over. The governor's strength wasn't what it once was, and there was always an endless line of people trying to get a few minutes of his time. Mike shook Wallace's hand, thanked him for listening, said his cordial goodbye, and turned to leave.

Then, as Mike was walking out the door, out of the corner of his eye, he saw Governor Wallace place the folder with the Lakeshore sports and recreation center proposal on the stack to his right.

12

REFINING THE VISION

Before Governor George C. Wallace's third term ended in January 1979, Lakeshore had its state-funding commitment to finance a new sports and recreation facility. In the years to come, even Mike would be amazed at just how much impact the facility would have.

The Lakeshore sports and recreation facility, to which George Wallace lent his support, proved to be the most exciting, most life-changing endeavor undertaken on the Lakeshore campus up to that point to improve the quality of life for individuals with physical disabilities.

Step by step, Lakeshore was becoming the rehabilitation campus envisioned by its original planners. As the 1970s drew to a close, Lakeshore was no longer a newborn. It was growing up and taking on a personality of its own.

On both Lakeshore's hospital side and its rehabilitation side, the patient census was steadily growing. As had been envisioned, some who came to Lakeshore had their initial rehabilitation at UAB's Spain Rehabilitation Center and then transferred to Lakeshore to continue that rehabilitation. However, more and more of the patients had never been at Spain; Lakeshore was their first stop in rehabilitation.

Mike Stephens said there were some obvious reasons why the demand for Lakeshore's services was climbing.

"We were attracting great staff, we had some innovative programs, and our facilities were really improving," said Mike.

He said that carefully designed renovations worked wonders with the interiors of the old stone buildings on Lakeshore's campus. "We ended up with the best of both worlds—the exterior charm of the historical structures, plus an interior that became functional and attractive."

And then there was Lakeshore's new construction—the new ancillary services building for which U.S. Senator Jim Allen had fought so hard.

"The truth was that, when Lakeshore first became a rehab campus in the early 1970s, our hospital was an ugly facility on the inside. Everybody wanted to go to Spain and nobody wanted to go to Lakeshore. We had the reputation of being this hole in the wall that took care of the dregs of society. But by the end of the 1970s, we were changing rapidly. We looked better, we had more to offer, and we were getting great results. Word was getting around that at Lakeshore we were changing lives for the better."

On the financial side, things were also looking up. Reimbursement would continue to be a challenge, because the whole rehab concept was new to many in the insurance industry. "But still, we had survived those horrible financial struggles in the mid-1970s," said Mike. "I so well recall the first time I went into a BMC corporate meeting when I was able to report that we were seeing financial daylight at Lakeshore Hospital. Things had been so bad out there financially, and now it was turning around. The executives at BMC couldn't believe what they were hearing!"

In November 1973, when Lakeshore accepted its first rehabilitation patients, then-administrator Dick Lind had released a statement to the news media about the scope of services at Lakeshore. Lind said that Lakeshore Hospital would have the basic services of a general hospital, but would not be required to provide an emergency room, obstetrical and gynecological services, and surgery. Arrangements had been made with other local hospitals to provide those services.

But as time went on, Executive Director Mike Stephens and Medical Director George Traugh and others at Lakeshore felt that original plan should be modified. In 1979, surgical services were added at Lakeshore Hospital. It was a sign of growth and of Lakeshore spreading its wings, a harbinger of things to come.

Lakeshore was also reaching out to the community and to its own staff. People bonds were being created.

A headline in the *Birmingham News* on October 26, 1977, told about one initiative: "Volunteers are needed for new programs and services at Lakeshore Hospital." In this article, Lakeshore leaders were calling for adult volunteers to help implement certain Lakeshore programs—to interact with both Lakeshore employees and patients. It was a way to stretch human resources at Lakeshore. It also was a way to spread understanding in the community as to what Lakeshore was all about.

At the same time, an esprit de corps was building with employees who worked on the Lakeshore campus. At the beginning, there were informal Lakeshore employee get-togethers. Then the get-togethers became more organized. In 1980, Lakeshore Hospital held its first picnic for employees and their families, with a day of fun and games on the Lakeshore campus, a day that included a cake bake-off and a rib-cooking contest. Cooking the ribs were Mike Stephens and George Traugh, and judging the ribs was Dennis Washburn, editor of the entertainment section and restaurant critic of the *Birmingham News*. In this fun contest, Mike was declared the rib-cooking champion.

WHEN LAKESHORE GOT its funding for the new ancillary services building, there was enough money in the package to build also a separate transitional living facility.

The transitional living concept had been a part of the original master plan for Lakeshore. It was a concept to which UAB rehabilitation medicine leader Dr. John M. Miller III strongly subscribed when he put forth his vision for Lakeshore in the early 1970s. It was a concept in which Michael Stephens strongly believed. In fact, when Mike completed his master's-degree healthcare administration studies at UAB, transitional living was his thesis topic.

The idea of transitional living was to provide an environment on a rehabilitation campus that was dedicated to helping an individual with a physical disability learn how to "transition" from life in an institution to independent life on the outside.

"We wanted Lakeshore to become an international model in how you could move patients out of a hospital environment into a college-like dormitory setting, and teach them skills of independence that would

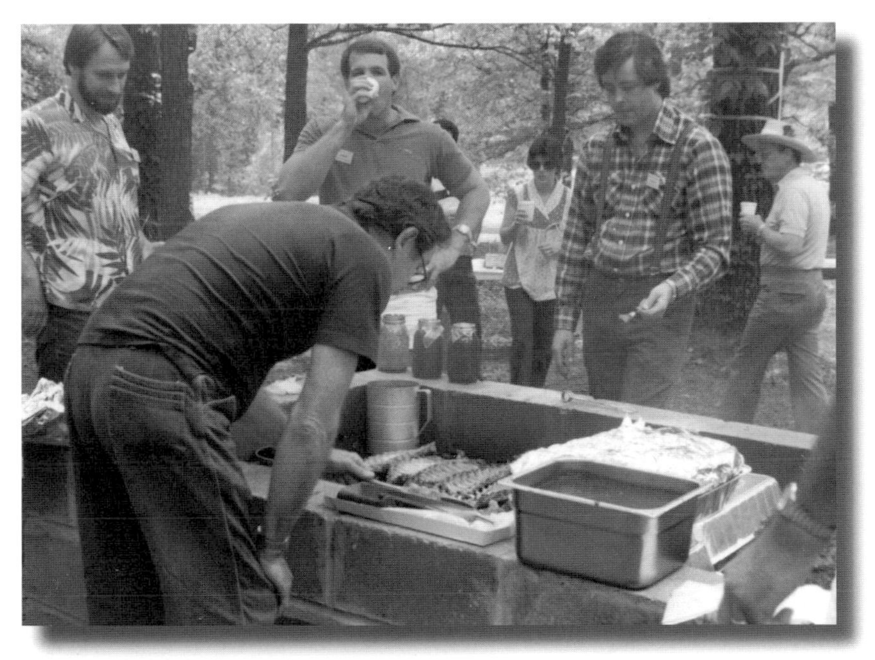

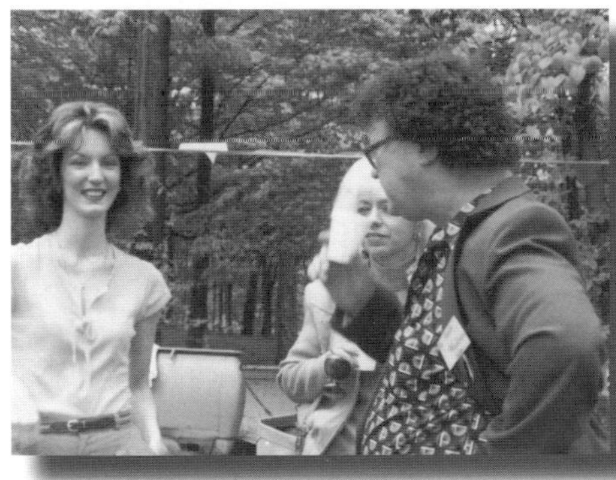

At a 1980 staff picnic, George Traugh (leaning over) and Mike Stephens (plaid shirt) had a ribs cook-off. **LEFT:** *Dennis Washburn (in apron) declared Mike the winner.*

let them for the first time really think 'healthy' instead of thinking 'sick,' " said Mike.

In the mid-1970s, Lakeshore had a makeshift transitional living section in its original hospital building. However, what that basically amounted to was dedicating some hospital facility beds for dormitory space and staffing them with transitional living instructors. Mike and his staff knew the setting was inadequate; they needed a separate transitional living unit, located away from the hospital environment and designed and equipped especially for teaching specific transitioning skills.

The new unit provided that, a facility dedicated to transitional living. The model program installed there was the first of its kind in the nation.

On June 15, 1979, Lakeshore's new transitional living unit was dedicated and named in memory of Dr. John M. Miller III.

However, another component of the original master plan—long-term residential living—was dropped, at the persistent urging of Executive Director Mike Stephens.

The original concept had included the building of a number of housing units on the Lakeshore campus where those with physical disabilities could live indefinitely after they finished rehabilitation. "From the time I saw that part of Lakeshore's plan, I thought it was a horrible idea, an absolutely horrible idea," Mike said.

As Mike knew from experience, one of the factors that had returned him to independence was getting reinvolved in the mainstream of society. That meant living in a home that was located in a traditional neighborhood in the community—in a neighborhood with able-bodied neighbors.

"Why in the world would you want to invest all these resources into transitional living, into teaching a physically disabled person how to live on his own out in society, if you're also going to say, 'Oh, you don't really have to learn how to function out in society. You can just live here on this rehab campus and depend on it forever!' Terrible idea," Mike said.

He was so opposed to the idea of long-term residential living facilities on Lakeshore's campus that he convinced the board of directors that it should not happen. He told board members, "We are not trying to turn Lakeshore into some kind of 'leper colony' in which we separate and segregate individuals with physical disabilities out away from the mainstreamed community. We are not here to say, 'If you have a major physical disability, if you are in a wheelchair, you can end up at Lakeshore and never get out!' That's not what Lakeshore is all about."

AS THE VISION for Lakeshore was being refined, there would be some who would not be happy. In a climate of escalating competition in the healthcare and rehabilitation industry, the competition factor was about to enter the Lakeshore story. As Lakeshore became more successful, it also began to be viewed by others in the healthcare and rehabilitation industry as being competitive.

The stage was being set for conflicts, including with leaders of the powerful entity that had helped birth Lakeshore and had helped design its original master plan—the University of Alabama at Birmingham.

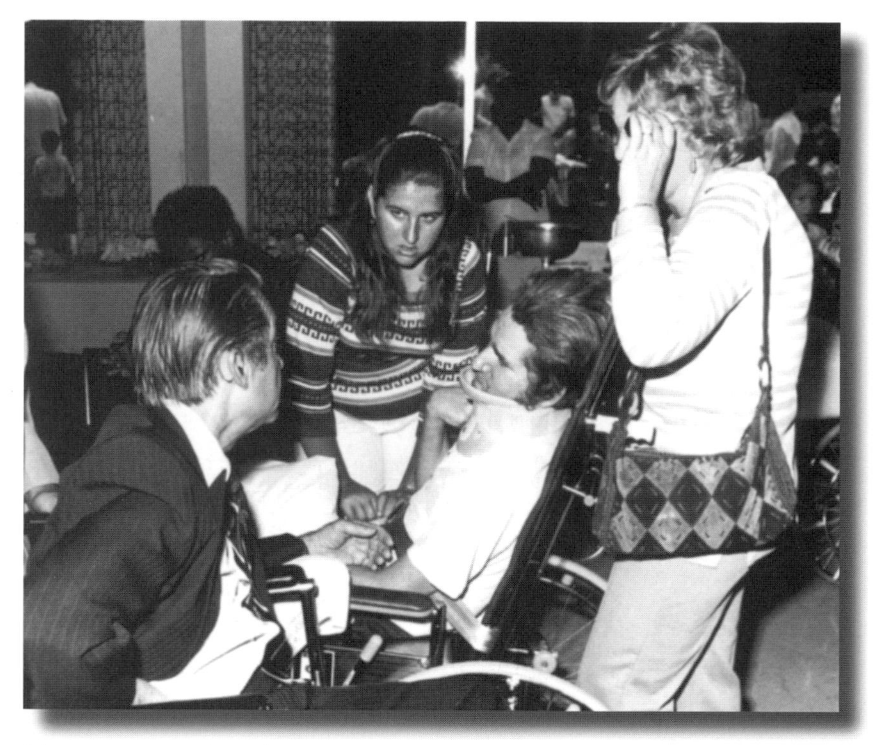

The suppport of Alabama Governor George C. Wallace—who was known to have a soft spot for sports and for those with disabilities—was crucial as Lakeshore began to expand its services.

Part III

Lakeshore Hospital Spreading Its Wings

13

A Governor's Empathy Births a Recreation Center

As described earlier, Mike Stephens went to Alabama Governor George C. Wallace in 1978 seeking state funding for a Lakeshore recreation center. The governor, himself paralyzed for life from the waist down, came through.

As Mike came to know this powerful man who would serve an unprecedented four terms as governor, he saw that Wallace was moved by the feelings and needs of those with disabilities. "George Wallace would spend literally hours talking on the telephone to others who, like himself, were confined to a wheelchair," said Mike. "Wallace would spend a lot of time talking on the phone to disabled individuals about issues in their lives. He set up a system at the Governor's Mansion in Montgomery to allow certain individuals with disabilities to bypass the usual tight screening system and get through directly to the governor."

As a result of Wallace's personal support, the Alabama Legislature generously funded part of the construction costs of a recreation center at Lakeshore. With the encouragement of Mike and Lakeshore's board, the state support inspired other donations from such entities as the Alabama Department of Education, Baptist Medical Centers, the Birmingham Quarterback Club, UAB and its Spain Rehabilitation Center, the Crippled Children's Foundation, and, very importantly, Lakeshore Hospital's board of directors.

The $1.24 million facility, part of the Lakeshore Rehabilitation Complex, opened in 1981 as a beautiful, barrier-free showplace designed for maximum function.

The recreation center would provide sports and recreation opportunities for thousands of individuals with physical disabilities. There was a full-sized gymnasium with a regulation basketball court and accommodations for volleyball and indoor racquet sports. There was a collegiate-size swimming pool, meeting specifications as a site for competitive collegiate events. Shower rooms and dressing areas were equipped for disabled use. The recreation center also provided a fitness facility, an arts and crafts center, and a space for social gatherings and games such as chess and table tennis.

AT THE DEDICATION ceremony of the George C. Wallace Recreation Center on June 15, 1981, the audience rose to a thundering ovation as Wallace was wheeled down a ramp to the speakers' platform. (Wallace's third term as governor had come to an end before the recreation center he championed had become reality; he would win an unprecedented fourth term the next year.)

The thrust of Wallace's message was that the new recreation center had been made possible by state and private funds; he stressed that many organizations and individuals had contributed. Looking out into the audience, Wallace said that the real supporters of the center "are you and also those who are not here—the people of Alabama."

As Wallace spoke, Mike Stephens watched with a sense of wonderment and fulfillment. Mike knew that something magical had been building during the weeks leading up to the opening of the recreation center, something that went far beyond the center itself. "I had noticed a growing level of community awareness, enthusiasm, and volunteerism that had not existed previously."

Because Lakeshore was continuing to operate on a tight budget, Mike was always looking for all the volunteer help he could get.The Lakeshore staff had worked to get the campus in tiptop shape for the Wallace Center dedication, and volunteers helped in every way they could, raking leaves and doing other cleanup projects around the campus.

With a smile, Mike recalled one of his favorite volunteer projects during this period: "Volunteers from the local Jaycees spruced up an

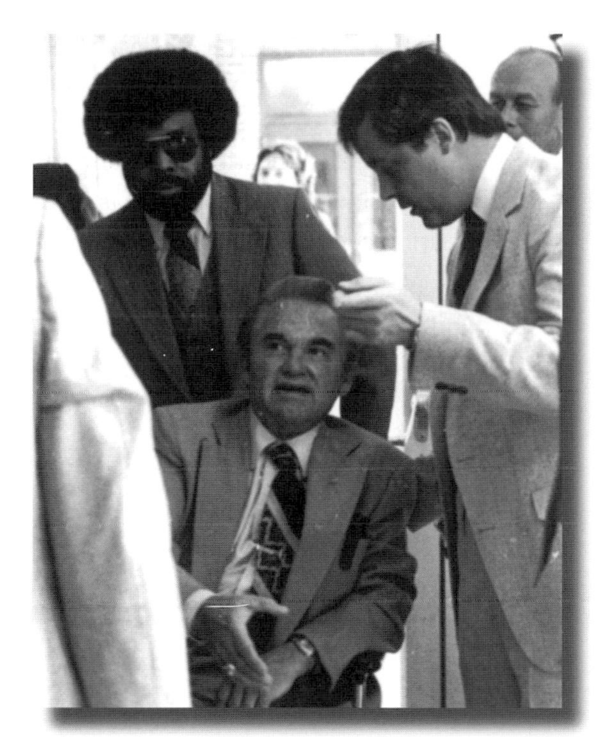

Mike Stephens with Governor Wallace at the dedication of the Wallace Recreation Center.

old military-surplus building we were using as a maintenance building. A graphic artist painted the building silver with an aviation-stripe design. By the time they finished, I'll have to say that was one of the best-looking buildings on the campus!"

Even though volunteers stretched Lakeshore's ability to accomplish necessary projects, Mike wasn't looking for volunteers solely because of the financial side of the picture. Volunteerism also brought in the public to interact with Lakeshore's patients.

"We had patients at Lakeshore who were frightened they would soon be reentering society, some for the first time since they had incurred physical disability," Mike said. "It wasn't unusual for a Lakeshore patient to be asking himself or herself, 'How am I going to face the public?' When patients could talk with these volunteers and see that the volunteers didn't view them as 'lesser people,' the patients felt more at ease, more self-confident."

Many times through the years after the Wallace Recreation Center

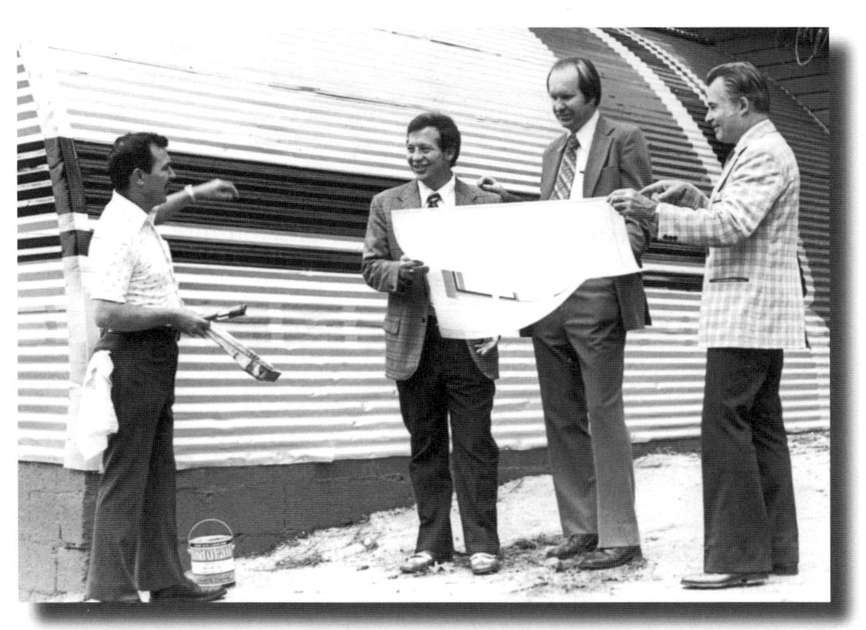

Volunteers from the Jaycees spruced up an old military-surplus Quonset hut that was being used as a maintenance building.

opened, Mike would reflect on a comment he made the day of the center's opening, during an interview with a news reporter.

"In your view, Mr. Stephens, what is Lakeshore trying to accomplish by opening this recreation center?" the reporter asked.

"Well, I guess what we're trying to do is to make somebody feel glad they're in a wheelchair!" Mike answered.

Mike admitted that to some people that might seem a strange, even insensitive, comment, but he strongly believed in its message. A similar sentiment was expressed by famous athlete Randy Snow—the first Paralympian to be inducted into the Olympic Hall of Fame—who said that after he became paralyzed he became motivated to achieve at a higher level than he ever would have as an able-bodied person.

"I was conveying, number one, that it doesn't have to be the end of the world for someone to end up in a wheelchair. I also was conveying that there are many individuals with disabilities who feel they have pushed themselves harder, have accomplished more, and have enjoyed life with more awareness and fulfillment than before they were disabled—because their disabilities actually have driven them to strive, to succeed, and to enjoy."

No one understood Lakeshore and its mission more than Mike Stephens. He lived and breathed Lakeshore. As a person who had a physical disability, Mike could get inside the hearts and minds of those who would use the Wallace Center and know what such a facility could mean to them.

But even Mike was overwhelmed by the extent to which those with physical disabilities were drawn to this center after word got around. People from a wide range of socioeconomic segments of society came to participate in or watch the sports and recreation programs. It was as though the center was reaching out and addressing a long-standing hunger and thirst in the lives of many of these individuals.

"Those of us who already had been participating in sports activities for the disabled—such as wheelchair basketball—had personally experienced how such activities could change participants' lives for the better," Mike said. "However, prior to the completion of the Center, never before in the Birmingham area had there been a well-equipped facility expressly built to house such programs."

More than just a place for fun and sports, the Wallace Center also provided a way to balance the lives of individuals with a physical disability. Many visitors had rarely been out of their homes for years. Mike noted that before coming to the center they "had this dark feeling deep inside themselves as if they really were already dead and all they wanted to do was sit around at home or go to bed."

Mike said the center also immediately started making a difference in the lives of a group of physically disabled individuals who had been diligent in pursuing various kinds of therapy but who had very little opportunity for recreation outside their therapy.

He noted that before the Wallace Center opened in 1981, the Lakeshore Hospital and Lakeshore Rehabilitation Facility could provide a wide range of services for individuals with physical disabilities. "We could get help for them with their medical problems. We could get them prostheses or other equipment to make their lives easier. We could provide them with driver's education and some kind of job training. We could help get them placed in jobs."

But those who guided Lakeshore's programs were painfully aware that many of Lakeshore's "graduates" were not enjoying overall long-term success with their lives.

"Even after we got people healthier and retrained them and placed them in jobs, we were seeing all too high an incidence of them quitting their jobs and going on Medicaid and Social Security disability rolls," said Mike.

What was missing, Mike explained, was the sports and recreation component. "These people were bored; their lack of involvement in something meaningful and stimulating tended to make them feel dependent on society," said Mike. "And in many instances they actually felt humiliated—like they were outsiders or outcasts of society. As individuals with physical disabilities looked around and saw this beautiful recreation center, they felt that the facility had been built for them. We were seeing people reconnect with energy they didn't even know they had, and start using muscles they had not used for a long time."

The recreation center also reached out to disabled athletes who had already been playing sports, some of whom proudly called the facility "our place."

The recreation center became the new official home court for the Birmingham Chariots wheelchair basketball team. "It was all the difference in the world," said Jim Wooten, who was already firmly entrenched as a star player for the Chariots when the recreation center opened. "We felt welcome and comfortable at the Wallace Recreation Center. Up until that time we had to beg and borrow for space and time to practice at other facilities. And we were using some facilities that were not wheelchair-accessible," said Jim. He said the Wallace Center was built so that athletes with disabilities could use it easily, and Lakeshore was generous in allowing these athletes to use it often.

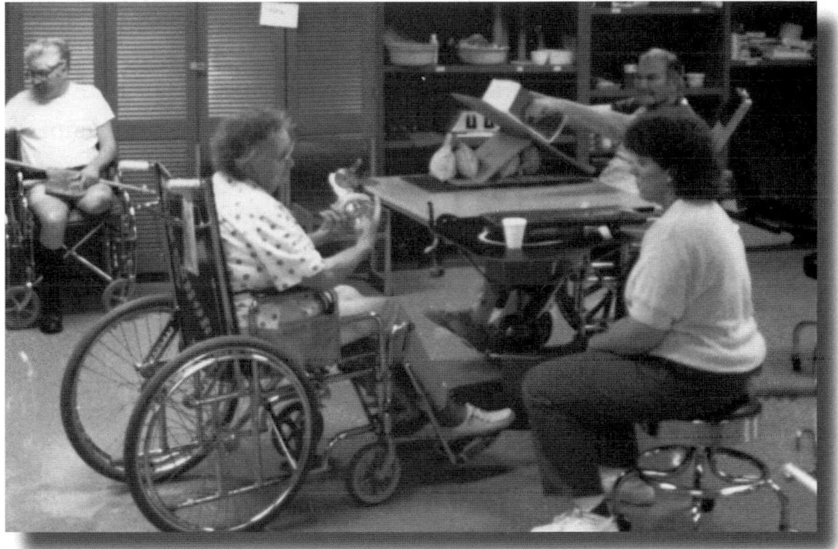

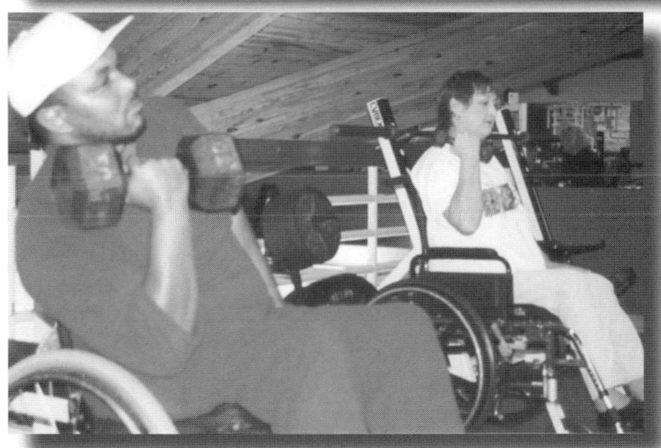

Lakeshore activities such as occupational therapy, weight lifting, target shooting, walking, and swimming gave purpose to people's lives.

The center was also a gift for spectators who had disabilities. Mike was particularly struck by one long-isolated, profoundly disabled man who was brought to Lakeshore by loved ones to be a spectator at a wheelchair basketball game. "This man had been isolated at home for so, so long. He had remained in much the same positions on a bed for so many years that his legs were frozen with contractions and curled and twisted up under him and even pointed off to the side," said Mike. "His loved ones rolled him around in a kind of steel roll-around cargo cart, the kind you might see in a commercial entity. But there he was,

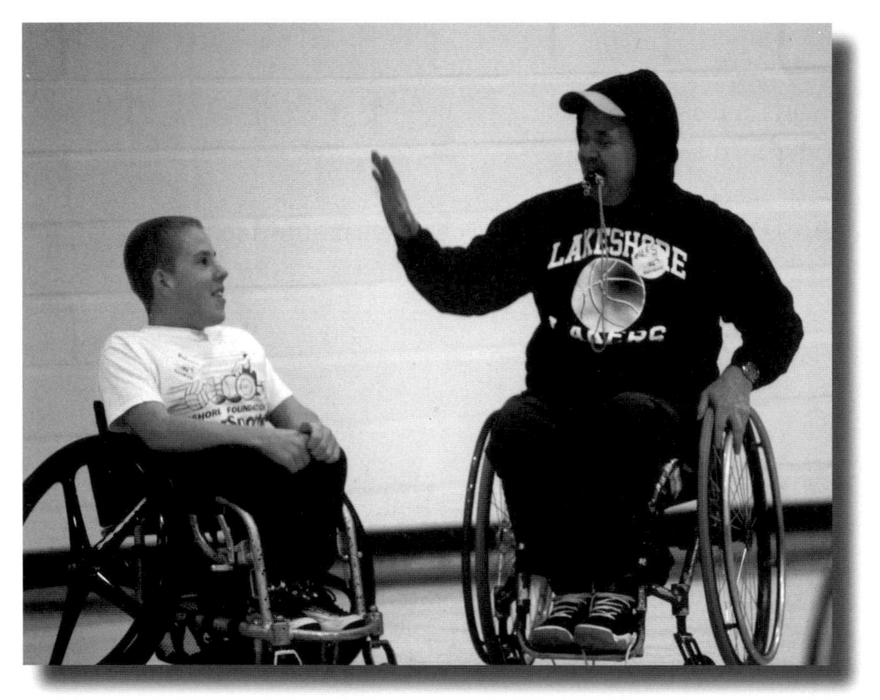

Professional staff members like Miles Thompson, himself in a wheelchair, motivated patients and clients to do more for themselves.

out in the world again—watching a wheelchair basketball game and enjoying himself!"

Mike said there was no doubt the Wallace Recreation Center filled a vital gap in the picture when it came to an enjoyable, productive way of life for individuals with physical disabilities.

NOT ONLY DID the energy generated by the Wallace Recreation Center touch the participants and spectators, but it also deeply touched the employees who helped make those activities possible.

From its start in the 1970s, Lakeshore attracted many employees who were driven by motivations to serve a mission higher than themselves. These employees were a mixture of able-bodied persons, never having had a severe physical disability yet driven for various reasons to help those who did, and disabled persons, motivated to serve those in similar positions as themselves. As time went by, there would be a number of staff members in wheelchairs, who would inspire Lakeshore patients and clients both by applying their professional abilities and by serving as role models.

Mike made sure to keep Governor Wallace informed about the huge impact that the Wallace Recreation Center was making. "It was important to me that George Wallace know just how special that recreation center was that he had made possible," said Mike.

It soon would become evident, said Mike, that the Wallace Center had become the first major step toward the establishment of the Lakeshore Foundation—a Foundation that would attract widespread positive attention for its prototype sports and recreation programs and facilities designed especially for those with physical disabilities.

Mike's head was filled with how important George Wallace's support had been and how it had planted seeds that would yield never-ending harvests. Mike repeatedly communicated to the longtime Alabama politician that the Wallace Recreation Center was more than just another building.

14

Bart and His Heroes

It started out to be a happy day. Children from a Birmingham church boarded a bus to travel to a church camp about 20 miles away.

Then there was the accident. The bus went down an embankment. There were injuries. The most serious injuries were dealt to six-year-old Bart Troxell—left paralyzed from the waist down and with nerve damage in his left hand.

"I was knocked unconscious," Bart would recall in adulthood. "I don't remember much about anything to do with the accident. Also, since I was so young when it happened, I don't remember much about being able to walk before the accident." Thus, to Bart Troxell, it would almost be as though he always had been in a wheelchair.

The accident occurred in 1981, the same year that Lakeshore's Wallace Recreation Center opened. Within a few months after he was injured, Bart's path would cross with Lakeshore, a facility that would cast a spotlight not on what was impossible for Bart, but on all the wonderful things that were possible.

"When disabled people are lucky, we often see that they are helped along in life by strong and capable family advocates," said Mike Stephens. "In that regard, Bart Troxell indeed was lucky. He had a great advocate in his mother, Norma Troxell. From the time Bart was injured, Norma was out there researching what could be done to help her child and following through on what she learned."

Mike recalled that Norma was on one of those missions when she came to Lakeshore one day and brought young Bart with her. "Some health professionals who had been taking care of Bart had suggested that he undergo a surgical procedure that Norma questioned," said Mike. "She came to Lakeshore to get a second opinion. At Lakeshore we in fact recommended against that surgical procedure—which proved to be a good call for Bart. While Norma was having this discussion with us, Bart was hanging out down in the Wallace Recreation Center, watching some of the guys play wheelchair basketball."

Those athletes—and their zest for life despite their disabilities—would light a fire inside this good-looking, dark-haired little boy with the infectious smile.

For Bart, that day was a beginning—the beginning of transformational roles that sports and recreation would play in opening tremendous doors in that boy's life.

As the years went by, Bart would speak of a number of athletes at Lakeshore who became his role models, including Joe Ray, a high-achieving, medal-winning physically disabled athlete.

Bart found a kindred spirit in Joe, who shared his interests in sports and cars.

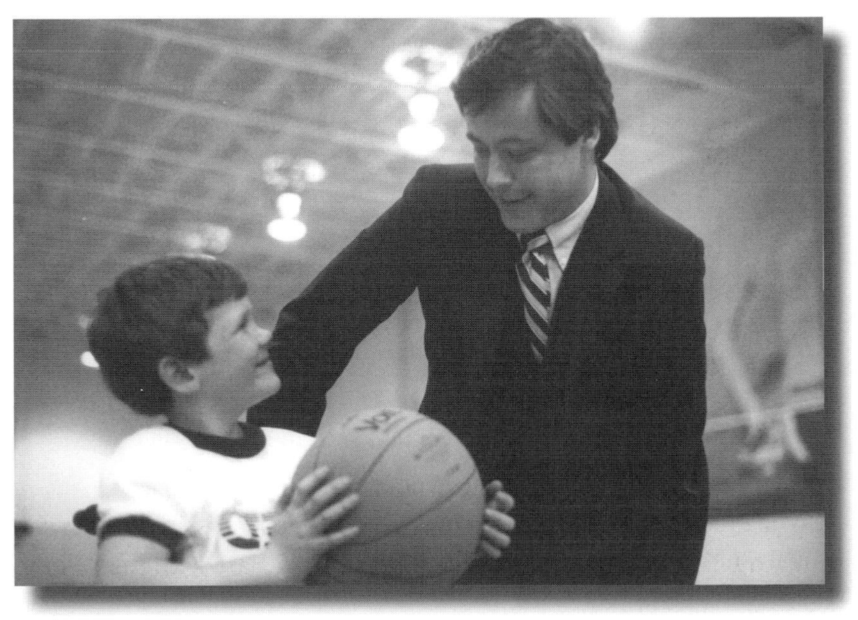

Young Bart Troxell gets encouragement from Lakeshore Executive Director Mike Stephens.

"My mom contacted Joe and he brought his Trans Am sports car over for me to see," said Bart. "I thought that car was the neatest thing!" Complete with hand-operated clutch, the car had been adapted so that Joe could drive it despite being paralyzed from the waist down. "Having that clutch made the car that much cooler," said Bart. "I mean, not many people in wheelchairs were driving a car with a clutch!"

Driving the "cool" Trans Am was typical of the "can-do" daredevil spirit of Joe Ray.

Joe, a native of Texas, was 20 years old when he was a passenger in a car accident that left him paralyzed from the waist down. By nature given to being spunky and feisty, Joe went forward with his life after he was left paralyzed. In 1979 he began taking computer training at the Lakeshore Rehabilitation Facility and got involved in wheelchair sports.

In the early 1980s, Joe became a vocal advocate of removing barriers that confronted those with physical disabilities, including that the majority of buildings were not wheelchair accessible and that most community sports events were not open to athletes with physical disabilities.

Joe attracted considerable attention when he was trying to convince the Birmingham Track Club to include wheelchair road racing as a division of road races the club sponsored. Members of the club wanted to proceed with caution and not open up activities that would be unsafe for participants in wheelchairs.

Joe Ray stirred real waves when he showed up at "the Vulcan Run," a highly popular race, to join in the race using his racing wheelchair, despite the race being open only to able-bodied participants. Joe recalled, "That day I thought, 'You know, I'm going to prove a point, because I know for a fact that I can safely run this race in my wheelchair!' "

Joe finished that race without suffering any injury. He had made his point. However, some of the race organizers were disturbed by Joe's brashness and his disregard for the current rules. Although Lakeshore wasn't officially sponsoring Joe in the race, Joe was identified with Lakeshore and Lakeshore Hospital Executive Director Mike Stephens caught some flack for what he did.

Mike recalled his thoughts at the time: "Even though Joe is causing problems with his 'I-don't-give-a-damn-what-anybody-tells-me' attitude, he's also calling attention to what disabled people can do instead of what they can't do!"

As a star athlete in sports for those with disabilities, Joe would set records and win world championships. He would be a member of a Lakeshore basketball team that would win a national championship. He would become proficient in road racing, track and field, and tennis and would win two world water-skiing championships.

As time went on, Joe would use his water-sports talents to help others through water-sports programs he led. He became executive director of a foundation called Adaptive Aquatics, which introduced the joys of water sports to many a person with physical disabilities.

One of those individuals was Bart Troxell. "I was around 12 years old when Joe got me up on water skis," said Bart. "I just knew that was the coolest thing I had ever done—ever!"

If attitude could be contagious, then the live-life-to-the-fullest attitude of Joe Ray and some of his buddies at Lakeshore was passed on to young Bart.

"I looked at Joe and the other athletes and saw the things they were accomplishing, and how they had adapted to situations. I was beginning to see the possibilities for my own life. You just have to stay focused and realize your potential," said Bart. "If you do that, there's not a lot you can't do!"

FROM THE TIME Bart sat on the sidelines watching the older guys playing wheelchair basketball at Lakeshore's Wallace Recreation Center, he felt drawn to wheelchair sports. For Bart, it would never be enough to sit on the sidelines; he wanted to be a participant. To do that, Bart needed a special wheelchair designed just for sports activity. After Bart was injured, there were many pressing needs draining the Troxell family's budget; it was difficult for that sports wheelchair to make it onto the priority list. "The racing wheelchair is more or less a luxury item, not a necessity," Bart's mom, Norma, told the *Birmingham News* in early 1983.

In response, Lakeshore and the Birmingham Chariots sponsored a fundraising event "Basketball for Bart," which raised money to purchase a sports wheelchair for Bart. The event was a rousing success. A crowd of some 600 gathered at the Wallace Recreation Center, clapping and cheering as the Chariots showed their wheelchair basketball skills against former Alabama and Auburn football stars and also against a team of physicians.

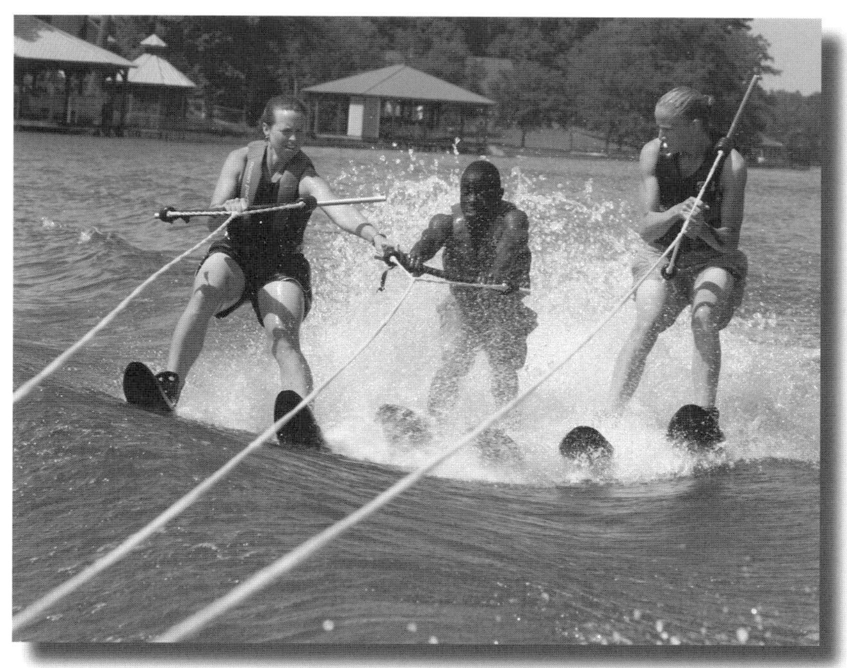

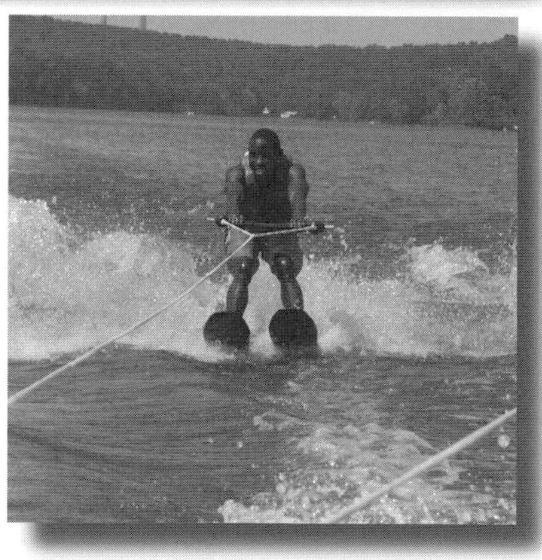

Bart Troxell learned to water ski on a mono-ski, or "ski sled." Others, like the young man pictured, could manage regular skis once staffers helped them up. (Photos at Lay Lake facilities partnered by Lakeshore and Adaptive Aquatics.)

In the days that led up to the "Basketball for Bart" event, Lakeshore had a forum to emphasize to the public the many opportunities open to athletes in wheelchairs. "There are very few things you can't do in a wheelchair," Lakeshore recreational director Sis Theuerkauf noted the week before the fundraiser. "Such sports as bowling, archery, hockey, square dancing, and track are all adaptable to wheelchairs."

The mounting community support for Lakeshore and wheelchair sports was also evident leading up to the event. At the time, Bart was undergoing treatment at the Shriners' Crippled Children's Hospital in Philadelphia, and the plane ticket home was too much for Bart's family to afford. The local Pioneers chapter (a telecommunications employees volunteer group) paid for plane tickets to fly Bart and his mother home in time for them to attend the Lakeshore benefit.

On the evening of the big event, seven-year-old Bart Troxell took center stage in the Wallace Recreation Center, and it was announced that Bart would get his sports wheelchair.

Bart's mother, Norma, was, as she put it, "overwhelmed by the interest and concern that Lakeshore has shown for Bart. . . . Lakeshore has really made a difference in our lives."

The sports wheelchair that came into Bart's life that night would be the beginning of Bart's entry into the world of wheelchair sports, including basketball, racing, swimming, and water skiing. Bart collected a growing batch of ribbons and trophies and models and just three years after he got that wheelchair, Bart would be named the outstanding junior male athlete at the 1986 Junior National Wheelchair Games.

As Bart grew into manhood, he continued to drink in life with zest. He took some college courses. He ventured into real estate. He had a home of his own in which he took pride. He continued to enjoy sports and cars.

Along the way in his journey, Bart had a chance to use some of his sports skills to bring joy into the lives of others, including his beloved mother, Norma, whom he took with him on a deep-sea diving trip to the Cayman Islands. This was Bart's chance to turn the tables on his mother, who had arranged so much in life that was good for him. He created excited experiences for her, including deep-sea diving, beyond what she could have imagined possible. For Bart, words alone could not describe what it meant to see the joy on his mother's face during that trip.

Bart remained close friends with Joe Ray, who was there for him after Bart lost his parents in 2007 and 2008. Bart and Joe were on a trip together out West when Bart met a young woman who became very special to him. They began making long-range plans for a life together. "She's an awesome person to have in my life," said Bart.

As he reached his mid-30s, Bart himself was moved to be of service to others. After losing his dad to the neurodegenerative disorder known as Huntington's Disease, Bart became an advocate for the Huntington's Disease Society of America. Bart felt he was honoring the memory of his soft-spoken, gentle father, who had given him such unwavering support.

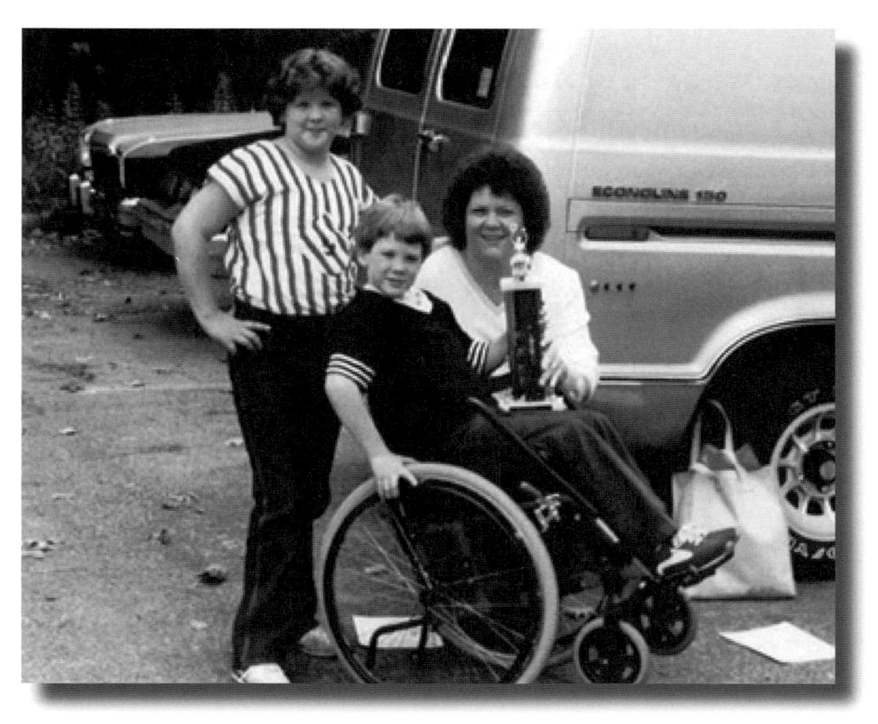

Bart Troxell with his sister, left, and mother, Norma.

Bart said that in the years after he sustained a physical disability, he learned lasting lessons about dealing head-on with loss and adversity, giving back to others, and living a rewarding, balanced life. He said he learned how to live a full life from his parents, from friends like Joe, and from his exposure to Lakeshore.

Bart was only one part of the circles of influence forming at Lakeshore—the families who supported, the individuals with disabilities who persevered, and one reaching out to help another.

From one to another, they are passing it on—the spirit of Lakeshore.

15

Riding the Momentum

It was as though the Wallace Recreation Center injected a super burst of steam into an engine that was already speeding down the track.

From the day the recreation center opened, it was put to high-profile use in sports and recreation. Too, the expansion was triggering enthusiasm that was helping to spur expansion in other areas of the Lakeshore campus. Lakeshore programs that already existed were growing, and new programs were taking root.

Lakeshore began to claim headlines as a state-of-the-art facility to host a wide range of sports activities for those with physical disabilities.

In February 1982, the Wallace Center hosted games sponsored by Southern Wheelchair Conference Basketball.

In April 1982, the 13th annual Wheelchair Games came to the Wallace Center under the sponsorship of Alabama Wheelchair Sports, Inc., a constituent organization of the National Wheelchair Athletic Association. The event brought to Lakeshore 40 entrants from three states—Alabama, Tennessee, and Georgia. Ranging in ages from 14 to 50, they competed in weight-lifting, table tennis, archery, tracks and field events, swimming, and slalom.

The Wallace Center also provided a place for athletes with physical disabilities to train intensively for competitive sports in various parts of the nation. Lakeshore athletes entered competitive events on an increasing basis and in a wide range of geographical locations, including wheelchair tournaments in Alabama, Georgia, and Minnesota.

In case after case, these Lakeshore athletes were returning with trophies and medals. In 1985, Lakeshore's impressive track and field cumulative results would afford an example: With 12 Lakeshore athletes participating, Lakeshore brought home 8 national records, 97 gold

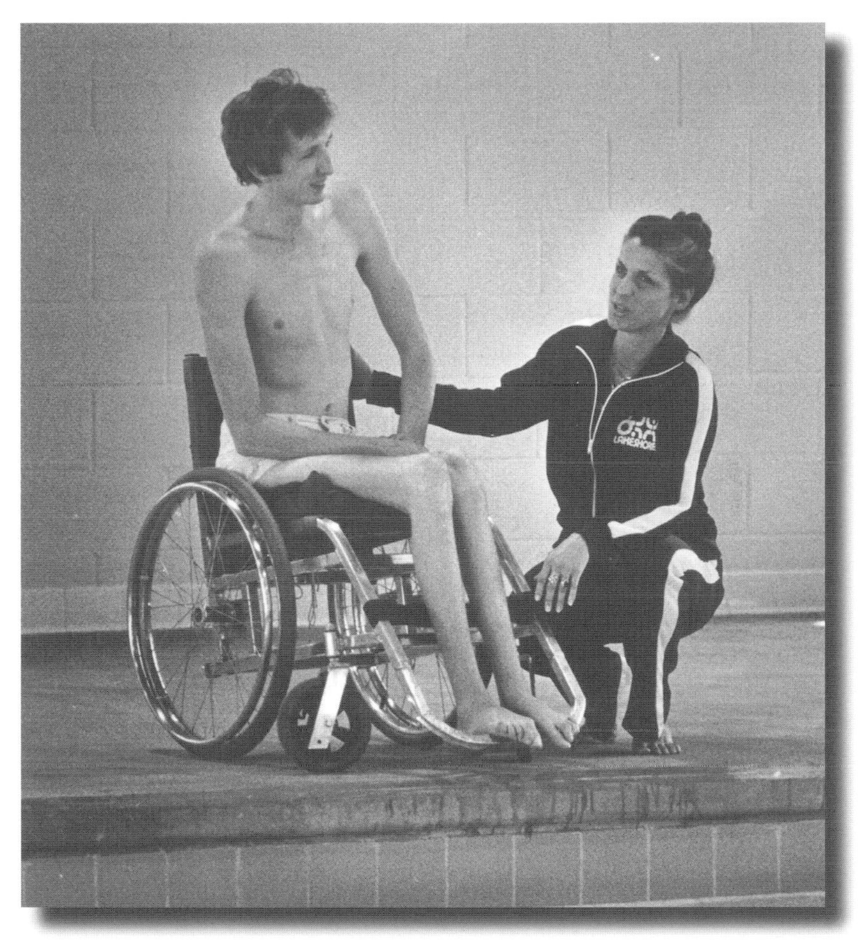

Joey Martin, here with recreational director Sis Theuerkauf, was one of Lakeshore's winningest athletes during his era.

medals, 45 silver medals, and 21 bronze medals.

TRAVEL FOR PARTICIPATING athletes was costly. Various groups in the community were pitching in to make participation at these sports competitions possible—including at international events.

One such example came in 1983, when Lakeshore and several civic clubs combined resources to help pay expenses for Joey Martin, a 23-year-old star swimmer from Clanton, Alabama, to participate in international wheelchair games in Bordeaux, France.

Joey Martin was earning medals in water sports even after a water-sports accident left him a quadriplegic. As a result of a dive that went bad, he was left paralyzed from the lower chest area down and without movement and strength in his shoulders and arms.

After the injury, Joey's breathing power was limited, and he no longer had the ability to cough up water out of his lungs. In order to return to swimming, Joey had to put forth a great amount of effort, and he had to exert extreme caution. Still Joey Martin persevered.

Joey did not disappoint the Birmingham area sponsors who had raised money to support his travel abroad to compete. He returned from France with six gold medals—earned in back freestyle, breaststroke, front freestyle, butterfly, individual medley, and as a member of a relay team.

The young athlete's mother, Inez Martin, told the news media in 1983 that she had seen something ironically positive occur with her son during the two years since he was injured. She said that before he was injured, Joey had not been very goal-oriented, but that since his injury he was achieving at a higher level than ever in his life. "I think about how changed Joey has been since the accident," she said, "and I think of those words, 'God moves in a mysterious way, His wonders to perform.' "

AS LAKESHORE RAPIDLY built its reputation, it increasingly became a place where sports celebrities sought treatment and rehabilitation for their own physical problems.

Grateful for the help that Lakeshore gave them, these well-known figures went out of their way to share their success stories with the public.

One such sports figure, veteran University of Alabama sportscaster John Forney, received help from Lakeshore at the beginning of the 1980s. After he suffered a stroke in 1980, at the age of 53, he underwent rehabilitation at Lakeshore for nearly a month. After making an almost miraculous recovery and returning to the broadcasting booth, John Forney was more than happy to tell fans about the speech, occupational,

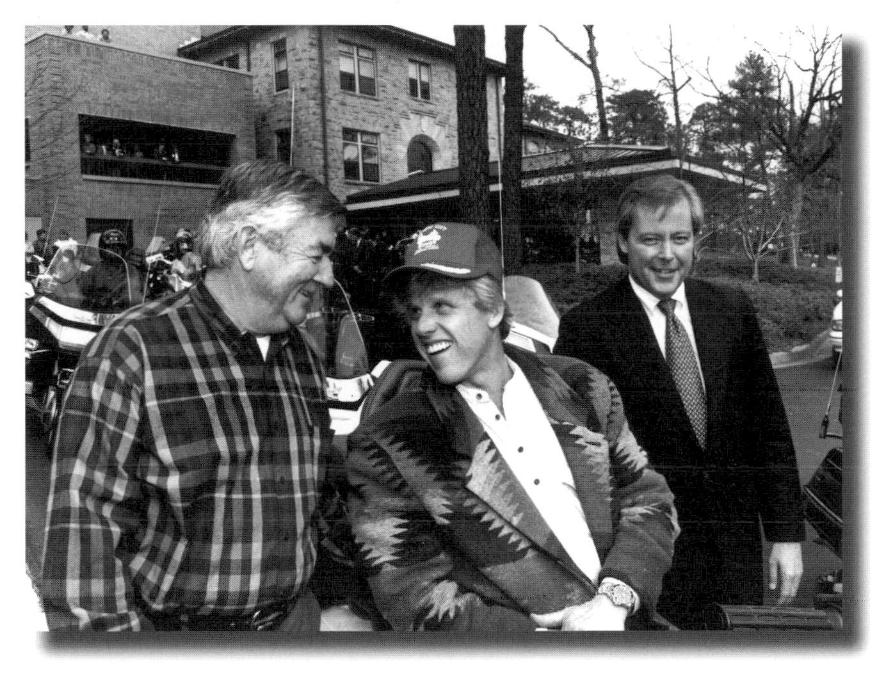

Lakeshore's rehabilitation services also helped famous athletes like Bobby Allison, left, shown here with actor Gary Busey (himself the victim of a brain trauma) and Mike Stephens, recover from serious injuries.

and physical therapy that had helped him so much at Lakeshore.

As for famed NASCAR driver Bobby Allison, he, too, would speak of the tremendous progress he made during his two months at Lakeshore after suffering a brush with death on June 19, 1988, in a car-racing crash. When he was admitted to Lakeshore, he was dealing with the debilitating aftermath of fractured ribs, three breaks to his left leg, and a brain injury; when he left, he walked with the aid of a cane.

Near the end of his stay at Lakeshore, Bobby Allison was able to deliver a very public message about how far he had progressed since coming so near to death. It was a Sington Awards Dinner, an event at which both able-bodied athletes and athletes with disabilities were being honored and funds were being raised to support wheelchair sports at Lakeshore. The Sington Award was named in honor of Fred Sington, a well-known Birmingham business and civic leader who was once recognized as a football "player of the century" for the University of Alabama. Sington had taken a special interest in the work of Lakeshore.

On this evening, Bobby's son Davey was receiving a Sington Award for his own racecar-driving achievements.Bobby's presence was not expected, since it was widely known that he was still in his rehabilitation at Lakeshore.

Then, in the midst of the evening's ceremonies, a dramatic phone call came in from Bobby Allison himself. Unknown to Davey and most of those in attendance, a telephone hookup had been arranged directly to his room at Lakeshore.

"During the program, Davey was told, 'There's somebody here who wants to talk to you,' " said then-Athletic Director Frank Burns, who had helped to organize the event. "Then the voice came on the loudspeaker and the audience could hear Bobby's voice booming out: 'Hello, Davey. This is your dad. I'm proud of you, son; I'm real proud of you.' Since his terrible accident, this event marked Bobby Allison's first public 'appearance,' his 'coming out.' There wasn't a dry eye in the place."

Beginning in the 1980s, there would be a series of these Sington Award fundraising dinners. Honorees would include the likes of Auburn University star athlete Bo Jackson, who went on to National Football League and Major League Baseball fame; Derrick Thomas, who made headlines first as a University of Alabama football player and later in the National Football League; and Alabama-born world heavyweight boxing champion Evander Holyfield. Nationally known emcees at the Sington Award dinners included sportscaster Keith Jackson and actor/comedian Tim Conway.

Funds raised at these events would fuel Lakeshore's wheelchair sports programs. Beyond that, the large amount of publicity and overwhelming public response generated by the events would further fuel Lakeshore's reputation.

AS LAKESHORE EXPANDED its sports and recreation programs, Mike Stephens and his staff made it clear that the programs were also de-

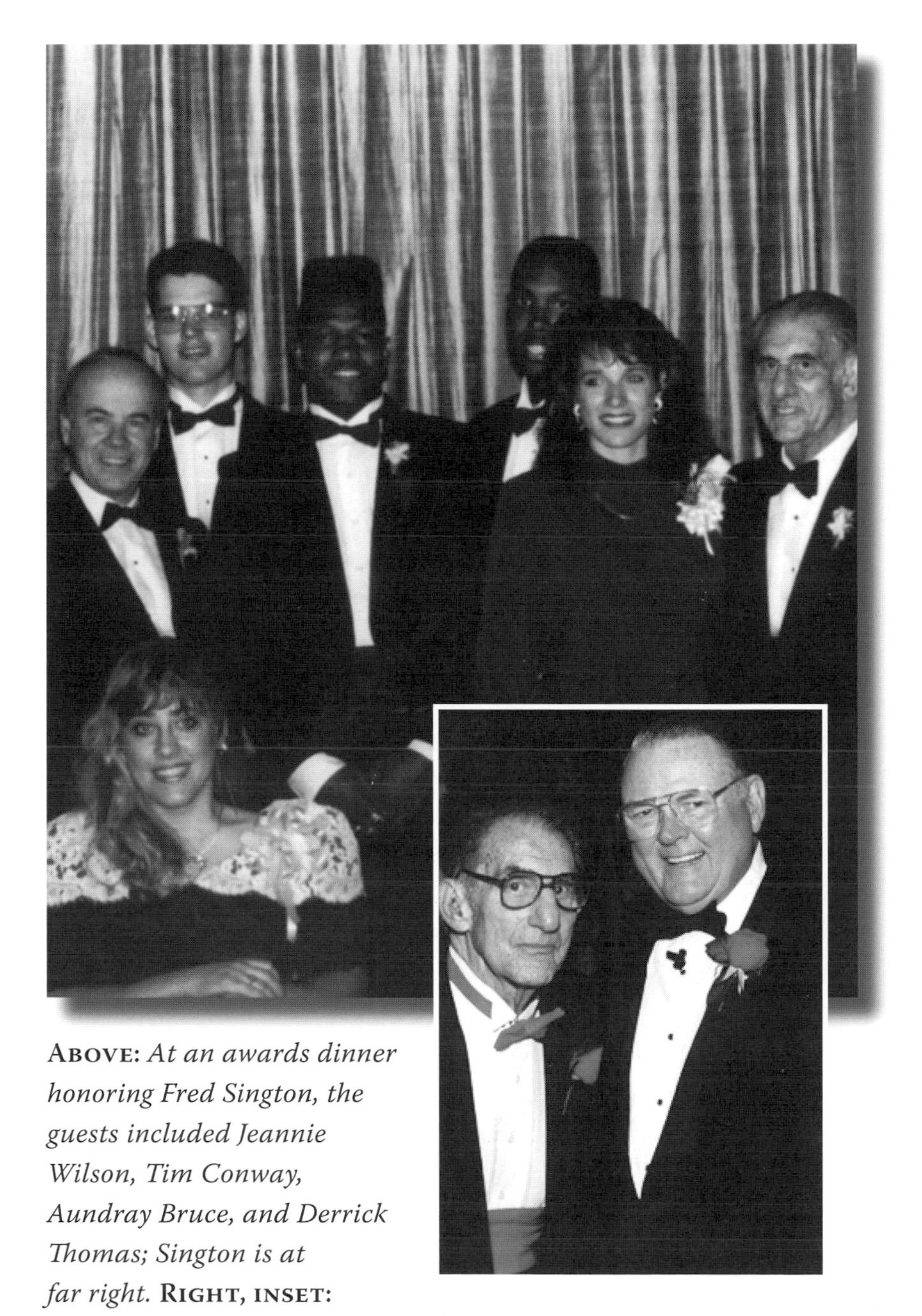

Above: *At an awards dinner honoring Fred Sington, the guests included Jeannie Wilson, Tim Conway, Aundray Bruce, and Derrick Thomas; Sington is at far right.* **Right, inset:** *Sportscaster Keith Jackson, right, was one of the celebrities who turned out for another awards dinner honoring Sington, left.*

signed for therapy, to help the body get stronger and to help improve attitude and motivation.

Therapeutic recreation was emphasized in arts and crafts programs in the Wallace Recreation Center. One woman told how she had regained much strength and flexibility in her crippled, arthritis-ravaged hands by using the skills she was learning in copper-tooling to fashion beautiful wall hangings for her home.

The theories behind therapeutic recreation Lakeshore-style were basically these: If a person with a disability could have fun and achieve in sports and recreation, he could see how he could have fun and achieve with life in general. From an emotional standpoint, he could be more motivated and self-confident, and learn to recognize his potential, to reach for opportunities, to ward off depression, to take care of his health, to expand his education, to hold down a job, and to be active in community service to help others. On the physical side, he was helping his body to become stronger and healthier by building his muscles, moving his joints, and stimulating his circulation.

LAKESHORE WAS EXPERIENCING growth across the campus in the 1980s. Both the hospital and outpatient census were going steadily upward. Hospitals both in Birmingham and out of town were increasingly transferring patients to Lakeshore for rehabilitation immediately after the patients received acute-care hospital services.

In 1979, Lakeshore added surgery facilities, and some patients began coming directly to Lakeshore for surgery and then staying for a time afterward for rehabilitation. New Lakeshore treatment programs were also being announced, including the first Center for Closed Head Injuries in the Southeast, established in 1983.

And, more and more, Lakeshore was adding the education element to therapy—teaching people how to improve their health in relation to physical disability and chronic illness. Lakeshore's new aerobics and aquatics classes—held at the Wallace Recreation Center—taught adults ages 55 and older how to strengthen their heart, lungs, and muscles and how to improve circulation.

Thus, feeding Lakeshore's increasing success was the fact that the Lakeshore campus offered such a variety of services to those with physical disabilities. For more and more individuals, Lakeshore was one-stop shopping for multiple services. It wasn't uncommon for a person with a disability to come to Lakeshore Hospital for some type of surgery following an accident, to remain at Lakeshore for occupational and physical therapy, to get an artificial limb and/or special braces designed by Lakeshore's prosthetics and orthotics specialists, to check into Lakeshore's transitional living facility to learn skills for independent living, to enroll in some kind of employment-training program at the Lakeshore Rehabilitation Facility, and then to get involved in some of Lakeshore's ongoing sports and recreation programs. In fact, the services at Lakeshore were so varied that, depending on what kind of services a person was receiving, he might be called "a patient" or "a client," "a Lakeshore athlete," or, at one time or another, he might be referred to by all three designations.

RECRUITMENT OF HIGHLY qualified key personnel was also helping to drive the Lakeshore train in the 1980s.

In 1985, Lakeshore recruited Frank Burns, a high-profile figure in sports programs for those with disabilities. This was a coup for Lakeshore.

Frank was an able-bodied man who had made a name for himself in coaching individuals with physical disabilities. Frank had developed a successful wheelchair sports program at Casa Colina, a rehabilitation facility in Pomona, California, about 40 miles east of Los Angeles. Then he had become associated with the University of Wisconsin-Whitewater, where he taught adaptive physical education and directed a wheelchair sports program.

Frank was recruited as Lakeshore's new athletic director. His job was two-fold—to develop and market Lakeshore's wheelchair sports program, and to develop a plan of action to raise funds to subsidize Lakeshore's wheelchair sports program.

Mike Stephens said the recruitment of Frank Burns sent out a loud-

and-clear positive message about Lakeshore.

"Since Frank had a national reputation in coaching wheelchair sports, the fact that he would leave Whitewater and come to Lakeshore showed, first of all, that Lakeshore had a serious intent to go in the right direction with sports and recreation," Mike said. "And, secondly, it showed that Lakeshore actually had things in place to develop a sports and recreation program that was worldwide in scope and reach."

Frank Burns said the Wallace Recreation Center, only four years old at the time, was one of the real drawing cards when he accepted his position. "Lakeshore had become one of the first rehabilitation centers to actually build athletic facilities on the same site as a rehabilitation hospital," Frank said. He was also interested in Lakeshore's plans to further develop and expand wheelchair sports programs.

Once he made the trip to Lakeshore, talked to Mike Stephens, and saw the Wallace Recreation Center, Frank said he knew he was hooked.

The Wallace Recreation Center was not the only construction project that helped to put Lakeshore on the map in the 1980s.

On Sunday, October 13, 1985, Lakeshore held dedication ceremonies for facilities that had been renovated and expanded through a far-reaching $11 million modernization project launched in 1983.

In addition to major inpatient and outpatient facilities, this project gave Lakeshore a new entrance, an improved road network, a new admitting entrance, and additional parking capacity.

At the rate Lakeshore was growing, it needed all these facilities and more.

And, in what was becoming a typical Lakeshore approach, the celebration of Lakeshore's big modernization project did not occur without a special touch to entertain and educate the public. This time, that special touch came in the form of an appearance by internationally known fitness and exercise guru Richard Simmons. During the weekend of the dedication ceremony, Lakeshore hosted an "exercise concert" led by Richard Simmons—featuring exercises designed for both the able-bodied and those with disabilities.

FROM HIS VIEW as executive director of Lakeshore, Mike Stephens could see that momentum was sweeping Lakeshore down the road in helping those with disabilities.

"We were using our growing sports and recreation programs to get physically disabled people active," Mike said. "For many of them, this was one of the steps in moving them forward to becoming gainfully employed.

"All in all, there is no doubt that, through Lakeshore's programs, we were making a positive impact on lowering the cost of taking care of some of these individuals by raising the bar for their success and productivity."

16

In the Competitive Arena

Not everyone was happy with Lakeshore's rapid expansion in the 1980s; some felt the expansion was stepping on their toes. Lakeshore was growing during a time when competition in the healthcare industry was raising its head as never before all around the nation—including in the Birmingham area.

Although healthcare entities had been competitive with one another for many decades, the competition became much more vocal in the wake of major healthcare-facilities expansions of the 1960s and 1970s. Academic medical centers found themselves competing against community hospitals, and for-profit institutions and not-for-profit institutions often waged their own competitive clashes.

In Birmingham, Lakeshore was in an area that was becoming one of the leading locations in the United States for rapid development of the healthcare enterprise. Some Birmingham area healthcare leaders could not believe how much Lakeshore had grown in the one decade since it had been established. For some, including the academic medical center that had helped give birth to Lakeshore—namely the University of Alabama at Birmingham—it was a little disturbing.

Back in the 1970s, Lakeshore started out as a sleepy little campus on a site that for decades had been home to the Jefferson Tuberculosis Sanatorium. Some who had input into the early Lakeshore vision had foreseen Lakeshore functioning in a laid-back, low-key manner in keeping with its serene, off-the-beaten-path wooded location—a location that had a peaceful rural feel, much in contrast to the urban buildings and busy traffic only a short distance away.

Dr. John Miller III, chairman of UAB's Department of Rehabilitation Medicine, director of UAB's Rehabilitation Research and Training

Center, and director of UAB's Spain Rehabilitation Center, had taken a key lead in envisioning Lakeshore in the 1970s.

Reportedly, Dr. Miller envisioned Lakeshore as a supplement to the Spain Rehabilitation Center. Since Spain was located in the same complex as UAB's hospitals and clinics, he thought Spain was an ideal place to provide rehabilitation services in the initial days and weeks after a patient suffered debilitating injury or illness. Then, the patient could be referred to Lakeshore for any necessary long-term therapy.

However, there apparently were no official documents that ever laid out such an agreement between Lakeshore and UAB. In fact, when Lakeshore opened in the 1970s it was touted by its proponents as a facility that would provide comprehensive rehabilitation services.

In the mid-1980s, Lakeshore initiated a move that stirred the anger of UAB. The move involved the establishment of a chain of satellite Lakeshore operations, located in various community hospitals in the Birmingham area.

Lakeshore's first satellites to open included those at Baptist Medical Center Montclair, established in October 1984, and at the main campus of Carraway Methodist Medical Center in July 1985. In 1988 Lakeshore would open another such unit at a Carraway hospital 15 miles to the west of Birmingham—at Bessemer Carraway Medical Center.

These hospital-based satellite units that Lakeshore would operate off its main campus would provide comprehensive acute rehabilitation—including full-time nursing care, social services, physical therapy, occupational therapy, speech therapy, and, something for which Lakeshore was building a signature reputation, recreational therapy.

Upset that Lakeshore was competing with the Spain Rehabilitation Center, UAB leaders requested a meeting with Lakeshore leaders.The meeting was held at UAB. Representing Lakeshore were Mike Stephens and Lakeshore Hospital board leader Jimmy Shepherd. Representing UAB were UAB President Dr. S. Richardson "Dick" Hill Jr., UAB Vice President for Health Affairs Dr. Charles A. "Scotty" McCallum, and UAB's University Hospital Chief of Staff Dr. Durwood Bradley.

"It was a heated meeting," Mike recalled. "Dr. Hill was a man noted for his gentlemanly approach, for keeping his cool. But he was obviously very disturbed about our satellite operations. When he first walked into the room for the meeting, he had something in his hand—a batch of papers, or a book—and he actually threw whatever he was holding. He said, 'Damn it! This is not what I wanted from Lakeshore!' "

Jimmy Shepherd said he had a lot of respect for the UAB leaders present at the meeting and viewed them as friends both before and after the meeting. But he said there was no doubt emotions ran high at that memorable meeting. "They jumped all over us, telling us that we were going off the initial vision for Lakeshore and leading it down the wrong road," Shepherd said. With a chuckle, he added, "Mike and I left the meeting with our tails between our legs, kind of like 'What in the world is going on here?' "

After that highly charged UAB meeting, it was Mike's opinion that the facts should be researched and that the facts should speak for themselves.

Mike had not been appointed Lakeshore's executive director until the Lakeshore plan was almost two years old. He asked Jimmy Shepherd to research the documents from the early 1970s that had led to the creation of Lakeshore—to see if there had ever been any formal commitment that Lakeshore would pursue a specific vision as it related to UAB.

"I researched those records and I could not find any place where any promises had been made by Lakeshore to UAB," Shepherd said. "I wrote a paper on my research, and I included that."

The participants in that first meeting at UAB agreed to have a second meeting, which took place on the Lakeshore campus. UAB sent one representative, Dr. Scotty McCallum.

"I knew Dr. Scotty McCallum and I had a lot of respect for him," said Jimmy Shepherd. "In fact, a lady who had once served as his secretary actually had become my wife [Frances Bell Shepherd]. But as soon as he walked into the room at Lakeshore for that second meeting, I started jumping all over him—telling him about my research and all these files I had that documented Lakeshore's original vision. Scotty immediately said, 'Hey, whoa, whoa. We're friends. We don't have any problems!' "

Jimmy Shepherd recalled this as a good meeting. "It worked out fine," he said, noting that in his view the Lakeshore and UAB story "became a case of people who sowed a friendship and worked together."

UAB was only one of the institutions left feeling threatened by Lakeshore's sudden expansion. At this time, it was getting harder and harder for the rehab hospital to please various referring hospitals that were competing against one another.

No tightrope-walking along these lines was more difficult for Lakeshore than when it was were caught in the middle between two Birmingham area acute-care hospital rivals—Baptist Medical Centers and Brookwood Medical Center—that were in competition for the same market of patients. Well-established, not-for-profit Baptist Medical Centers, with its decades of experience in healthcare, was none-too-happy in the 1970s when newly built Brookwood Medical Center opened its doors as the unwelcome for-profit new hospital kid in town.

Lakeshore's position in this particular competitive scenario was particularly sticky. While Lakeshore was getting rehab referrals from both Baptist Medical Centers and Brookwood, Lakeshore had a unique history with Baptist Medical Centers. When Lakeshore Hospital first began operating in the 1970s, Lakeshore had a management contract with Baptist Medical Centers. In fact, Mike Stephens was actually recruited to go to Lakeshore by Baptist Medical Centers, and in his initial years as executive director at Lakeshore, he reported to Baptist Medical Centers as one of its vice presidents.

Brookwood resented that early close relationship between Lakeshore and Baptist Medical Centers. Periodically when it seemed to Brookwood that Lakeshore was particularly catering to the Baptists, Brookwood would threaten to cut off its referral of patients to Lakeshore.

"Brookwood would complain, 'You're in bed with the Baptists, and we're not going to send you any patients!' " recalled Jimmy Shepherd.

The Lakeshore Board of Directors decided to hire Mike so that he no longer had to report to the Baptists.

DURING THIS PIVOTAL Lakeshore transitional period, outstanding leadership was crucial, Mike recalled, in order to make sound decisions about the path Lakeshore would follow.

Lakeshore was fortunate at that time to have some very wise businessmen and community leaders serving on its board of directors, including James W. "Jimmy" Shepherd, a real estate executive who served for two terms and who would become one of the four original members of the board of trustees to oversee the Lakeshore Foundation.

"Jimmy Shepherd was a capable leader, a much-needed leader who was visionary," said Mike. "The way I saw it, Jimmy Shepherd's last name was very appropriate, for he indeed was the one who helped 'shepherd' Lakeshore through a very transitional period. Jimmy had a quiet manner, he had strength, he was very knowledgeable, and he was careful to pull his facts together to make sure that what we were doing at Lakeshore was right. Jimmy Shepherd was a man who just had good hunches; he pushed us through in the right direction so that truth prevailed. And, as a great asset, Jimmy was not influenced by healthcare politics—which was very important for Lakeshore at the time."

From the view of Jimmy Shepherd himself, the hostility that Lakeshore faced from some of its competition came as a surprise. He was a successful businessman who had experienced competition in conventional business. Shepherd had to get accustomed to the fact that open competition had arrived in the healthcare industry as well. "I had just never realized how competitive hospitals could be!" he said.

As Mike Stephens would look back on the 1980s at Lakeshore, he would say that it was particularly crucial that Lakeshore not cave in to its opposition.

The 1980s proved to be a significant transitional period for Lakeshore, a time when Lakeshore was spreading its wings and expanding into something bigger and broader than many had ever thought possible. "Lakeshore was feeling the strength of the programs it had incubated," Mike said. "And Lakeshore was emerging from the shadow of UAB."

In the end, Lakeshore continued on its path. It never slowed down.

17

Roots of a Company and a Foundation

The year 1985 would mark the biggest turning point at Lakeshore since Lakeshore Hospital had first opened its doors to rehabilitation patients in late 1973.

For it was in 1985 when the Lakeshore Board of Directors, under the direction of Mike Stephens, authorized an extensive reorganization involving the establishment of seven distinct corporations. The multi-corporation system would operate under the umbrella of a parent holding company, Lakeshore, Inc., with Mike as the holding company's president and chief executive officer.

One of the driving forces behind this significant milestone was reimbursement.

Prior to 1985, Lakeshore Hospital was operating a hospital, outpatient clinics, a sheltered workshop, a transitional living facility, a prosthetics shop, among other service entities. The restructuring allowed Lakeshore Hospital to put these in different corporations to get maximum and fair reimbursement from Medicare, Medicaid, and insurance companies.

This restructuring would lay the groundwork for Lakeshore Hospital to become the model institution for establishing and growing an entire rehabilitation company from a single institution.

Lakeshore Hospital would serve as the flagship facility—the prototype, the model—as a network of rehabilitation facilities in several states would be developed.

In 1984 and 1985 the Lakeshore Board of Directors authorized Mike Stephens and the staff he supervised to operate rehabilitation facilities in Huntsville, Alabama; to develop plans for a comprehensive outpatient facility in Mobile, Alabama; and also to proceed with plans for a 50-bed rehabilitation hospital in Macon, Georgia.

Mike Stephens was at the helm of the private, for-profit company that would oversee this tremendous growth. The company would first be known as Lakeshore System Services, and later as ReLife, Inc.

ONE OF THE seven corporations that emerged as a result of Lakeshore Hospital's 1985 restructuring was a tax-exempt, not-for-profit foundation to raise funds for Lakeshore's growing sports and recreation programs for the physically disabled.

The foundation, called simply the Lakeshore Foundation, Inc., was founded by Mike Stephens. Original officers of the board of trustees of the foundation included Chairman Lathrop Smith, Vice Chairman William Billingsley, Treasurer James "Jimmy" Shepherd, and Secretary James Hughey.

Mike later would say that when he conceived his vision for Lakeshore Foundation in the mid-1980s, he did not have a long-range plan for all the foundation could achieve. Instead, he just had very specific thoughts about the need for such a foundation and about its potential.

As he devoted hours to thinking about it in 1984 and 1985, a recurring set of thoughts drove his resolve. "In the past several years, I have seen sports and recreation programs weave miracles in the lives of many individuals with disabilities who have come through the doors of Lakeshore," Mike said. "With a foundation totally dedicated to such programs, I think there is no limit to the miracles we can help bring about in people's lives. Deep down in my heart, I know it's the right thing to do to establish the Lakeshore Foundation. "

Part IV

Reaching Out to Serve the Children

18

Response to a 'Yearning'

Lakeshore would become known around the world for its innovative and life-molding sports and recreation programs for children. Mike Stephens said that much of the vision for these youth-oriented programs was simply a series of creative responses to need.

"What we were doing at Lakeshore in the early to mid-1980s was responding to needs as we saw them," said Mike. "Rather than coming up with a grand plan and fitting the needs into it, we were allowing needs to present themselves to us and then trying to be practical, effective, and progressive in the programs we tailored to address these needs. Children's programs were being requested by parents and in many cases by kids themselves. There weren't a lot of sophisticated programs then in existence to address the sports and recreation needs of children who had physical disabilities. So we were coming up with our own blueprints."

Mike said that he and staff members at Lakeshore began to see more than just a need for sports and recreation programs designed especially for children; they saw a kind of "yearning." Children and their parents were seeking for children the same kind of sports and recreational activities that were doing so much for older teens and adults.

"The first time I recall seeing this was back when I was playing and coaching wheelchair basketball, years before we had the Wallace Recreation Center, back when we were still playing in borrowed community centers. I began to see some disabled youngsters and their parents who got real fired up by watching our adult wheelchair basketball games. We heard comments such as 'Gosh, it would be great if we could have sports programs like this for children.' "

THE GROUNDSWELL OF interest in sports and recreation programs for disabled children intensified as a result of Lakeshore's much-publicized 1983 "Basketball for Bart" fundraiser to raise funds to purchase a sports wheelchair for seven-year-old Bart Troxell, who had been paralyzed in a bus accident.

Opportunities that Lakeshore opened for Bart went far beyond just the fundraising event that honored him and resulted in a sports wheelchair entering his young life. Lakeshore introduced Bart to the joys of wheelchair sports and to mentors who would inspire him—young people with physical disabilities who were achieving and experiencing a fulfilling lifestyle, with the help of wheelchair sports.

"What Lakeshore did for young Bart became a symbol to many people of how an injured child's quality of life can be transformed for the better by connecting to wheelchair sports," said Mike.

Mike himself was touched deeply by seeing how Bart responded and benefited. First of all, Mike was happy for Bart. As time went by, the boy's success story tugged at Mike's heartstrings.

Second, Bart became a motivational symbol for Mike. He could see this happy and energetic child as he maneuvered his wheelchair in sports activities. Mike could see how sports ultimately led to Bart's winning medals, and, far beyond that, how these activities led to Bart being able to have a more fulfilling life.

If wheelchair sports can inspire and motivate a child as they have young Bart, Lakeshore can do that for other children as well.

BY THE LATE 1980s, the time was ripe for the founding of Lakeshore programs for children with physical disabilities.

First, Lakeshore recruited a key facilitator named Randy Snow.

Randy came to Lakeshore in two roles—as a member of Lakeshore's staff, and as an athlete continuing his training at Lakeshore for his own ongoing participation in competitive sports at national and international levels. As a Lakeshore staff member, Randy served as assistant athletic director and became the first director of Lakeshore's organized sports programs for children with physical disabilities.

Randy's personal story was typical of the reality that most severe accidents occur within a matter of seconds but alter the victims' lives forever.

In the mid-1970s Randy was 16 years old and working a summer job with a hay-baling outfit in Paris, Texas, not far from his hometown of Terrell, Texas. "My job was to drive a tractor and retrieve large bales of hay and stack them in a designated area," said Randy. "I attempted a shortcut, and it got me in trouble." A 1,000-pound bale of hay came crashing down on the teenager, permanently paralyzing his legs.

Randy had grown up in a family that loved the outdoors and sports. Hunting and fishing was a way of life for Randy, and he also excelled at tennis. At the time he was injured, the teenager already was a ranked junior tennis player.

But Randy's big athletic success was yet to come.

After his legs were paralyzed, Randy continued to excel in sports—not in one sport, but in three: tennis, wheelchair basketball, and wheelchair racing. Randy Snow would develop into such a worldwide athlete-superstar that in 2004 he would become the first Paralympian to be inducted into the Olympic Hall of Fame.

Randy would tell the world that in a sense his crippling injury had served him well—by motivating him to work harder, reach higher, and excel at a level far beyond what he felt he otherwise would have reached had his injury never occurred.

Randy's rise in wheelchair sports bloomed during his college years. After high school, he entered the University of Texas at Austin, where he led in trying to start a wheelchair basketball team. He sought the help of a coach who also had a physical disability and was in a wheelchair. This was a coach who would become an internationally known agent of change in wheelchair sports—Coach Jim Hayes of the University of Texas at Arlington.

Hayes already was creating new opportunities in wheelchair sports. After graduating from and then going to work for the University of Texas at Arlington, he created an Office for Students with Disabilities and organized teams in both wheelchair basketball and wheelchair tennis. At UT Arlington, Hayes would go on to coach the championship wheelchair basketball team, the Movin' Mavs. A successful athlete himself, Hayes also won medals as a wheelchair racer.

When Randy Snow asked Coach Hayes to come to UT Austin and advise him about wheelchair basketball, the coach agreed. Randy was so drawn to Hayes's enthusiasm for wheelchair sports that he followed him to UT Arlington, where Randy ultimately earned a baccalaureate degree in business.

With Coach Hayes as his role model and mentor, Randy participated in athletic programs that the coach created and led. Randy played wheelchair tennis and wheelchair basketball, and became expert as a wheelchair racer. He would credit Coach Hayes as being "the first person who brought the Trojan horse of wheelchair sports into my life." Randy also would say that wheelchair sports became such a force in

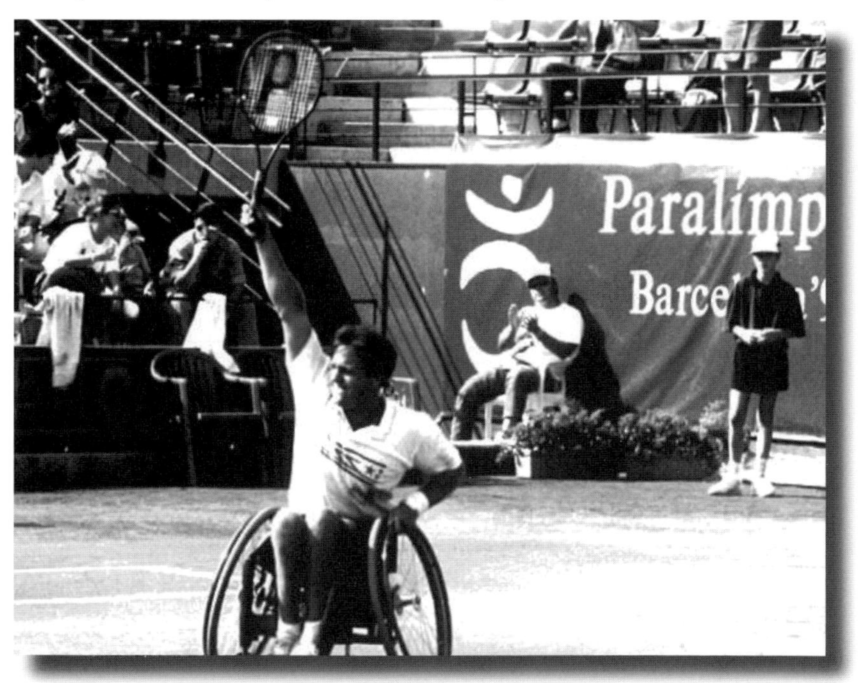

Randy Snow, whose recruitment as Lakeshore's first director of organized sports programs for children with physical disabilities, was a turning point for him and the institution.

his own rehabilitation that it was "like a rescue boat came to get me."

IN TERMS OF high-profile public interest in wheelchair sports, a major turning point occurred in the summer of 1984. Randy was a part of that history-making event. With a large audience cheering him on, he won a silver medal in wheelchair racing.

The occasion was a men's 1500-meter wheelchair race that was added to the Summer Olympics as an exhibition event—part of the centerpiece for what was the first track event for disabled athletes in the history of the Olympics. It was a groundbreaking event—giving athletes in wheelchairs unprecedented access to a large live audience in Los Angeles and to widespread television coverage.

The response was electrifying. The live audience gave a standing ovation to these athletes who raced like the wind in their wheelchairs. Millions more were tuned to their television sets in sheer wonder.

This 1984 wheelchair racing event would prove to be a milestone in securing for Paralympic sports a permanent spot on the Olympic landscape. At an individual level, the 1984 wheelchair racing event gave silver-medal winner Randy Snow yet another boost on his road to becoming an international star in wheelchair sports.

Four years after the Paralympic event in Los Angles, Randy came to Lakeshore.

When Lakeshore Athletic Director Frank Burns went to Lakeshore Foundation's founder Michael Stephens with the idea of recruiting Randy, they agreed that the timing was good. They believed Randy had the potential to make a significant contribution to Lakeshore's rapidly expanding programs in sports and recreation.

Randy was in his late 20s when he arrived at Lakeshore. Years later he would look back on his time at Lakeshore as some of the most pivotal, constructive years of his life.

And Mike and Frank would look back on Randy's recruitment as part of the beginning of something unbelievably big in the development of Lakeshore's sports and recreation programs for children with physical disabilities.

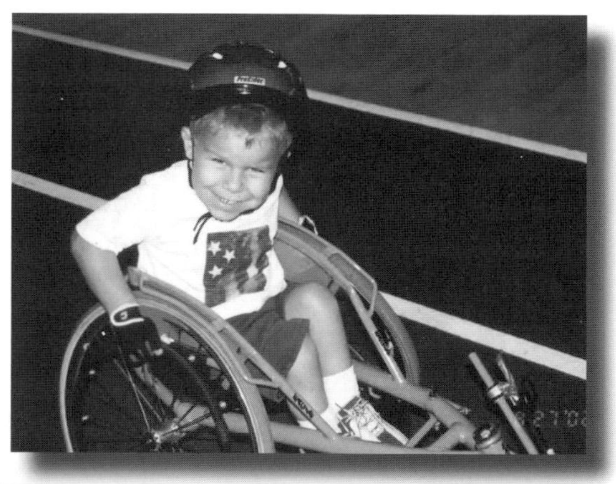

Lakeshore programs such as Super Sports Saturdays changed the lives of children such as Abraham Hausman-Weiss (see page 289). Abraham is at right, and, a few years later, chasing the ball below.

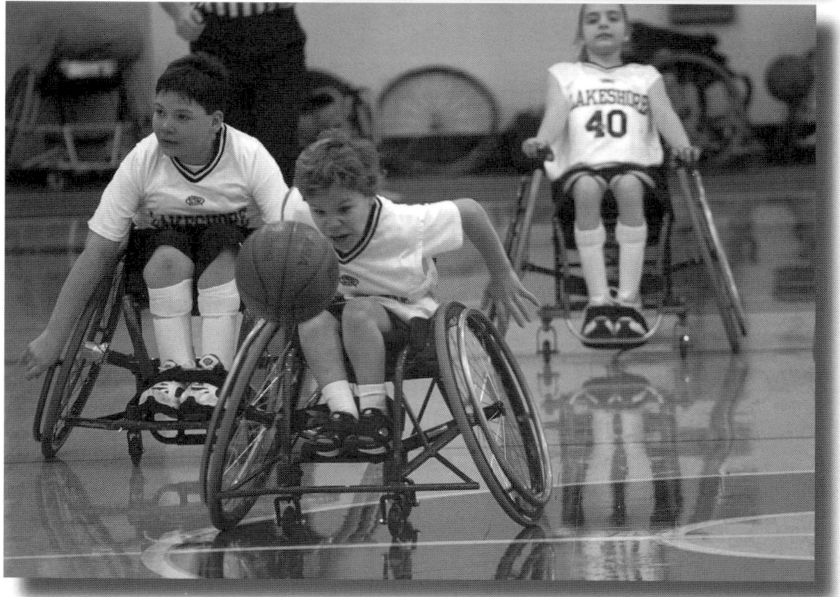

"I credit Frank Burns for making this match," said Mike. "Frank knew Randy, and he could see that in addition to Randy's extraordinary skills in sports he also possessed a natural charisma. Frank believed that Randy could inspire and motivate the kids, and that proved to be the case."

On Saturday, June 27, 1988, the first Super Sports Saturday was held at Lakeshore's Wallace Recreation Center.

This was to become a regularly scheduled all-day sports camp for children with physical disabilities. With Randy Snow as the program's director, Super Sports Saturday also made use of coaching-and-mentor services provided by several other wheelchair athletes.

Children worked closely with their athlete role models as they ventured onto the basketball court or into the swimming pool of Lakeshore's well-equipped Wallace Recreation Center. With their mentors guiding them, the children learned swimming strokes or how to maneuver a sports wheelchair while at the same time mastering the basketball basics of dribbling, shooting, and passing.

In September 1988 interviews with the *Birmingham News*, supporters of this new children's program expressed their views.

Gratitude came from Sharon Kamber, the mother of a seven-year-old boy who had been among the first youngsters to participate in Lakeshore's Super Sports Saturday. Through the program, her son had discovered that just because he used a wheelchair didn't mean he had to miss out on the fun of sports and recreation. "If there wasn't a program like this, he wouldn't be able to participate in sports," the mother told the newspaper reporter. "My child doesn't get invited to other kids' houses because people don't want to be responsible for him."

From Ben Hunter, a 25-year-old wheelchair athlete who served as one of the role-model teachers for Super Sports Saturday, came a statement about one of the driving tenets in the program. His message was that children with disabilities could benefit from sports and recreation at a very young age: "You need to start with kids early!"

THE PROGRAM FOR children that Randy Snow initially headed was destined to grow and flourish and, as decades went by, to change for the better the lives of many children.

Randy was proud of the role he played in that program's formative years. As the years went by, he was well aware that this program injected enjoyment and motivation into the lives of many. Randy knew that Lakeshore's programs for kids with disabilities became key to rehabilitation for many a child.

However, in an interview for this book, Randy said it would be an omission if he did not state how Lakeshore also had given him a second chance.

In addition to the successes and high-level athletic medals that had come his way since he was injured at age 16, Randy said he also had problems with substance abuse. After being recruited to Lakeshore, he said the time came when he "fell off the wagon."

He said he was given a second chance by Mike Stephens and Frank Burns. "Rather than saying to me, 'You're not wanted,' Mike and Frank said, 'Randy, go take care of yourself. Here at Lakeshore we are about second chances, about rebuilding. That's what rehabilitation is.' " Randy said he availed himself of a rehabilitation program for his substance abuse and then resumed his work at Lakeshore.

"Lakeshore leaders demonstrated to me that same great Lakeshore spirit that Lakeshore has demonstrated to so many others," said Randy.

IN ADDITION TO Randy's contribution to the initiation of Lakeshore's sports and recreation programs for children, his star-power as a wheelchair athlete helped Lakeshore promote wheelchair sports to the community.

"At the time, Randy was a number-one ranked wheelchair tennis player," said Frank Burns, Lakeshore's athletic director during the time Randy was at Lakeshore. "One of the reasons for bringing Randy to Lakeshore was to position him to be a spokesperson for Lakeshore's Wheelchair Sports Program. We could promote Randy's athletic achievements, and Randy was a very good spokesperson."

Randy Snow's effectiveness as a spokesperson inspired financial contributions from the community that contributed to the building of tennis courts on Lakeshore's campus.

Mike Stephens often would say that he viewed Lakeshore as a kind of incubator that developed people. "Some stay a long time; some come and stay a brief time. But, whichever way it goes, I believe strongly that there's a two-way benefit. Those who come to Lakeshore benefit from their stay at Lakeshore, and, on the other side of the coin, Lakeshore benefits as well. It's all a part of passing along that Lakeshore spirit."

Randy was among those who came to Lakeshore, stayed awhile, and then went on to other opportunities. When Randy Snow left Lakeshore in the early 1990s, he left to further his sterling athletic career and then to write books and establish his own motivational-speaking company.

He continued to make news as a top achiever in three sports—tennis, wheelchair basketball, and wheelchair racing. He especially continued to win tennis match after tennis match—in all, ten US Open tennis singles titles. In the 1992 Summer Paralympics in Barcelona, Spain, he won gold medals in singles and doubles tennis.

In 1996, Randy was selected to receive the Paralympic torch from President Bill Clinton to launch the Atlanta Paralympic Games. In those games, the same high-achieving Randy Snow who became a seven-time member of the USA wheelchair basketball team also became a bronze-medalist in wheelchair basketball.

Randy became the first athlete in history to compete in three different summer Paralympic Games and earn medals in three different sports. And then he made history in 2004 as the first Paralympian to be inducted into the Olympic Hall of Fame.

As Randy went beyond that achievement to write books and establish his Texas-based motivational speaking company, he shared with many audiences his track record of converting adversity into success. To audiences ranging from children and youth to corporate executives, Randy would combine his natural charisma, his speaking ability, and his life experiences into a platform for inspiring others.

As is true of many who claim a national and international spotlight, Randy Snow often became a motivator to individuals he had never met. One he inspired from afar was a teenage boy in Illinois—Kevin Orr, who would grow up to succeed Randy in continuing the development of Lakeshore's sports and recreation programs for children.

There it was again, that Lakeshore *spirit*.

19

Kevin Orr, Role Model and Mentor for Kids

In the small town of Algonquin, Illinois, just outside Chicago, 16-year-old Kevin Orr was sound asleep when his mom rushed in to urge him to watch something on television.

"Kevin, wake up! Wheelchair racing is on television!"

On that day in the summer of 1984, Kevin's eyes soon were glued to the TV screen. He was mesmerized by the wheelchair racing he saw during the Summer Olympic Games in Los Angeles.

I can do that! I can do that!

Kevin spoke these words to himself as he watched athletes racing their sports wheelchairs with great speed and no inhibitions—to the applause and cheers of the audience.

In the years ahead, Kevin would become a high-level competitor in wheelchair racing and other wheelchair sports. He would win medals. Then one day he would be working as a staff member at Lakeshore, serving as a mentor for others—furthering the children's sports and recreation programs that Randy Snow had helped get started.

Unlike Randy, Kevin had not become disabled in an accident. Kevin Orr was born with a disability that limited the development and function of his leg muscles to the point he had to get around with crutches and braces. In his late teens he started using a wheelchair instead of the crutches "because getting around in a wheelchair was a lot easier."

The official term for Kevin's birth defect is *arthrogryposis.*

Despite his disability, Kevin grew up "with the belief that I could do things!" He had two able-bodied brothers who were very athletic—Kevin's twin brother and a second brother 14 months older. Kevin found ways to take part in athletic activities with his brothers and to participate in some community athletics as well. "Talk about role-modeling and mentoring!" said Kevin. "I had two brothers who did not have disabilities who served as my mentors."

When Kevin was in the sixth grade, he convinced his mom to let him take part in a community wrestling program, competing against able-bodied contenders. Kevin's able-bodied dad had been a standout high school wrestler, and Kevin wanted to follow in his dad's footsteps.

Kevin was relentlessly determined to compete just like any able-bodied kid. He made good grades and had aspirations of becoming a chemical engineer. He was an outgoing boy who was a social success. Since he was successful in other aspects of his life, why not in athletics?

Even after Kevin broke a leg while wrestling as a high school freshman, he returned to wrestling and made the varsity wrestling team, continuing to compete against able-bodied opponents. CNN spotlighted him as a disabled teenager who was "a gutsy kid." But, rather than feeling complimented by that praise, Kevin was bothered. He didn't want to be looked upon as a disabled kid who was succeeding; he wanted to be viewed as a kid who was succeeding.

So it was that Kevin's own goals already included athletic achievement by the time his mom summoned him at age 16 to the television set to watch that 1984 wheelchair racing exhibition. That televised wheelchair racing—the first Olympic track event ever held for wheelchair athletes—would alter the direction of young Kevin Orr's life.

"One of those wheelchair racers who inspired me that day was Randy Snow," said Kevin. "On that day, Randy won a silver medal for his wheelchair racing."

In addition to being inspired by the wheelchair racing that day, Kevin also saw the related television feature about a progressive collegiate wheelchair sports program in his own state, at the University of Illinois at Urbana-Champaign. This was a program headed by Dr. Brad Hedrick and Marty Morse, whose names were becoming synonymous with encouraging and coaching award-winning wheelchair athletes at

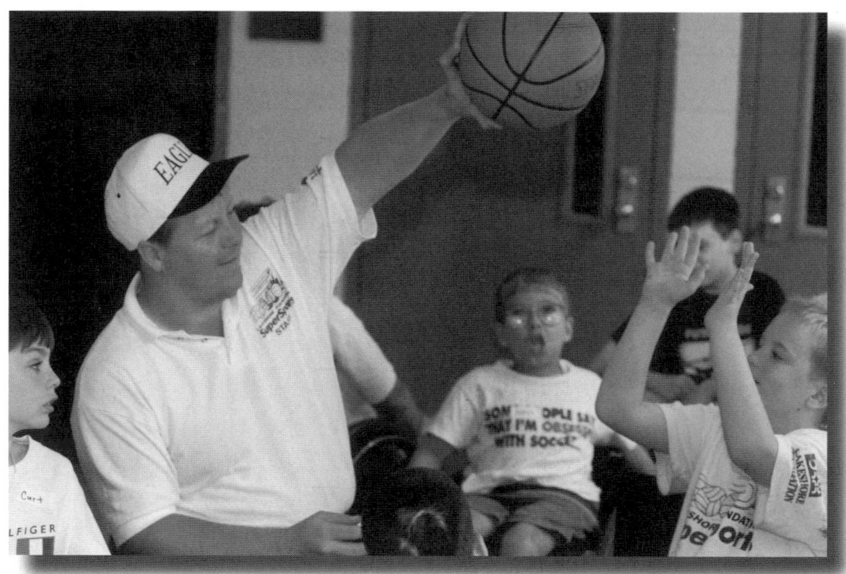

Former Lakeshore Foundation staffer Kevin Orr was a master at interacting with children with disabilities.

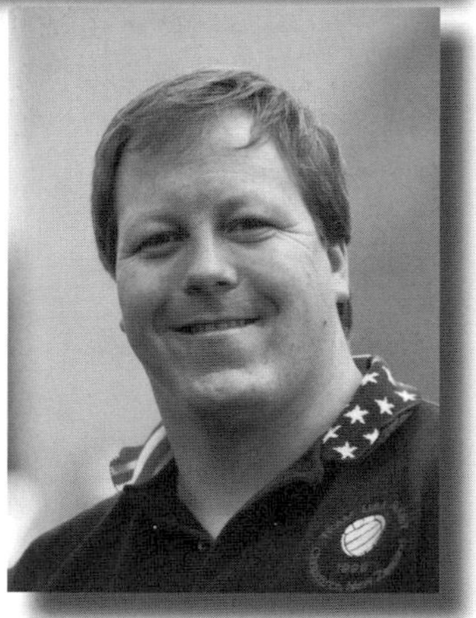

national and international levels. Hedrick was an expert wheelchair basketball player who would coach the women's gold-medal winning USA Paralympic wheelchair basketball team in 1988 and the men's bronze-medal winning Paralympic wheelchair basketball team in 1996; he was married to widely known wheelchair track star Sharon Hedrick, who had been coached by Morse.

Without having an appointment with anyone, Kevin made a trip to the University of Illinois. Director of Recreation and Athletics Dr. Brad Hedrick greeted Kevin warmly and spent 3½ hours with the teenager.

In the fall of 1986, Kevin enrolled at the University of Illinois. He said that being around Hedrick and Morse was like "having the influence of a Coach Bear Bryant at the University of Alabama."

Kevin the high school wrestler became Kevin the college wheelchair basketball player and teenage track star.

Even at his young age, Kevin recognized the significance of the mentoring that he was receiving from Hedrick and Morse. They not only molded Kevin's athletic career but also planted a seed that would change his mind about his career plans. "I had wanted to be a chemical engineer," he said. "After seeing the impact that Brad Hedrick had on so many people, including myself, I decided, 'I want to be like that! I want to be like him!' "

Kevin launched into a career as a coach and mentor in wheelchair sports. As a start, he earned a University of Illinois baccalaureate degree in leisure studies, with emphasis in therapeutic recreation. As he was earning that degree, he consistently excelled in wheelchair basketball and wheelchair racing.

During his years of playing wheelchair basketball at the University of Illinois, Kevin was a four-time national champion and was Most Valuable Player in his senior year.

As a wheelchair racer, Kevin held five national records between the ages of 18 and 21. In Paralympic trials in wheelchair racing, he even beat Randy Snow. And, under the international spotlight of the 1988 Paralympic Summer Games in Seoul, South Korea, as a member of Team USA, Kevin became a bronze-medal winner in both the 800-meter and 5000-meter track competition. He was only 20 years old.

IN WHEELCHAIR RACING, Kevin became a top contender not only on the standard track but also in road races in cities around the United States. He was an especially fierce hill climber, a knack which eventually brought him to Birmingham to compete in the hilly annual Vulcan Run.

That trip to Alabama also introduced him to Lakeshore. He already had heard of Lakeshore and of Lakeshore Foundation founder Michael Stephens. He had heard that Lakeshore had a commitment to developing something special with youth sports and recreation programs. Since Kevin already knew that he wanted to work with children's and teens' sports and recreation programs as a part of his career, he was intrigued.

Touring the campus, he was impressed with Lakeshore's Wallace Recreation Center with its well-equipped gym, swimming pool, and weight room "that were dedicated facilities for people with disabilities." Kevin was elated to find these topnotch facilities that the disabled didn't have to share with the able-bodied world. Kevin was well aware of how difficult it was for children and teens with disabilities to find space where they could enjoy recreation and athletics, because they often had to wait for "leftover time" when able-bodied people were not using the facilities. That wasn't true at Lakeshore; these facilities were there for them, whenever they wanted.

Kevin felt an instant connection with Lakeshore. He really wanted to help kids with disabilities. "I was like, 'Man, Lakeshore is the place where I could do that!' "

Kevin quickly connected with what he learned of Mike Stephens's vision. "I thought, 'What's here at Lakeshore all falls in line with what I've always wanted. And I believe the vision that Mr. Stephens has for Lakeshore comes from the fact he has been there and he knows what is needed!' I knew that Mr. Stephens had been a patient in rehabilitation, and that he thus understood the needs of someone in rehabilitation," said Kevin. "I knew that Mr. Stephens had been involved in wheelchair sports, that he had played and coached wheelchair basketball—that he knew what wheelchair sports could do for people with physical disabilities. Also I knew that Mr. Stephens was aware of the gaps, the things that were lacking in sports and recreation programs for people with physical disabilities."

As Kevin looked around, he could see that Lakeshore was leading the way in filling in some of those gaps. Years later, Kevin would still be talking about how he was impressed from the start with the Lakeshore vision and how his belief in that vision had continued to grow. He would say that, in his view, the firsthand insights of Mike Stephens were key to "both the success of Lakeshore Hospital and to the success of the Lakeshore Foundation that Mr. Stephens founded."

In being introduced in his early 20s to the Lakeshore campus, it was as though Kevin had been introduced to a new friend. The young man made it a point to get well acquainted.

He made use of the Wallace Recreation Center, doing some training, and hanging out and chatting with wheelchair athletes who used the center both for serious athletic training and for just plain fun.

Kevin also helped out with Super Sports Saturday activities at Lakeshore—interacting with the kids and with one of his own heroes—Randy Snow, the international star wheelchair athlete on Lakeshore's staff who directed the Super Sports Saturday program.

Soon Kevin had arranged an internship experience at Lakeshore. In August 1990, he moved to Birmingham.

When Kevin arrived at Lakeshore, he had a clear-cut goal: *Yep, I can go to Lakeshore, and there I can make a difference.*

Later he would look back and smile at his 22-year-old brashness. Yet, again, Kevin Orr was correct. He would stay at Lakeshore for 19 years. And he indeed would make a difference.

When Kevin started out as a Lakeshore intern, he immediately took on several roles. He was helping Randy Snow with Super Sports Saturday. He began coaching track and field. He also had a job in Lakeshore Hospital as a recreational therapist.

As Randy Snow left in the early 1990s to further his career as a medal-winning Paralympic athlete, Kevin found himself entrusted with increasing responsibilities in Lakeshore's sports and recreation programs for children and teens.

Before long Kevin embarked on a quad rugby project at the Lakeshore Foundation. At the time, quad rugby was a sport still in its early years in the United States. Rapidly drawing growing interest, quad rugby was a version of the fast-paced rugby sport that was played by athletes in wheelchairs—athletes who had impairment in both their upper and lower extremities.

Kevin had become excited about quad rugby in 1989, when he had observed the sport at the University of Illinois. He became a volunteer with the quad rugby team. In his usual ambitious style, he wanted to do a lot more. When he arrived at the Lakeshore Foundation, his goal was to establish and coach a quad rugby team. He would achieve that goal.

However, Kevin's first step at Lakeshore was with the kids. He had two early goals: One goal was to expand the number of opportunities through Super Sports Saturday. The other goal was to create a structured, disciplined approach with the kids—to teach them skills and to make them more independent.

Gradually the Super Sports Saturday opportunities expanded from being held a few times a year to being held around 24 times a year.

To make the kids more independent and skilled at a young age, Kevin had a tough-love approach. His mission was not to coddle the kids; his mission was to help them.

The "Kevin Way" of working with children and teens in Lakeshore's sports and recreation programs:

—Convincing parents to allow their disabled children to try when it came to sports and recreation. "The number one barrier in these kids reaching their potential was the over-protectiveness of their parents," said Kevin.

—Pushing for children with disabilities to achieve bowel and bladder control to make them more independent.

—Expecting more from the physically disabled children and teens, so they would expect more of themselves. To Kevin, a number-one priority in this area was to expect kids to push their own wheelchairs instead of others doing it for them.

—Teaching to young boys and girls who had physical disabilities the same basic athletic skills that able-bodied athletes learned. "If you're going to teach people, you're going to have to teach them the fundamental skills of whatever sports activity you're trying to teach," said Kevin. "You just need to teach them to do all these things that are necessary for them to strive for equality, because it's not going to be given to them."

Kevin was convinced that it was a "gift" from a mentor to a disabled child when that mentor set a high expectation for the child. He was further convinced that if a coach or trainer could set the stage for a child to achieve on a basketball or tennis court, or while racing around a track, or while practicing strokes in a swimming pool, this could raise the child's performance in school and in life.

As a mentor and coach for children with physical disabilities, Kevin considered himself a teacher. "People might say, 'Well, you're just involved in sports with these kids. You are not really a teacher,' " said Kevin. He strongly disagreed. "Well, yes, you are a teacher! You are a teacher with these kids in sports and recreation. They learn how to dribble a basketball and they taste success there, and that removes an 'I can't' attitude from their view of how they can dribble a basketball. So what you are doing as a teacher in sports and recreation is that you are converting more of their 'I can't attitudes' into 'I can attitudes' in terms of what they can do in life."

ONE OF KEVIN'S first major successes as a mentor and coach was with two little boys, Jeremy Campbell and Brad Lawler.

Jeremy was seven when Kevin first met him at a Super Sports Saturday event at Lakeshore. The boy had been born with spina bifida, in which some of the vertebrae overlying the spinal cord were not fully formed. On the day Kevin first saw him, young Jeremy was leaning on his crutches as he stood in the Wallace Recreation Center; his whole demeanor conveyed his burning desire to get involved in wheelchair sports.

"So we got Jeremy into a little wheelchair, and he just started buzzing around in it," said Kevin. "I was like, 'That's cool. He reminds me of someone.' " Kevin had been there; he understood what Jeremy was feeling.

It took a bit of explaining and demonstrating to convince Jeremy's mom, Cindy, that her son was capable of some of the athletic endeavors Kevin had in mind for him. Soon the mother began to see the potential; a spark of enthusiasm lit up for her, and she wanted more sports activity for her son. She asked Kevin if he would work with Jeremy not just at Super Sports Saturday events but also during some afternoon hours following school. Kevin agreed.

Brad Lawler, who also had spina bifida, became another of Kevin's

THIS PAGE, BELOW: *The humble beginnings of Lakeshore's quad rugby program—a bunch of guys in wheelchairs in a parking lot at Brookwood Mall.* **THIS PAGE, BOTTOM:** *The Lakeshore Wheelchair Football League, with sponsors, arose next.* **FACING PAGE, TOP:** *Today, the Lakeshore Foundation serves as the national governing body for wheelchair rugby; teams based at Lakeshore, like the one shown here in the Lakeshore fieldhouse, have won many national championships.* **FACING PAGE, BOTTOM:** *And, as Bryan Kirkland has just demonstrated to a hapless opponent, quad rugby ain't beanbag.*

LAKESHORE
Lakeshore Wheelchair Football
SPONSORED BY
AUTO PRIDE CAR WASH

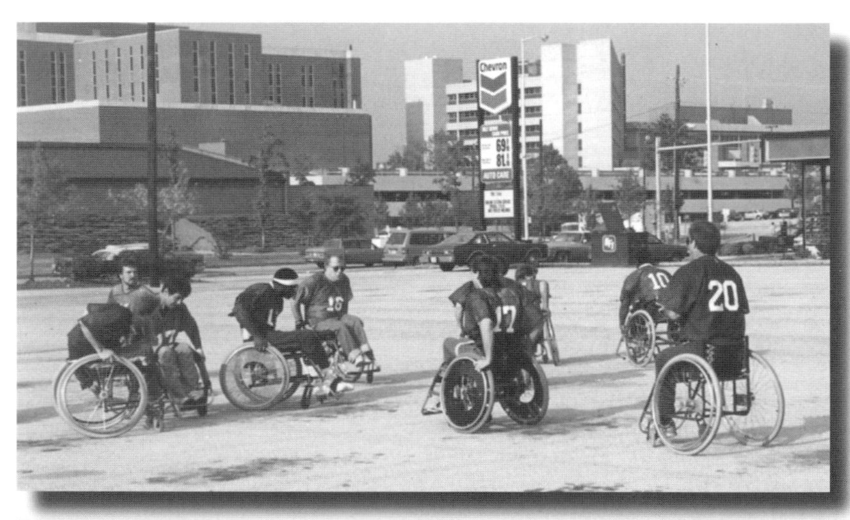

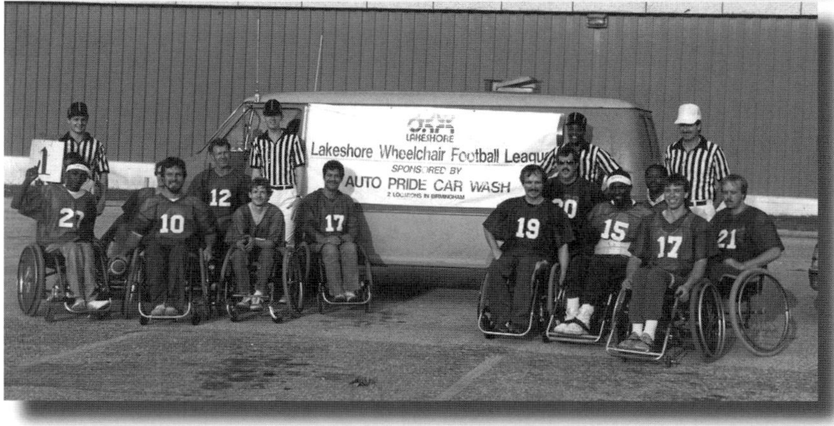

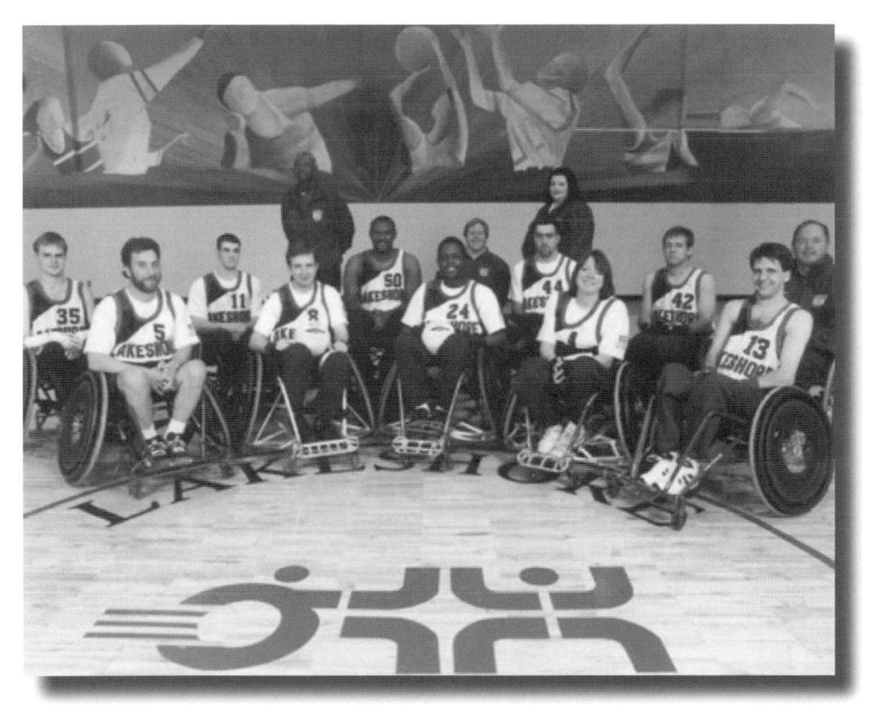

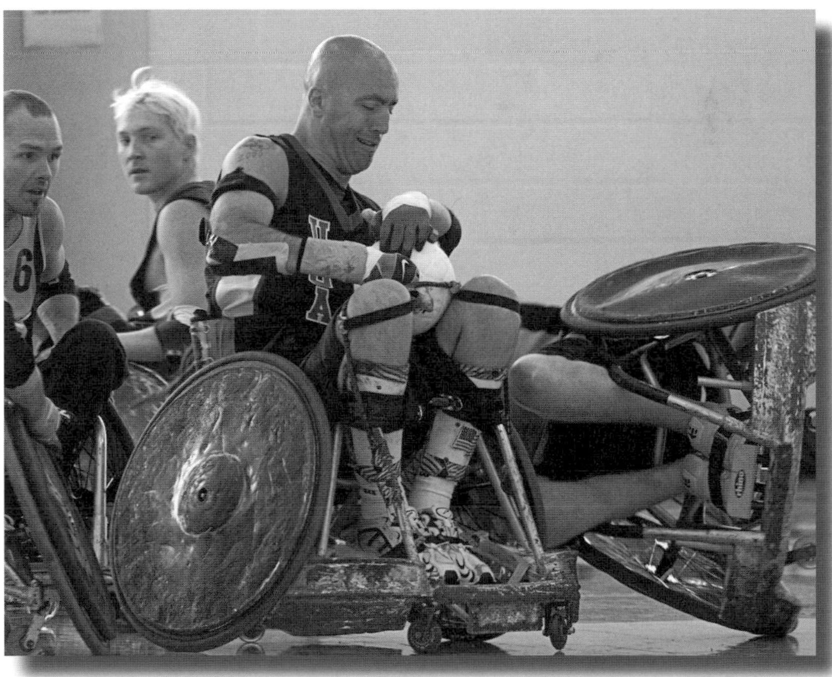

athletic students. Brad was nine years old when Kevin met him. Brad had first become exposed to Lakeshore through Super Sports Saturday under Randy Snow's direction.

After Kevin got to know Jeremy and Brad, both boys soon were coming to Lakeshore two to four days a week to learn athletic skills.

Kevin was serious. He pushed Jeremy and Brad like a coach would push kids in able-bodied sports. He focused on teaching skills, having the boys practice the same skills again and again: "I would work with Jeremy and Brad on basic mechanics of dribbling a basketball for 15 to 30 minutes—using both hands, left hand, right hand, behind the back, working on passing mechanics—set, pass, follow-through; set, pass, follow-through; until they were perfect. At first we didn't shoot baskets, we didn't play basketball, we didn't run up and down the court. We just worked on mechanics."

In Kevin's view, the boys were in training. And that included pushing laps—putting forth the rigorous physical effort to push themselves in their wheelchairs up and down hills on the Lakeshore campus. "I would yell at them, 'Push up the hill. Come on, you can do this!' " said Kevin.

Kevin said sometimes bystanders would give him harsh looks. "To some people I know that it seemed that what I was doing with these kids was cruel and unusual punishment," said Kevin. "But it was for the boys' own good."

As time went on, Kevin's life as a Lakeshore mentor and coach was becoming so all-encompassing that it was reducing his ability to maintain the intense training and travel schedule that went along with his being a competitive athlete. He found it difficult to devote the necessary hours to his increasingly demanding work at Lakeshore and still find the hours to train and compete.

Gradually Kevin was leaving behind the competition element in his life in order to devote full time to his career as a mentor and coach. In the meantime, his personal life was blossoming. Kevin would marry and become the father of two daughters.

Also, increasing administration and supervision duties were being added to Kevin's roles. He would become director of youth programs at Lakeshore. Then, as Lakeshore's adult and children's programs became more intermingled, he would become associate director of athletics for both the children and adult programs.

In one innovative program after another, Kevin was joining with other Lakeshore staff members to make a difference.

He had a role in many adult programs and none was more rewarding to him than the quad rugby team he started.

In the kids' arena, he would see Super Sports Saturday expanded and after-school programs added, along with a sports skills program in the summer, overnight sports camps, and a career-connections initiative. He would take pride in Lakeshore kids' programs in which he

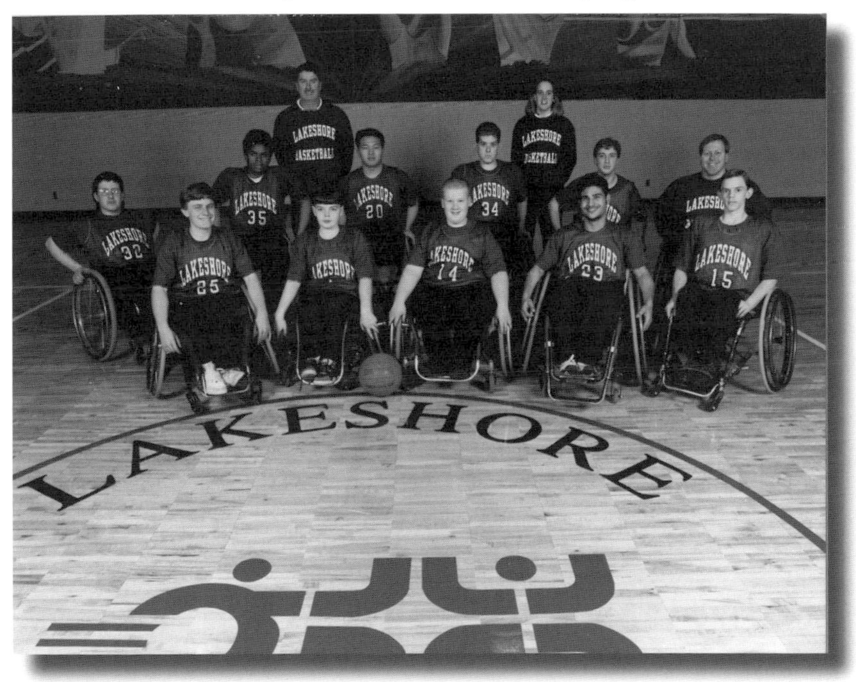

The original youth wheelchair basketball team in the new fieldhouse, with the Lakeshore logo painted on the court. That's Jeremy Campbell and Brad Lawler on the front row, second and third from the left, respectively. Coaches Frank Burns and Allison Morrow (Stephens) are standing at the back.

was not directly involved, such as a kids' outdoor adventure program and a learn-to-swim program. As additional staff joined Lakeshore, the athletic teams for kids would expand—Team Lakeshore in track and field, the Lakeshore Sharks prep league basketball team for kids 13 and under, and the Lakeshore Lakers high school basketball team. In years to come, Kevin would be among Lakeshore staffers taking a lead in Lakeshore's participation in a Paralympic Academy, aimed at the youth population with disabilities and also aimed at the general public—to spotlight Paralympic opportunities that were opening up for athletes with disabilities.

Meanwhile, Brad Lawler went on to college in Arizona. And Jeremy Campbell also went to college at the University of Wisconsin-Whitewater—on an athletic scholarship.

Not long after Jeremy arrived on the Wisconsin campus, there was a campus website feature in which some of the students were answering this question: "Who is your hero?"

Jeremy Campbell's answer was Kevin Orr.

In his website posting, Jeremy wrote that "Kevin told me that wheelchair basketball could be my ticket to getting a college education."

Kevin Orr—right once again.

20

Making a Difference for Each Child

In the eyes of Mike Stephens, the success of kids' sports and recreation programs at Lakeshore could be measured in how these programs were impacting each individual child who participated. The difference manifested itself in the improved quality of life for many a child and teenager in their present-day lives. The difference also manifested itself as an investment for many of these kids in their future lives.

"There's just no question that you can turn things around for the better for a physically disabled child by exposing that child to quality sports and recreation programs where the child can have fun, be active, and achieve," said Mike.

"Disabled kids exposed to these programs are no longer sitting on the sidelines watching able-bodied kids have all the fun. And once we get them off the sidelines and involve them in sports and recreation, we often see them get off the sidelines of life. Kids see what they can achieve in sports and recreation, and they begin to believe in themselves in terms of achieving in school, going on to college, and pursuing a career. It's like a snowball."

Sports and recreation can made a difference in the life of a child or teenager with a physical disability, regardless of how long he or she has been disabled, said Mike. However, the issues can be very different. There can be one set of issues for the kids who had physical disabilities from the time they were born. There can be still another set of issues when a child had lived a few years of life as an able-bodied person and then was stricken with an illness or injury that left behind a permanent disability.

For kids disabled since birth, one of the big issues can be over- protective parents, Mike noted. For parents who have never seen their disabled child participate in any structured sports or recreational activity, the idea can be scary. Parents can fear for their child's safety and wonder if it is a good idea to let him or her take part.

"Too, when it comes to birth defects, the parents' guilt element can come into play," Mike said, "Parents often blame themselves for a birth defect in their child. They might ask themselves questions that feed the guilt: 'Did my child's congenital physical disability happen because I drank something? Did it happen because I smoked? Did it happen because I have the wrong DNA?' If you already have parents who feel some level of guilt about their child's birth defect existing in the first place, then those parents can be taking extreme precautions to overprotect the child from birth going forward."

Mike said he could see a gradual lessening of these overprotective attitudes in parents as a positive spotlight began shining on recreation and athletic programs for physically disabled children—such as the programs at Lakeshore.

"Many parents saw what could be done for other children and they began to embrace these programs for their own children," he said.

At the same time, as sports and recreation programs for kids with disabilities were increasingly successful, professionals in the rehabilitation industry had to learn to deal with the opposite attitude in some parents. "We saw some impatient parents who expected these programs to bring about unattainable overnight success with their disabled kids," said Mike. "There has to be a balance."

MIKE NOTED THAT it is crushing for any able-bodied person, regardless of age, to have his or her world turned upside down by a permanently disabling illness or accident. To go from being able to walk and run to living life in a wheelchair can be overwhelming.

"For a child this can be particularly devastating. A kid lives the first few years of his or her life in the culture of the able-bodied; he runs and plays with his siblings and schoolmates. Then he incurs a physical disability that puts him on the sidelines. That's horrible for the child! He's old enough to remember when he was able-bodied but at the same time still awfully young to assimilate and make sense of the differences that have come into his culture, into his world."

In these cases, sports and recreation can help the child see that his life did not end when the physical disability presented itself—that exciting outlets and opportunities are still out there for him.

It's important to insert quality sports and recreation as soon as possible into the life of a child who has a physical disability, said Mike. When this happens, a child begins to have fun and perform and excel before he gets so much of the "I can't" view in his life.

"Sports and recreation can give a physically disabled child a positive view of how he fits into the overall 'puzzle' of the life in which he lives," said Mike. "In essence, we all live in a puzzle. Some pieces are easier to figure out than others. For children, sports and recreation can help them figure out the puzzle pieces of their lives—both the easier pieces and the more difficult pieces.

"If you are an able-bodied kid, you might have your problems with issues such as pimples or flunking a test, but you are not likely constantly struggling to figure out where you fit into the overall puzzle of 'normal' life. But if you are a disabled child, and you're held back because you're told you can't do this and you can't do that, you don't know where you fit. A disabled kid can easily say of his home life, 'Well, my brothers and sisters are all running around, and there I sit in the wheelchair, with nothing to do.' And he can easily say of his school life, 'When it comes recess time, I'm either sitting outside watching the other kids play, or I'm inside, watching them out the window.' This child can easily believe that he does not fit in anywhere. If you can take that same disabled child and put him in an environment of wheelchair sports and recreation, and he's out there participating, then he can begin to make better sense of the pieces of his own puzzle and where he fits in.

"He finally feels that he is beginning to know a place in the puzzle where he does fit—a good place, one that he can enjoy, and where he feels comfortable and also motivated. And this begins to give him a foundation of who and what he is—and, very important, it begins to give him a foundation of who and what he can become."

AS TIME WENT on with the Lakeshore Foundation sports and recreation programs for kids, Mike was aware that tremendous progress was being made. He knew about the growth of the programs, the phenomenal increase in the numbers of kids who participated. He knew the high level at which Lakeshore's young athletes were achieving—the impressive winning records that kids from Lakeshore were racking up in various sports. He also could see the rising numbers of kids who were coming to Lakeshore just to participate in fun recreational activities, with little or no aspirations for structured athletic competition.

At no time did the true meaning of all this come closer to home for Mike than one day in 2004 when he attended a career-day program for kids at Lakeshore.

On that day, a little five-year-old boy in a wheelchair caught Mike's eye. The boy handled his wheelchair like an expert, rolling it around Lakeshore's indoor track as he laughed and took part in all the exciting activity that was going on.

"And there running along beside the little boy in the wheelchair was his brother, an older able-bodied child around nine years old," said Mike. "You could just look at that able-bodied boy and know this had come to be a natural thing for him—running and playing alongside his brother in a wheelchair. Both of those boys had a common-ground place in the puzzle of life. The brother in a wheelchair was no longer an outsider. And the able-bodied brother felt comfortable in his disabled brother's world of sports and recreation."

Mike said he choked back tears that day. "I knew that what Lakeshore had started for kids back in the late 1980s was paying off."

Part V

Lakeshore Hospital Inspires a Company Called ReLife

21

Creating a Successful Rehabilitation System

Lakeshore's growth and success, and its ultimate reorganization, became the seed in the mid-1980s for Lakeshore Hospital to become the "flagship" facility for a rehabilitation company called ReLife, Inc.

Just as Lakeshore's development had been led by Michael E. Stephens, ReLife was Mike's brainchild. He pushed for the development of the company, and then he led it as president and CEO.

"In ReLife we moved to protect the referrals coming to the flagship hospital, by developing what we would call a hub-and-spoke network," said Mike. "We were driven by our feeling that the environment at Lakeshore and its subsidiaries would be further strengthened through this network. We also believed that through this network we could offer exceptional service to patients—bolstered by the years of experience we already had in rehabilitation and by ReLife's system of multilevel service that was not matched by our competitors."

ReLife was founded as a for-profit company because Mike felt he had little choice if he wanted to continue to lead a progressive, cost-effective rehabilitation operation.

"There was a trend in the 1980s for healthcare providers to specialize in rehabilitation," said Mike. "The companies set up as for-profits had an advantage over the not-for-profits such as Lakeshore—because the for-profits had access to investor capital and the not-for-profits did not."

As the move toward a for-profit structure was being contemplated, thoughtful consideration was given as to how Lakeshore Hospital would fit in. Lakeshore's board saw the hospital's mission as that of a community provider. Board members did not want to expand across state lines, operate a complex multilevel corporation, and have Lakeshore Hospital itself become a for-profit facility. Mike came to the hospital's board with an alternative plan: that Mike on his own would found ReLife as a for-profit company, and Lakeshore Hospital would remain a not-for-profit institution operating as a flagship hospital under the ReLife umbrella.

"I went forward on my own, and I'm glad I did," said Mike. There was considerable risk involved, including Mike's investment of his own money. "At the time, it was scary," he said.

By 1991, five years later, the ReLife network of facilities included:

—Both rehabilitation hospitals and outpatient facilities in Birmingham and Huntsville, Alabama; Macon, Georgia; Baton Rouge, Louisiana; and Chattanooga, Tennessee.

—A day treatment center in Birmingham and a skilled nursing facility scheduled to open soon in Fort Valley, Georgia.

—Rehabilitation units located in acute-care hospitals in Birmingham and Bessemer, Alabama; Nashville and Knoxville, Tennessee; and Kinston, North Carolina; with another soon to open in Charleston, South Carolina.

There were other elements as well. Examples included ReLife's two rehabilitation-equipment entities. Also, to ensure that a multilevel system was in place, ReLife would buy out several related entities—such as the Brown Schools, which specialized in brain injuries.

In 1991, Mike led ReLife to a highly successful public offering, setting the stage for even more phenomenal growth.

ReLife grew rapidly and generated high-quality results, as measured on several fronts. From a clinical perspective, ReLife's growth would bring model-program results in the treatment of rehabilitation patients. From a business perspective, the growth would bring ReLife recognition as a thriving enterprise. And, as measured by national media attention and special honors, Relife was a blue-ribbon standout.

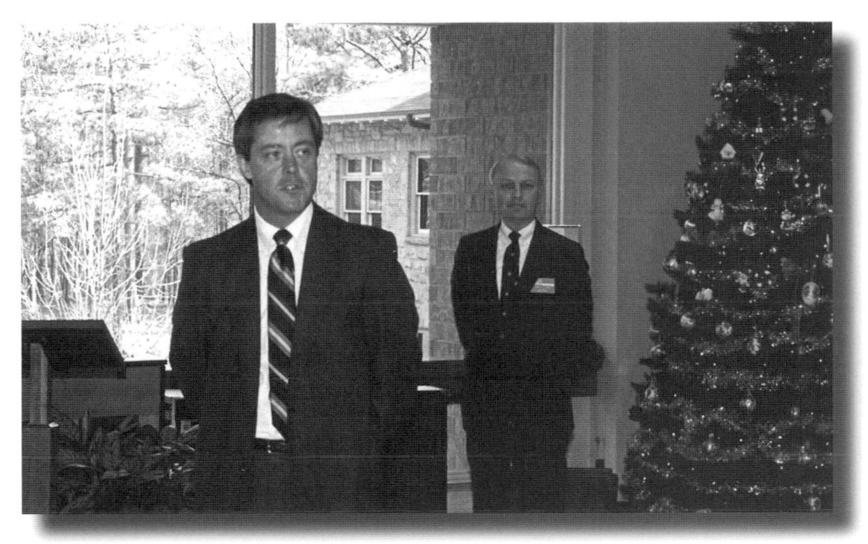

Mike Stephens speaking to ReLife employees about the mission and philosophies of the company's rehabilitation services. The occasion was a staff Christmas party.

THE NEEDS OF individual patients were the core of the ReLife mission. From the time the company was established, founder Michael E. Stephens based ReLife on two guiding lights—what he had learned personally as a rehabilitation patient, and what he and his staff had established for patients at Lakeshore Hospital.

ReLife's official organization year was 1986. However, Mike said its concepts were grounded in philosophies dating back to Lakeshore Hospital's beginnings in the 1970s.

"Lakeshore Hospital was the model for ReLife. As we developed and operated various types of facilities through ReLife, we offered some services beyond those that Lakeshore offered. Yet, no matter how far ReLife expanded services, the inspiration gained from Lakeshore Hospital continued to be the overriding spirit of how we touched and impacted people. That Lakeshore spirit was embedded in ReLife."

The concepts used in ReLife also were heavily driven by Mike's own personal experiences as someone who had sustained a severe physical injury and had gone through rehabilitation.

Those experiences were evident time and again in his writings during the years he led ReLife. Some of those writings were highlighted in his column entitled "Message from Michael" that appeared in ReLife's newsletter *Team Conference.*

"When I first came to Lakeshore, I had a dream, which came from a nightmare of going through rehabilitation without support," Mike wrote in 1992. "I prepared for my dream as much as possible with an education, but then I just started. It's interesting that when you take the first step, you know what the second step should be. And now that dream has resulted in the ReLife system we have today."

THE PERSONALIZED RELIFE approach was based on a comprehensive four-level package of services. All four levels were interrelated to ensure that the patient did not fall between the cracks at any stage in his or her rehabilitation. Often called the "hub-and-spoke" system by ReLife Leaders, the program consisted of (1) early intervention, (2) intermediate care, (3) community reentry, and (4) outpatient services.

ReLife's mission was based on being able to tailor the level of care to the needs of each patient and on being able to adapt and adjust treatment quickly as the patient's needs and situation changed.

In addition to the many facilities that ReLife operated directly, the company forged partnerships with acute-care hospitals and trauma centers to complete a circle of care.

If one byword drove Mike in his leadership of ReLife, it was "outcomes." Mike often said that ReLife was not driven by process, that it was not driven by competing with other rehabilitation companies, that it was not driven by doing battle with state and federal legislators, insurance companies, and healthcare providers. Instead, ReLife was driven by the goal of attaining set outcomes for each patient. He said that key measurements of ReLife's success were the outcomes produced in patients' lives.

In a 1990s speech to his peers in the rehabilitation industry, Mike stressed the importance of outcomes: "As long as you are looking at what's best for that patient outcome-wise, and I don't care if it's where you're dealing with the competition or where it's dealing with the legislators or where it's dealing with providers, once you go in and sell that outcome—it's the reason we are all here—you're going to be successful."

However, being successful was about to become more difficult because, Mike believes, the insurers got greedy. In the first few years of ReLife's existence, Mike felt that a system was in place that could keep patient needs front and center. But then the tide began to shift. The pressing issues had to do with increasingly strict limitations on how much insurers would pay for services rendered to rehabilitation patients. As the situation worsened, Mike had to question whether he even wanted to run a rehabilitation company.

By the early 1990s, ReLife was touching the lives of thousands of patients with its "tailored-services" approach. "I felt that ReLife had accomplished a turning point in healthcare," said Mike. "We actually were approaching each patient's case with a personal tailoring of his or her care based on the patient's needs and ReLife's projected outcomes in caring for the patient."

To reach this point and make it work with the insurance companies, ReLife had engaged actuarial firms to predict cost of care.

Mike gave an example of how the system worked: "We could actually call up an insurance company and say, 'We will take this patient. For X dollars in insurance reimbursement, we can take him and rehabilitate him, teach him how to drive, put him in an educational program such as a computer programming course, and make him employable.'

"There were other companies in the rehabilitation industry at that time that were placing patients in a regular rehab program and then just releasing them back into society. However, our ReLife system—which included crucial elements such as education—was designed to strengthen patients' ability not only to reenter society but to function productively. As we increased our patients' successes, we were contributing to society's financial picture as well as serving individual patients—by reducing patients' future hospital admissions and by keeping them off welfare rolls."

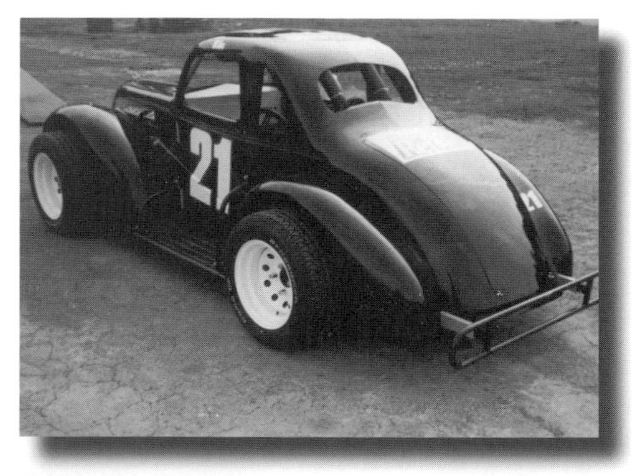

Below: *Mike Stephens watches production of a ReLife TV commercial.* **Right:** *ReLife's only other advertising was its logo on the back of a ⅝-scale Legends car that Mike raced.*

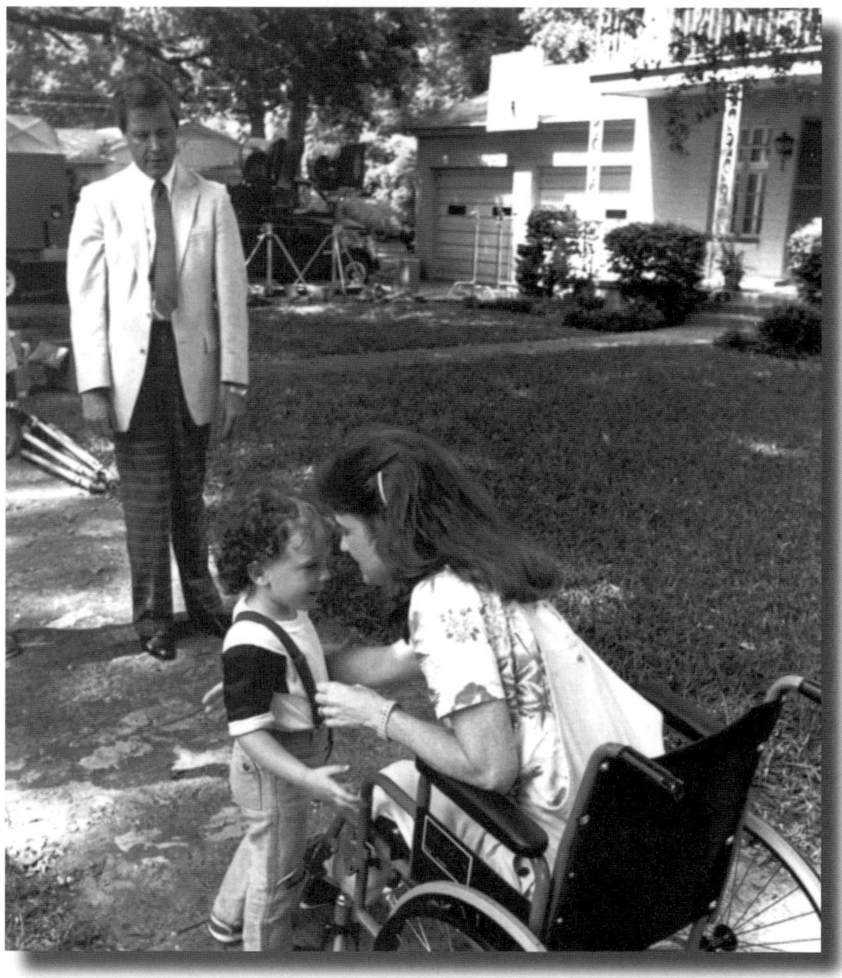

Through ReLife's tailored-services approach to treating each patient, Mike saw positive differences being made in the lives of even some very severe cases, such as patients who were quadriplegics and those who had suffered traumatic brain injuries.

"Based on information from our actuaries, and based on tests and other workup in which our ReLife staff had great expertise, we could negotiate with the insurers to arrange a total circle of care for a patient within our system," said Mike. "We had a place for each patient within our ReLife system, regardless of the individual route the patient took in progressing through the system."

Along the way with this individualized system, Mike's ongoing goal and theme, as always, consisted of "outcomes, outcomes, outcomes!"

THE RELIFE SYSTEM had tremendous benefits for the patient and his family, said Mike.

"Since ReLife had such an efficient network of facilities specializing in various services and spread out over a wide geographical area, we could provide the patient with (a) the type of service he needed at the level he needed, and (b) as close to the patient's home as possible.

"And, of the utmost importance, with our tailor-made services specifically to each patient's needs, we felt we could maximize the chances that each patient would recover to the extent that was possible for him."

Mike strongly believed the ReLife tailored-services approach also held benefits for the insurers.

"Since we were willing to take the progressive step of using actuarial models in computing costs, we were willing to take the uncertainty of cost predictions off the backs of the insurance companies," said Mike.

"We had devised a progressive system of ReLife care through which we had the willingness and the capability to combine our knowledge and expertise with the formulas of actuary models to predict such outcomes as whether a given patient would come out of a coma, and whether a given patient would walk again. We were willing, and capable, of making such predictions even for complex cases such as closed head injuries."

Those ReLife projections basically would take a given patient's case, predict how the patient would progress, match the care to those outcome goals, and then attach a cost for the services.

If the patient's recovery could be maximized, the insurance companies stood to gain for a long time to come, said Mike, because many patients would require less costly health services down the road.

WHILE THE INSURERS bought into ReLife's tailored system for a time, the tables began to turn.

"The insurers got greedy," said Mike. "They began to back off their support of ReLife's comprehensive treatment for each patient. Instead, they wanted to follow a limited pre-set program, regardless of whether the proposed program was a fit for the patient.

"Under the system that the insurers wanted, the insurers' idea was, for example, that we had a few weeks to teach a severely paralyzed person how to manage basic bowel and bladder, skin care, and how to transfer to and from a wheelchair. Then, as I saw it, after these basics were accomplished the insurance company was finished with what it would approve for that patient!"

Mike had suffered a paralyzing injury and had been a rehabilitation patient; he could identify with what a patient actually needed to become the best he or she could be. He knew how difficult it was to be in the patient's situation in the first place. And then insult and further damage could be added to initial injury when a patient's insurance company was limiting payment for vital services.

After several years of proudly running ReLife to serve patients, Mike now felt that insurers were tying his hands. His mind began to race with thoughts that were agonizing to him.

In my view, there are some rehab companies out there that are mainly focused on the company's bottom line rather than on the patient. I can't run a rehab company that takes that view.

If the insurance companies are going to force us to use a general system approach rather than an individually tailored approach to deal with all patients, how can we strive for the maximum outcome for each individual patient and really find out what a given patient can accomplish?

For example, if we apply this system approach to all paralyzed patients, with no regard to individualizing their care, how can we really assess which patients have the potential to walk again and which ones do not?

I can't help but think back to my own situation after I was injured. Following my injury and my stay in an acute-care hospital, if all I had received immediately afterward in rehab had been the basics of bladder and bowel management, skin care, and transfer in and out of a wheelchair, I would have never walked again. I mean, at that time nobody even hoped I would walk again. Thus, if I had received the bare minimum of rehabilitation services, in my view the low expectation for what I could achieve would have become a reality. I would not have received enough rehab services to have reached the point to find out what I actually could achieve, which for me thankfully turned out to be that I indeed walked again.

The reason I wanted to set up a rehabilitation company was to serve the patients. Now I feel these insurer-driven changes are placing ReLife in an environment that does not serve the patient the way I feel the patient should be served. With the way insurers' payments now are being viewed, it appears to me that the goal is much more to keep costs down than it is to provide the patients with the services they need.

Where ReLife is concerned, I don't understand the point of this. At ReLife we are achieving both our goals: We are focused on the patient as our mission, and also ReLife is a profitable business. I just strongly believe that profit should come as a by-product of the quality of service or product that a company is providing.

Since I have been in the position of being a rehabilitation patient, the very thought of having to participate in this changed environment digs at the core of my conscience. I simply cannot see myself at the helm of a company that can't place the patients' needs front and center.

22

A Merger for ReLife

After eight years of leading ReLife, Mike Stephens was in a frame of mind that a few years previously he could not have imagined. Frustrated by restrictions imposed by insurers, Mike was open to the idea of merging ReLife with another rehabilitation company.

"I realized the harsh reality that we had reached the point in which the insurance companies were dictating what had to be done for our patients rather than the patients' care being determined by the patients' needs and the recommendations of our rehabilitation teams," said Mike.

"When I saw that was how it was going to be—that the insurance companies were not going to permit individualized tailored care for the patients—then I knew I needed to get out of running a rehabilitation company," he said. "It wasn't that I had an attitude of 'Well, they won't do it my way, and thus I'm not going to play.' Instead, I had the feeling of 'If I can't serve the patient in the way that I think will serve him best, then I can't play this game.' "

In an interview a decade and a half later, Mike would reflect, "You know, there is no such thing anymore as tailor-made healthcare. I guess, in believing so strongly in that approach back in the 1980s and 1990s, I was a member of a dying breed."

Ironically, in the very time period when Mike Stephens became willing to consider selling ReLife, the company was enjoying tremendous success and was attracting strong, positive national media attention.

By this time, ReLife had gone through two successful public offerings. It was positioned to compete with larger and larger companies in the rehabilitation industry.

As it attracted one accolade after another, Relife won the prestigious Jemison Venture Award for Success. In a 1994 issue of *Forbes* magazine, in the "Up and Comers" section, Relife was listed among "Best Small Companies in America." In that same year, Relife appeared in a similar listing in *Business Week* magazine.

"ReLife was in a strong enough position that we could have gone out and bought another company rather than selling out to another company," said Mike. "But I told our ReLife board, with the climate in this industry headed the way it is, rehabilitation companies are going to be forced by the changing policies of insurers to provide reduced services to patients. Providing reduced services to patients is not what ReLife has stood for from the time it was established, and we should not be operating a company that's a part of such a strategy in the future."

As Mike decided he was ready to sell ReLife, the rehabilitation industry was ripe for merger deals. There were several rehabilitation companies on a fast track of expansion. Leading the pack were Pennsylvania-based Continental Medical Systems, Inc., and Alabama-based HealthSouth Corporation.

Since HealthSouth was headquartered in Birmingham, Alabama, as was ReLife, HealthSouth had a particular interest in ReLife—including a keen interest in ReLife's much-respected flagship, Birmingham-based Lakeshore Hospital.

In 1994, ReLife merged with HealthSouth.

By the time of the merger, ReLife had grown to include 46 rehabilitation facilities that spanned 12 states.

OUT OF THE merger with HealthSouth came an altered direction for two entities that carried the name "Lakeshore."

For Lakeshore Hospital, the merger meant that it would go forward, through a lease agreement, under the HealthSouth banner.

And for the Lakeshore Foundation, the merger became a phenomenal boost. In fact, the ReLife merger would help pave the way for a tremendous surge forward.

Meanwhile, Relife founder and Chairman/CEO Michael E. Stephens was being asked a provocative question by HealthSouth Corporation founder and Chairman/CEO Richard M. Scrushy.

"Mike, when we get this merger finalized between ReLife and HealthSouth, what role do you want with HealthSouth?" Scrushy asked during a conversation in 1994.

There was no hesitation to Mike's response.

"Richard, I don't want any role in HealthSouth," he said. "I want to focus on further development of the Lakeshore Foundation that I started back in the mid-1980s. Lakeshore Foundation is where my heart is."

THERE WERE THREE basic reasons why Mike turned down the offer of an executive role in HealthSouth—which was becoming considerably bigger after gaining access via merger to ReLife's multistate network of facilities.

One reason was that Mike did not believe that his philosophies about rehabilitation of physically disabled patients would match with HealthSouth's. "In my view at that time, HealthSouth subscribed to the 'widget' approach of taking care of patients, whereas I could not move away from my basic commitment to the 'tailor-made' approach," said Mike. "By the time I reluctantly gave in to the idea of ReLife merging with HealthSouth, I had faced the reality that insurance companies would no longer reimburse for the approach to which I was so committed. That realization played a big role in my decision that it was time to turn loose of ReLife. Now, since I had just gone through the painful process of making that decision—and it was painful—why would I want to become an executive in a company that would be using an approach I didn't subscribe to in the first place?"

A second reason that Mike did not want to become a HealthSouth executive was that he believed rehabilitation companies were facing a rough road.

"By the mid-1990s, the rapidly changing landscape in healthcare delivery and the rigid attitudes of the third-party payers were closing in financially on the rehabilitation companies—even if the companies did subscribe to what I call the 'system approach' that payers favored," said Mike. "In my last months as chairman/CEO of ReLife I saw that encroachment and erosion escalate. If you're running a for-profit rehabilitation company, and you have a responsibility to turn a profit for the investors, you're headed for real problems if your reimbursement base continues to decline. From where I was sitting, I could see a growing risk that in the not-too-distant future the whole system could implode. To me it looked like a snowball headed to hell, and that was another reason why I wanted out of the rehabilitation business."

(And indeed the rehabilitation industry did evolve, because of limited reimbursement, to the point of fragmentation—including nursing home rehabilitation, hospital step-down units, and freestanding rehabilitation hospitals.)

Mike's third reason for not wanting an executive position with HealthSouth simply had to do with what he told Richard Scrushy: He wanted to focus his attention on Lakeshore Foundation, because he believed the one-decade-old Foundation could accomplish even greater things to change many lives for the better.

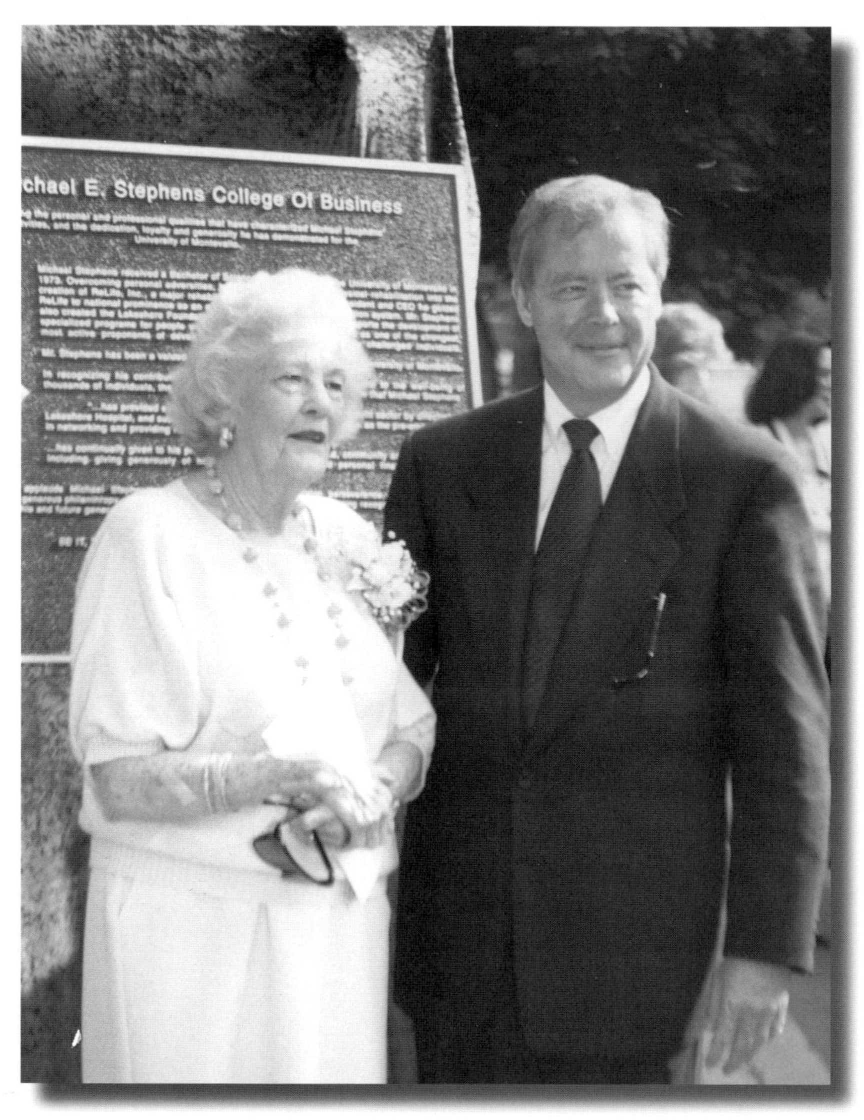

Things change. The former bad boy of the University of Montevallo returned to school, applied himself, graduated, realized his dream of becoming a hospital administrator, then succeeded beyond his imagination as a healthcare entrepreneur. Today, his alma mater honors him with the Michael E. Stephens College of Business. He is shown here at its 1997 dedication, with his mother, Gee Gee Stephens.

Part VI

Milestones for Lakeshore Foundation

23

Giant Leaps for Lakeshore Foundation

What happened with the Lakeshore Foundation in the mid-1990s would play out almost like a fairy tale. But it was no fairy tale; it was very much a true-to-life saga.

When the dust had settled by the end of 1994, there would be no doubt that the formerly tiny Lakeshore Foundation had grown up to be the "Big Man on Campus."

Even though the major developments in this chain of events would take place in 1994, groundwork already had been laid by a series of Foundation-related developments in the years leading up to 1994. Several years previously, Lakeshore Hospital had given Lakeshore Foundation an endowment of $1 million, and some of those resources were used to hire an original Foundation staff of three. Also, during a 1990 retreat held by the boards that oversaw both Lakeshore Hospital and Lakeshore Foundation, plans had been explored for the future of the Foundation. During the retreat, board members had taken a close look at the Foundation's strengths, weaknesses, and opportunities, as well as obstacles to the Foundation's future.

This detailed planning for the Foundation's future was evidence of the faith that board members had in the successful programs of sports and recreation that the Foundation already was providing with limited resources. The 1990 board retreat was the beginning of stepped-up program development by Lakeshore Foundation and also the beginning of increased board-member involvement in the Foundation's future.

Then came the Lakeshore Foundation's banner year of 1994—when two developments took place that would change the Foundation forever. The first was a massive restructuring of Lakeshore Foundation. Then, within a few months, there was the ReLife/HealthSouth merger.

When the restructuring took place, all of the assets of Lakeshore's holding company were transferred to the Lakeshore Foundation. Up until that point, the Foundation had been a small player on the Lakeshore campus and Lakeshore Hospital had been the "Big Daddy." Then, in 1994, the old legal structures were dissolved and were replaced by a new Foundation that became the parent not-for-profit entity.

Just before the 1994 restructuring, the Foundation had assets of $1.1 million. At the end of the restructuring, the Foundation had assets that included the 45-acre tract of land comprising the Lakeshore campus and all buildings on campus, including the hospital buildings. The Foundation was now the landlord of the campus, and anyone leasing space in any of those buildings would pay rent to the Foundation. The Foundation also became the owner of the Certificate of Need to operate the 100-bed Lakeshore Hospital. In terms of oversight, the Lakeshore Hospital and Lakeshore Foundation boards were merged.

Then, a few months later, Lakeshore Foundation grew significantly financially stronger due to the merger between ReLife and HealthSouth. Some $15 million came into the Foundation coffers as a result of ReLife stock that was held by the Foundation. Another $10 million came to the Foundation as a result of an up-front payment for an agreement that HealthSouth made to lease buildings housing the former Lakeshore Hospital—a hospital that HealthSouth now would operate.

All in all, at the end of 1994, Lakeshore Foundation had some $60 million in cash and assets. For the first time since Mike Stephens had conceived the vision for the Foundation in late 1984, it had the resources to run world-class sports and recreation programs for those with physical disabilities.

And, as the Foundation went forward following the ReLife/HealthSouth merger, Mike Stephens had a front-row seat in his role as a member of the board that oversaw the Lakeshore Foundation.

At the core of Mike's enthusiasm for Lakeshore Foundation was the opportunity to focus on the mind and the spirit of an individual with physical disabilities.

"During my years working in the rehabilitation field, and before that as a rehab patient, it had occurred to me time and again that the whole rehabilitation process got so caught up in dealing with the patient's body—his physical being—that often there was too little attention given to the patient's mental and emotional state," said Mike.

"You know, if you can put more emphasis on the mind of a physically disabled individual—attention aimed at improving this person's attitude, his enthusiasm and zest for life, his motivation, his belief in himself, his determination—then that can go a long, long way in improving his future. By the time Lakeshore Foundation had a tremendous opportunity to expand in the wake of the ReLife/HealthSouth merger, I already had seen years of evidence as to what Lakeshore's programs in sports and recreation could do to improve the mind and the spirit. Beginning in the mid-1990s at Lakeshore Foundation, we had a great opportunity to expand our sports and recreation programs in far-reaching ways never before possible for us. As a Foundation board member, I was excited to take part in that process."

So it was that in 1994 Mike's mind was filled with reasons why he felt so gratified that Lakeshore Foundation would reap significant financial benefits from the merger of ReLife with HealthSouth.

It has been important to me that Lakeshore Foundation benefit on a long-term basis from what ReLife has accomplished. Somehow that's only fitting. It was the spirit and patient-care model of Lakeshore Hospital that provided an inspiration for ReLife. It was Lakeshore Hospital that provided the umbrella under which Lakeshore Foundation operated in its early years. Now, as the ReLife/HealthSouth merger takes place, the not-for-profit Lakeshore Hospital as we knew it is disappearing and will be replaced by a for-profit facility operated by HealthSouth. Yet, the not-for-profit Lakeshore Foundation continues to survive and thrive and serve its community, carrying forward the same spirit that was embodied in the Lakeshore Hospital that in the 1970s was born in buildings once occupied by an old tuberculosis sanatorium.

In future years, Mike would also recall his 1994 mindset that related to the concept of "winners." Those thoughts were capsuled in what went through Mike's mind in the form of his own private, unspoken message to HealthSouth CEO Richard Scrushy:

Okay, Richard, through the merger of the network of ReLife facilities into HealthSouth, you have won a battle. But, in this current difficult healthcare environment, there's not just a battle under way; there's a war! And the objective of the war is to survive and maintain excellence. With this merger between ReLife and HealthSouth, there will be a win-win, a survival on more than one front. HealthSouth will survive in a new environment, that will include the addition of ReLife facilities and a new HeathSouth presence on the Lakeshore campus. And, with the help of revenues generated by this merger, Lakeshore Foundation will gain an unprecedented strong base to continue and expand its programs—to carry forward with the Foundation's spirit of serving the physically disabled through sports and recreation.

24

Jeff Underwood Takes on a Leadership Role

The first employee hired specifically to work fulltime for the fledgling Lakeshore Foundation had a well-rounded resume when he was hired in 1991 as executive director.

"I came to my position at Lakeshore Foundation in a sort of roundabout way," said Jeff Underwood. "I had some governmental experience. I had academic medical center experience. And I had a little political experience." Along the way, he had come to know the Birmingham area community well.

It was a good professional background for his role as the Foundation's president. Later, in the midst of the restructuring and subsequent growth in the mid-1990s, his title would convert to president and CEO of the Lakeshore Foundation.

During his undergraduate college years at the University of Alabama, Jeff majored in economics, with emphasis on municipal government, urban planning, and regional development.

He first put his urban-planning studies to work in the planning department of the City of Montgomery. Then—after earning a graduate degree in public administration from Auburn University in Montgomery—he returned to the Birmingham area where he had grown up, working in Jefferson County's new Office of Planning and Community Development.

In the course of his work in Jefferson County, Jeff came to know longtime elected official Ben Erdreich, who served as a Jefferson County commissioner before being elected to Congress from Alabama's Birmingham-based Sixth District. In the early 1980s, Erdreich recruited

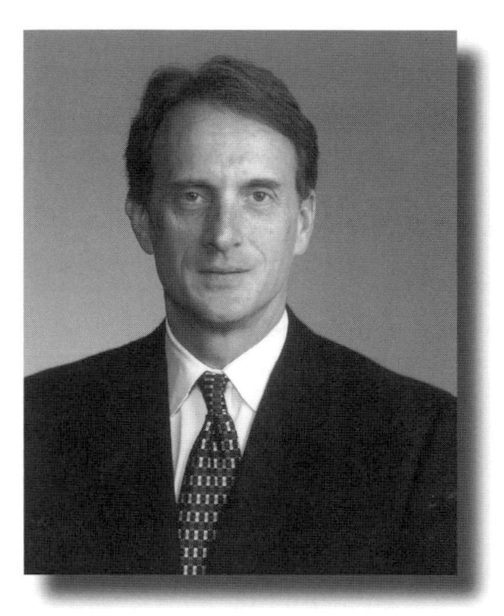

Jeff Underwood.

young Jeff Underwood to come to Washington and work for him as a legislative assistant.

From his position in Washington beginning in 1983, Jeff had a glimpse from afar of the Birmingham-area community. "I was involved in a lot of correspondence for Congressman Erdreich—keeping in touch with the people back home," said Jeff. "It was an exciting period."

After his stint in Washington, Jeff again returned home to Birmingham to take a position as director of community affairs for the Comprehensive Cancer Center at the University of Alabama at Birmingham (UAB). In that position, he was helping to expand community awareness of the Cancer Center.

Soon, in addition to his UAB job, Jeff took on a role in local government. In 1986, he ran for and was elected to the city council of Homewood, his hometown, the small suburb located just south of Birmingham. Jeff was following in the footsteps of his dad, Ferrell Underwood, who also had served on the Homewood City Council. In 1990, Jeff became the council president.

The early 1990s also brought Jeff the opportunity to serve as an elected official at the state level. When a state senator from Jeff's district, Jim Bennett, became Alabama's Secretary of State, Jeff ran for and won Bennett's unexpired term. That gave him a couple of years of experience in the Alabama Legislature. It was a rewarding experience, he said, and he learned from it. "I gained a firsthand close-up inside working knowledge of state government—how the process works," he said.

WHEN JEFF WAS invited to interview for the position of executive director of Lakeshore Foundation, he felt drawn by the possibility of going to work for a small foundation that had a big purpose. The more he learned about the Lakeshore Foundation, the more he admired this organization that already was changing lives, and that had the potential to grow and change many more.

Since Jeff had grown up in Homewood, where the Lakeshore campus is located, he could recall when it was a tuberculosis sanatorium. "As a kid growing up in Homewood, I saw the TB sanatorium as a place that had a real aura of mystery to it, because outsiders really weren't allowed on the property," he said.

Jeff could appreciate the stark contrast between the use of the 45-acre site for a TB sanatorium and its later use as the home of Lakeshore Hospital and Lakeshore Rehabilitation Facility, and later the Lakeshore Foundation.

When it became official in July 1991 that Jeff had the job as Foundation executive director, his first office was in one of the historic stone buildings that had formed the center of the old Tuberculosis Sanatorium campus and then later was at the center of the Lakeshore rehab campus.

AS AN ABLE-BODIED individual who became executive director of a foundation dedicated to the needs of the physically disabled, Jeff was introduced to a whole new culture when he came to Lakeshore.

He said he was amazed at the drive, determination, and positive attitudes of individuals he met who had severe physical disabilities—including paralysis, debilitating head injuries, and loss of limbs.

"I heard from several individuals who had suffered extensive injuries in accidents who actually said their lives had become better since they had become disabled," said Jeff, explaining that they told him they had pushed themselves harder and had achieved more since being motivated by their disabilities.

The father of two daughters, Jeff said he was personally inspired by the commitment he saw in parents of physically disabled children—children who had been disabled all their lives due to birth defects or who had incurred disability early in life as a result of injury or illness. "I met parents who lived a considerable distance from the Birmingham area who would travel two to three hours each way, as much as three times a week, to bring their kids to take part in programs sponsored by the Lakeshore Foundation," said Jeff. "I found myself going, 'Wow!' "

As executive director, Jeff was charged with managing a foundation that was growing by leaps and bounds.

Being a part of such an organization brought a special satisfaction, said Jeff. As time went by, and as the staff grew, Jeff said it was easy for him to see why so many people—both able-bodied and disabled—wanted to work at Lakeshore.

"The Lakeshore Foundation is a place where every day you can see the value in what you are doing," said Jeff, explaining that every day lives are being changed for the better at Lakeshore. "When you can see every day that your work is reflected positively in the lives of the people you serve, that's a wonderful thing. Lakeshore Foundation is a place where you can make a difference. That's what we do at Lakeshore Foundation; every day, every single day, we make a difference."

As Lakeshore Foundation recruited more and more staff members,

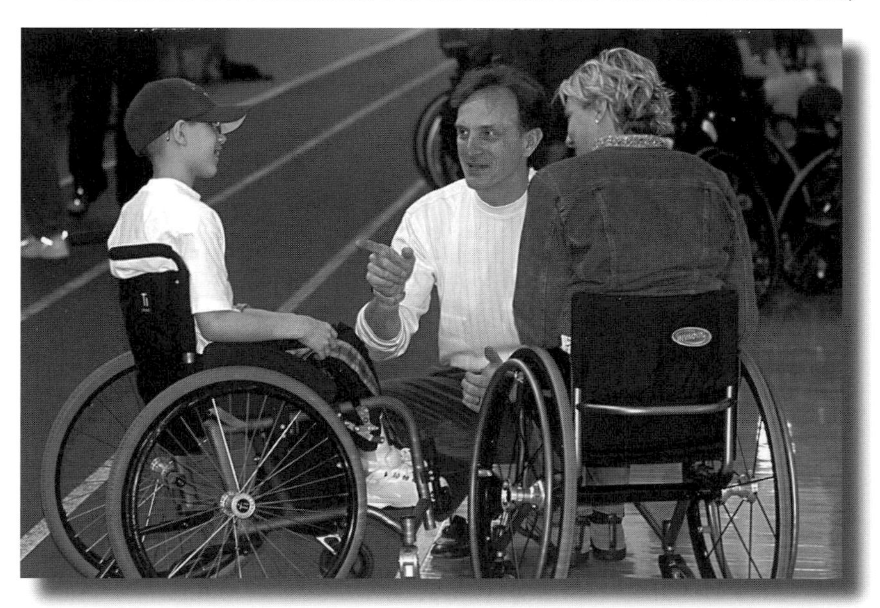

As an able-bodied director of a foundation dedicated to those with physical disabilities, Jeff was introduced to a whole new culture.

Jeff was impressed both with the credentials and the caring nature of those who came to work for the Foundation.

By 2011, the Lakeshore Foundation staff numbered around 100 full-time and part-time workers.

In keeping with the Foundation's focus as a facility for sports, recreation, and fitness, staff jobs included recreation specialists, exercise physiologists, personal trainers, aquatic specialists, coaches, and lifeguards. Lakeshore Foundation's respected international reputation helped the Foundation attract employees who had strong backgrounds in both education and experience.

"Something that really has impressed and touched me about our staff as a whole is that there is a spirit among them to push our clients to push themselves," said Jeff.

"Staff members are very aware that we see many physically disabled individuals come to the Foundation for services who in the past have been exposed to environments of low expectations. Because these individuals have disabilities—in many cases, severe disabilities—often they have not been setting high goals for themselves and, in addition, others have not been setting high goals for them. However, our Lakeshore Foundation staff members do set high goals for those they serve, and they want those they serve to set high goals for themselves. Our staff members are often hard to please; they are not satisfied with the status quo. They don't buy into the notion that just because individuals have disabilities they can't achieve."

In his role as Lakeshore Foundation president, Jeff saw ongoing examples of Foundation staff making a difference by pushing the Foundation's clients. He saw the Foundation aquatic instructor teaching the basics and the joys of swimming to a child who had been diagnosed with cerebral palsy at birth. He saw the Foundation coach helping a paralyzed person learn sports skills. He saw the exercise physiologist designing a tailored program to help a stroke victim to regain strength. He saw the personal trainer leading strenuous workouts for adults and kids on Lakeshore Foundation's sports teams and also directing specifically designed conditioning sessions for Paralympic and Olympic hopefuls who came from around the nation. He saw the recreation therapist showing disabled children and adults what it was like just to have fun getting involved in activities in the fieldhouse, pool, and outdoors.

A driving force behind the Foundation staff's pushing of clients to get involved, have fun, and achieve was that the staff cared so much, said Jeff. "Our staff members realize that Lakeshore Foundation is unique, that the Foundation has services designed to benefit the physically disabled that our clients are not able to find anywhere else. And the staff wants our clients to benefit as much as possible from those Foundation services. Actually, our staff members draw their inspiration from those they serve—in seeing Lakeshore Foundation's clients improve, do more, and just get better and better!"

IN SERVING AS president of a foundation that steadily grew in productivity, and also grew in stature around the world, Jeff Underwood found opportunities coming his way to take on leadership roles at high levels.

At the Olympic/Paralympic Games in Beijing, China, Jeff held the distinct honor of serving as "Chef de Mission" for the U.S. Paralympic Team—a role that placed him high in leadership for the United States' entire select group of Paralympic contenders who were competing in various athletic events in Beijing. This role for Jeff both paralleled and mirrored the heights that Lakeshore Foundation had reached as a recognized model for Paralympic training, the Foundation having been named as an official Olympic/Paralympic training site of the United States Olympic Commission (USOC).

Then Jeff served on the U.S. Paralympic Advisory Committee.

With Lakeshore Foundation also rendering more and more widely recognized service at local and state levels, Jeff took on additional leadership roles on home ground. For example, he was selected to serve a year's stint in Leadership Alabama.

As these opportunities and honors came his way, Jeff made it a point of saying they were a reflection of what Lakeshore Foundation was achieving, through the dedication of its staff and its board of directors.

He said he learned every day—from the Foundation's staff members, and from its board members. And he said that every day he felt pride in Lakeshore Foundation.

"It makes me incredibly proud of Lakeshore Foundation when I hear officials of the USOC speak of Lakeshore Foundation as a leader in the Paralympic movement," said Jeff.

"It also makes me very proud of Lakeshore Foundation when we have distinguished individuals from around the world who come to visit, in order to learn more about the Foundation's progressive programs and how they work." Jeff cited an example of five Washington, D.C., visitors who represented the office of the chiefs of service of the four branches of the United States armed forces—the Joint Chiefs of Staff. Drawn to Lakeshore Foundation to learn more about the Foundation's growing programs of sports, recreation, and fitness for injured military personnel, this delegation of visitors was led by Colonel David W. Sutherland, a special assistant to Admiral Michael G. Mullen, chairman of the Joint Chiefs of Staff.

In 1991, when Jeff was getting ready to leave UAB to take the job with the Lakeshore Foundation, he received somewhat of a warning from a fellow employee at UAB who was aware of the visionary, always-striving-for-excellence reputation of Michael E. Stephens—who had led Lakeshore Hospital as executive director, had become the founder of the Lakeshore Foundation, and then had become founder and chairman/CEO of ReLife, Inc.

Mike Stephens had the reputation for uncompromising high standards when it came to ministering to the needs of those with physical disabilities. He had the reputation for showing little to no patience with those who came up short in achieving quality and addressing needs when providing services for the physically disabled.

Jeff said he appreciated the alert and wouldn't forget it.

At that particular time, Mike was heading Relife and Lakeshore Hospital was the flagship hospital in the multistate ReLife system of hospitals, clinics, and various other rehabilitation facilities to serve the physically disabled. At the Lakeshore Foundation, where Jeff Underwood would function as executive director and later president, it was Mike Stephens who was founder of the Foundation and who, from its beginning, had defined the core vision for the Foundation's mission.

At the same time, Jeff said his UAB colleague's comment about Mike also gave him a reassuring sense that he was about to go to work in a high-quality setting where there indeed were high expectations and far-reaching goals for achievement. "Because of what was said to me, I got this feeling that very serious goals existed on the Lakeshore campus, along with a very serious sense of responsibility and accountability."

As Lakeshore Foundation grew and Jeff's role evolved, he would have increasing opportunity to get an up-close view of Mike Stephens's vision and passion for Lakeshore Foundation and what had been accomplished as a result.

Jeff would come to know Mike first as founder/chairman/CEO of ReLife. In later years, he would come to know him as a Lakeshore Foundation board member who was generous in his support of the Foundation.

There would be many times when Jeff would be working side-by-side with Mike in helping the Foundation to stretch its wings toward even higher goals—goals that had not even been dreamed a decade previously. That would include Mike and Jeff journeying together to Salt Lake City, Utah, along with then-Foundation President William P. "Bill" Acker III, to successfully push for Lakeshore Foundation to be designated, in 2003, as one of the USOC's small number of very carefully selected Olympic/Paralympic training sites.

In the course of his interaction with Lakeshore Foundation and Mike Stephens, Jeff developed a clear picture of, and a high respect for, the tremendous ongoing impact Mike had on Lakeshore Foundation and its success.

Jeff said that his view about the impact Mike Stephens had on Lakeshore Foundation could be summed up in one sentence.

I don't think there would be a Lakeshore Foundation today if there had not been Mike Stephens!

Jeff noted that as Lakeshore Foundation had developed its international reputation for sports, recreation, and fitness for the physically disabled, groups from far and near had approached the Foundation for advice, wanting to know, "How do we build a facility like Lakeshore Foundation?"

He said he told these groups that there were various ways to approach the founding and developing of a facility with a mission similar to the Lakeshore Foundation. However, Jeff said he would tell them that he was convinced the main key to Lakeshore Foundation's success has been having "a champion."

"Lakeshore Foundation's champion has been and continues to be Mike Stephens," Jeff said in 2011. "Lakeshore Foundation's champion is a man who has awakened morning after morning with the Lakeshore mission as a priority. He is someone who has understood Lakeshore Foundation's programs instinctively. He is someone who knows why Lakeshore Foundation's programs are life-transforming. All those things are true of Mike Stephens, the champion of Lakeshore Foundation."

Jeff said the core part of the Foundation's mission continued to be based on filling gaps that Mike had seen back in the 1970s and 1980s when he was executive director of Lakeshore Hospital: "Mike saw the need for sports, recreation, and fitness programs for the physically disabled as he headed a rehabilitation hospital where disabled patients were being admitted and readmitted for health problems such as severe decubitus ulcers—often because they were sitting around in their wheelchairs day after day with nothing to keep them occupied!"

From the mid-1990s forward, as Lakeshore Foundation attained increasing stature as a prototype facility for sports, recreation, and fitness programs for the physically disabled, Mike Stephens was serving on the board of directors that guided the Foundation. In that role, Mike visited the Foundation often, for meetings and special events. During many of those visits, Jeff said it had touched his heart to see how Mike took the time and interest to interact on a personal level with clients served by the Foundation.

Jeff said he had observed this interaction firsthand—when Mike would pause to have informal conversations with Foundation clients.

"I have seen Mike approach some of the Foundation's clients while they were sitting in their wheelchairs at our entrance, waiting for the bus to transport them back home," said Jeff. "I've seen him go up to them and just start talking to them—about themselves and their experiences at Lakeshore Foundation. When Mike does this, he is very low-key. He doesn't go up and say, 'I'm Mike Stephens, the guy who founded this place and a current board member.' He just says, 'Hi, I'm Mike Stephens.' More often than not, these individuals have no idea about the critically important roles Mike has held and continues to hold, the great contributions he has made and continues to make, at Lakeshore Foundation."

These impromptu conversations often would result in Mike's taking follow-up actions to pave the way for expanded Lakeshore Foundation opportunities for Lakeshore Foundation clients he had met. "For example, sometimes I will receive a phone call from Mike, or he will place calls to various members of our staff," said Jeff. "In these phone calls, typically Mike will be telling us something to this effect: 'Hey, I met a guy today who might need some help with a scholarship in order to afford to participate in some of the Foundation's programs. I don't want to see someone who could benefit from certain Lakeshore Foundation services to end up falling through the cracks due a lack of funding.'

"Mike just keeps on taking a personal interest in the people who come in and out of the Lakeshore Foundation building," said Jeff. "He just wants to see people helped."

As Jeff had served in his role as Lakeshore Foundation's president, he said it had been incredibly fulfilling to him to work with Mike Stephens in moving the Foundation forward. "Mike and I have similar interests at heart," said Jeff, "because both of us have Lakeshore Foundation's interests at heart."

DURING HIS YEARS with Lakeshore Foundation, Jeff Underwood had encountered many individuals who had faced significant health-related crises. In 2009, he came face-to-face with his own health crisis. At age 57, he was diagnosed with a life-threatening cancer of his left tonsil.

Driven by their knowledge that cancers of the head and neck are particularly hard to treat and can be deadly, physicians who treated Jeff used aggressive treatments. Jeff had surgery; he had seven weeks of radiation treatment; he had three rounds of adjuvant chemotherapy.

Jeff submitted himself to these treatments because, with them, he stood a stronger chance of beating the cancer on the long-term. As is true for most cancer patients who undergo aggressive treatments, the months following his diagnosis were grueling.

When he was taking radiation, he became intensely claustrophobic when he was loaded into a tube-like machine while wearing a mask—an approach designed to make the radiation delivery very precise.

Some of the treatments made it so difficult for Jeff to swallow that he had to be fed for two months by a feeding tube.

The fatigue was overwhelming. The weight loss was major. One treatment side effect was some hearing loss—leading to Jeff's wearing hearing aids. His taste buds were jolted, resulting in negative taste changes regarding certain foods he had once enjoyed. His saliva production also was permanently lessened, raising the chances of tooth decay and leading to daily fluoride treatments.

Despite the downsides, Jeff said again and again that he felt very fortunate.

He said he felt fortunate that state-of-the-art treatments were available for him within a few miles of where he lived in the Birmingham area—an area known around the world for its progressive approaches to fighting various cancers. Jeff actually went for treatment to the same renowned cancer-fighting institution where he had worked just before coming to Lakeshore Foundation—to UAB's Comprehensive Cancer Center, one of a national chain of federally-designated cancer-fighting complexes.

Jeff felt fortunate for his faith that helped sustain him during his difficult cancer battle. He felt fortunate to have wife Melinda and their two daughters for support. And, when he was able to return to work, he felt very fortunate that he was returning to the Lakeshore Foundation.

Lakeshore Foundation was, as Jeff had said many times, "a place where you can make a difference." He returned to work at a time when Lakeshore Foundation was busy expanding its programs for injured military personnel, when the Foundation was working with UAB to set up a chair in rehabilitation research, and when the Foundation was embarking on crucial strategic planning that would help mold its future directions.

When Jeff returned to work, he said he could feel benefits flowing on a two-way street. On the one hand, he was glad to be back working and serving. On the other hand, he said he was much aware that this same Foundation that had helped build strength in so many now was helping to build back strength in Jeff Underwood. He could feel his strength being fed by the inspiration of people around him whom he viewed as having faced and conquered much more than he. "Lakeshore has become therapeutic for me," said Jeff.

In 2011, as Jeff looked back on his rigorous cancer-fighting experience, he said there was no doubt that the experience had forever changed his life—including the way he viewed his life, and even his willingness to discuss his life.

One of the ways in which Jeff knew he had been changed by his cancer experience was that he had become more willing to open up and share personal feelings and experiences.

As one who had been president of Lakeshore Foundation for years, and also as one who had held public office at state and local levels, Jeff had done considerable public speaking and had answered questions in many news-media interviews. Standing at a podium or speaking in an interview came naturally to him. At the same time, until Jeff confronted cancer, he had remained a very private person about his own feelings and experiences. When he made speeches or gave interviews, he addressed the causes and programs he represented and not the very private feelings or experiences of Jeff Underwood. He just didn't feel comfortable talking much about himself.

Then it came to be that Jeff felt a media spotlight on his personal feelings. After it became public knowledge that the president of Lakeshore Foundation was battling cancer, Jeff was asked to talk about the very personal aspects of fighting this very serious disease that had invaded his body and his life. Surprising to him, he found he could talk about it; more than that, he wanted to talk about it.

Jeff gave an extensive interview to writer Jeff Hansen for the *Birmingham News*—telling Hansen about the support he had received from so many sources, including Lakeshore Foundation.

As he revealed very specific details of his cancer battle in the newspaper interview, Jeff told writer Hansen about days when his mouth had ached so badly from the treatments that he didn't feel like talking, when he was so exhausted that he could not concentrate and chose to retreat to the solitude of his bedroom. As he poured out his experiences, Jeff said to writer Hansen, "I'll have to admit, it surprises me that I am so willing to talk about it. I am not one to quickly share my feelings."

Then, months later, as he spoke in this interview for a book on Lakeshore Foundation, Jeff again shared his innermost feelings—this time also talking about how specific individuals at Lakeshore Foundation had inspired him during some of the lowest points during his cancer battle.

As he went through his months of treatments, and then more months of rebuilding his strength, Jeff said he thought of specific clients who had come through the doors of Lakeshore Foundation, and also of specific Foundation staff members, who had persevered no matter what the obstacles.

One of those Foundation staff members who inspired him was Bob Lujano—a man who, despite having amputations on both arms and both legs, had helped thousands of disabled individuals and had become an internationally acclaimed athlete.

"I see Bob working here at Lakeshore Foundation every day, making such a difference as he does his job of ministering to others," said Jeff. "Bob always has this big grin on his face; he's always looking on the positive side. I look at Bob and I tell myself, 'So how could I ever complain?' "

The inspiration of another individual who flashed into Jeff's mind time and again was longtime Lakeshore Foundation client Fred Ostroy.

Jeff had a special insight into the positive spirit of Fred Ostroy because he had known Fred both before and after Fred incurred severe physical disability. Jeff had met Fred back in the days before a stroke had ravaged his body and before he starting coming regularly to Lakeshore Foundation to rebuild his strength in the Foundation's fitness center and pool.

Fred had earned a PhD in biophysics and had worked in a research position at UAB's Comprehensive Cancer Center at the same time Jeff was employed there. Versed in information systems, Fred later held a faculty position in UAB's Department of Health Services Administration and taught graduate-level courses there. Then, when Fred was only in his mid-50s, a massive stroke ended his rewarding career and took a major toll on his mobility, speech, and eyesight. Year after year following the stroke, Fred came to Lakeshore Foundation to make his strength as good as it could be. He used the strength and energy he could muster to continue his interests in music, computers, investing, and even slapstick comedy.

Fred maintained a connection with Lakeshore Foundation for the rest of his life, which, in 2011, ended when he was 69. "Over the years, as Fred came to the Foundation, I would see him there in the pool area or in our fitness center," said Jeff. "I would stop and chat with him, and we would recall our days when we both worked at UAB's Comprehensive Cancer Center." Even before Jeff was diagnosed with cancer, he said that Fred had become an inspiration to him; after cancer entered Jeff's life, he felt even more inspired by Fred. "I thought of how Fred had remained engaged in life and with those around him, despite what had happened to him with his stroke," said Jeff. "I also thought of what Lakeshore Foundation had done for Fred, how much the Foundation had meant to Fred."

In speaking of Bob Lujano and Fred Ostroy, Jeff said he was just singling out two among many of those at Lakeshore Foundation—both clients and staff members—from whom he had drawn inspiration.

Even before his own cancer-fighting experience, Jeff had always felt a deep admiration for people he had come to know at Lakeshore Foundation who had met major adversity and dealt with it.

"However, since my experience with cancer, my admiration is on such a personal level," said Jeff.

One reason for his deepened personal connection was that Jeff strongly believed there were so many at Lakeshore who had gone through so much more than he had faced.

"I've given a lot of thought to this," said Jeff. "When I was taking my treatments, I would think from time to time, 'Well, here I am going through a few months of sheer you-know-what, but then, if things go well, after that I will be better." If things went well, said Jeff, he stood a good chance of returning to close to the same health status he had before, without suffering major permanent losses. That was in stark contrast to many clients served by the Lakeshore Foundation who had learned to deal well with major permanent loss. "At Lakeshore Foundation, we see people who for the rest of their lives will be dealing with paralysis, or the loss of a limb, or the effects of a stroke or a chronic disabling disease or condition. That puts my own situation into a great deal of perspective. I have a lot to be grateful for—a lot."

25

A New Building

By the late 1990s, it was apparent that the time had come to plan toward a new building to house Lakeshore Foundation's rapidly growing sports, recreation, and fitness programs for those with physical disabilities.

Those programs had entered a growth spurt that had begun with the 1981 opening of the Wallace Recreation Center on Lakeshore's campus.

That growth spurt seemed to have no end in sight.

Planning toward a new Lakeshore Foundation building went forward full-steam ahead in 1996 and early 1997, leading up to presentation of these plans at a 1997 retreat of the Lakeshore Foundation Board of Directors.

Although Mike Stephens was heavily involved in pushing the new building forward, he was functioning in a different role from when the Wallace Recreation Center was being planned years before, during the time when he was executive director of Lakeshore Hospital. At that point, it had been Mike who had led the push for the Wallace Recreation Center, including his visit early on to Alabama Governor George C. Wallace to seek the governor's support of the building project.

Now, when a new home for the Lakeshore Foundation was under consideration in the late-1990s, Mike's role was that of a Lakeshore Foundation board member. "By this time, I had pulled away from day-to-day operations, and details of the new building project would be handled by current Foundation staff members under the direction of Jeff Underwood," said Mike. "At the same time, from a board of directors' perspective—and as Lakeshore Foundation's founder—I took a heavy interest."

Mike knew the construction of this new building was a real milestone in positioning Lakeshore Foundation to reach its future potential. He was pleased that the architectural work for the building was being conducted by Gray Plosser and his colleagues at KPS Group, Inc., of Birmingham and Atlanta. Mike had worked previously with Plosser and KPS in projects related to his ReLife company. Mike knew the architectural firm was progressive and that the Lakeshore Foundation design would be both functional and beautiful. He knew that KPS understood Lakeshore's mission and had the ability to plan with the future in mind. Also, it pleased Mike that KPS was expert in site planning and thus would make the most of the serene wooded acreage of the Lakeshore campus.

"As planning went forward, it mattered to me that the site chosen for the building was at the highest point on Lakeshore's 45-acre campus," said Mike. "That location within itself was a symbol. The location sent a message about the preeminent position now held on the campus by the Lakeshore Foundation (which, in the wake of the ReLife/HealthSouth merger, had become the landlord of the Lakeshore campus). The site chosen for the Foundation's new building was ideal for a facility that could be the crown jewel of the Lakeshore campus."

After the Lakeshore Board of Directors sanctioned plans for the building at the board's 1997 retreat, work proceeded in an orderly fashion. "That 1997 board retreat laid the groundwork," said Lakeshore Foundation President Jeff Underwood.

Months before plans for the new building went to the Lakeshore Board of Directors for intensive review, Lakeshore staff members had major input into planning for the building.

High value was placed on obtaining input from Lakeshore Foundation staff members—staff members who actually worked closely with children, teenagers, and adults with physical disabilities who benefited from the Foundation's sports, recreation, and fitness programs.

One of those Lakeshore staff members who took part in planning for the new building was Wynn Harris, who, by the time the planning took place, had been working on the Lakeshore campus for a decade and a half. She had come to the campus in 1982, the year after Wallace Recreation Center opened, to do an internship in therapeutic recreation as a part of her studies at the University of South Alabama. Then she went to work at Lakeshore Hospital as a therapeutic recreation specialist and got involved in the hospital's fledgling wheelchair sports programs and aquatics programs. After the ReLife/HealthSouth transition, Wynn ultimately would become director of aquatics, fitness, and recreation for Lakeshore Foundation.

Wynn recalled the Wallace Recreation Center as being a treasure in the 1980s: "It was state of the art!" She recalled the joy of watching that center become a place where so many lives were changed for the better: "Our programs in Wallace Recreation Center grew and grew. Finally we got to the point where the only limitation that we had was literally the bricks and mortar that surrounded us. We outgrew the facility, could not expand programs further, and were having to turn people away. Then we started planning for the new Lakeshore Foundation building."

The enthusiasm of the staff in helping to plan the new building was something that Wynn said was beyond words to describe. "We were able to take all of our knowledge from over the years—what had worked, and how we could do things better for those we served. Being a part of all that was so exciting!"

As the Foundation's new building took shape through the construction process, observers soon saw that the new building indeed was the product of those who dreamed and planned big.

Almost a decade after the new building opened in October 2001, Jeff Underwood said he still was seeing visitors utter gasps of awe and admiration when they first entered the facility.

"Lakeshore Foundation's building would continue to have that 'Wow!' factor," said Jeff. "In fact, I would constantly need to voice this reminder: 'Yes, this Lakeshore Foundation building is great. But you have to keep in mind that the building would be nothing without the incredible work of our staff who have made sure these great facilities are put to good use to serve the people we are here to serve.' "

The two-level brick and glass facility, totally accessible to individuals with physical disabilities, would be constructed at a cost of some $22 million. There would be many who had reason to have personal pride as donors, since the cost was covered not only by Lakeshore Foundation resources but also by the generosity of donors that included other foundations as well as corporations and individuals.

Just the imposing size of the facility—some 126,000 square feet—would draw many "oohs and aahs." The sweeping, open, aesthetically appealing architectural touches also drew praise. Gray Plosser and his colleagues at KPS Group had designed the building as a showcase for the striking Lakeshore campus. There were areas in which the glass walls extended upward for the full two levels of the building, creating a stunning view of the wooded areas beyond.

The areas within the building designated for various programs were spacious, functional, and aesthetically appealing. Those areas would become beehives of activity. During tournaments, the huge fieldhouse would be packed with athletes and spectators as competitors in wheelchairs filled all three hardwood courts. There would be times even on a non-tournament day at Lakeshore Foundation when one could see sports and recreation activity on all three courts plus on the 200-meter track that surrounded the courts.

After a visitor entered the front door of the building, it wasn't long before his eyes opened wide in admiration to the sight of the new home for the Foundation's aquatics center—two expansive side-by-side pools (a lap pool and a therapy pool). No stone had been left unturned to adapt these pools to the needs of the physically disabled who used them—the zero-grade entry level, steps, ladders, chairlifts, etc. As was true of the fieldhouse, the aquatics center had users who were young children and teenagers, and it had users who were adults. Those who enjoyed and thrived at the aquatics center came with conditions such as spinal cord injury and visual impairment, with birth defects such as cerebral palsy and spida bifida, and with physical challenges dealt later by health problems such as multiple sclerosis, stroke, cardiac problems, arthritis, and diabetes.

The building also was equipped with a 6,000-square-foot fitness center, a rock climbing wall, a 10-lane archery and marksmanship range, community meeting rooms and other meeting areas, plus convenient locker rooms and assisted dressing rooms.

WHEN THE WALLACE Recreation Center had opened in 1981, wheelchair athlete Jim Wooten was among those who had felt both happiness and pride in knowing that those with physical disabilities finally had a place of their own for sports and recreation.

Jim had participated in early-day wheelchair basketball in the Birmingham area—a talented and aggressive player who earned the nickname of "Danger" on the basketball court. He could recall when Birmingham area wheelchair athletes had to beg for use of gymnasium or community-center space where they could practice and play their games. He painfully remembered those difficult days when he and his teammates had to literally drag themselves and their wheelchairs and equipment up the steep steps of non-accessible community centers where they were unwanted visitors. And, then there were the insults—the times when able-bodied athletes would make fun of the athletes in wheelchairs and urge them to hurry their practices and games and get out of the borrowed space as soon as possible, or sooner.

After the Wallace Recreation Center opened on the Lakeshore campus, Jim had said that he would wheel his chair into the facility and think to himself, "Wallace Recreation Center is our place."

By the time the Lakeshore Foundation's new $22 million facility opened in 2001, Jim Wooten still was associated with Lakeshore. He still was playing competitive wheelchair basketball; he was beginning to do a little coaching at Lakeshore.

One day at one of the events to dedicate the new building, Mike Stephens spotted Jim. The two of them had journeyed down some of the same paths with Lakeshore. In fact, in the early days of Lakeshore competitive wheelchair sports, Mike had coached a basketball team on which Jim had played. "Well, Wooten, what do you think of Lakeshore Foundation's new building?" Mike asked Jim.

Just as had been true with the Wallace Recreation Center, Jim "Danger" Wooten was filled with pride and enthusiasm. Although he usually was a man of few words, he was exuberant in his response to Mike.

"You remember way back yonder when those able-bodied guys out at the community center in Ensley would refer to us disabled guys as 'crips' and tell us we needed to get out of their center?" said Jim Wooten. "Well, nobody can tell us to get out of this building!"

Mike had to grin.

"As Jim 'Danger' Wooten looked at that beautiful new building, you could see it in his eyes," said Mike. "It was like, 'We've come a long way. Yeah, man, we've come a long, long way.' "

Lakeshore's Expanded Campus and World-class Facilities

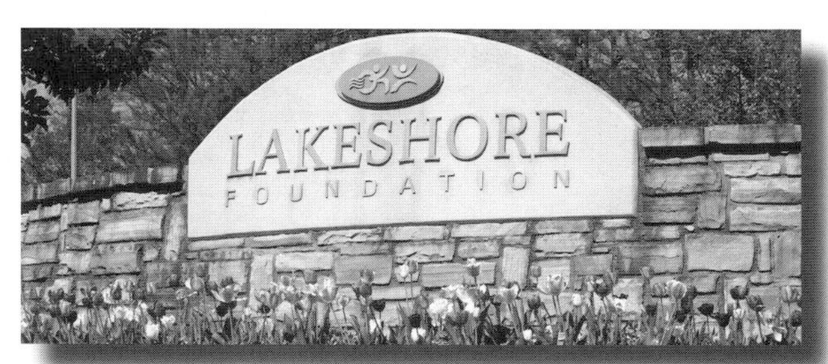

Signage off Highway 31 in Homewood, Alabama.

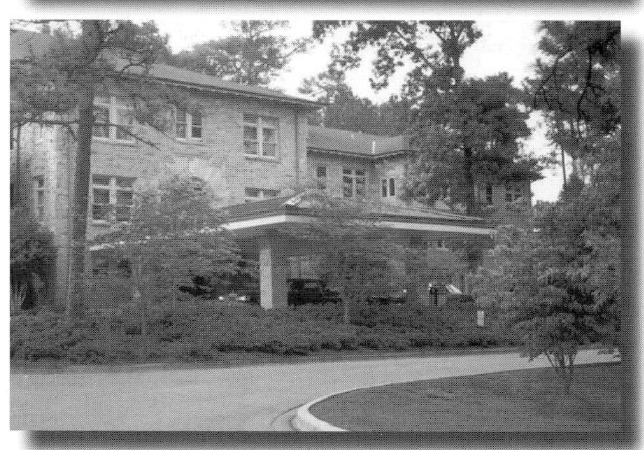

Right and below: *Renovated older stone buildings and new, modern architecture harmoniously blend on the campus.*

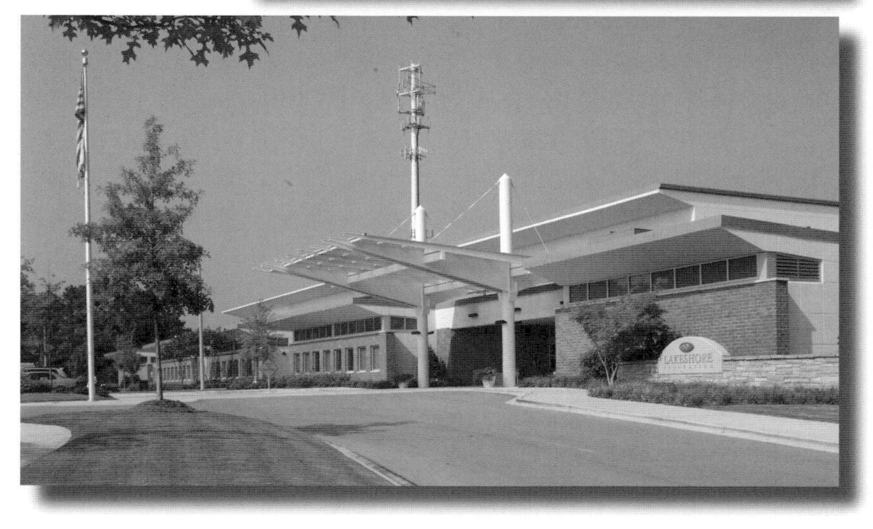

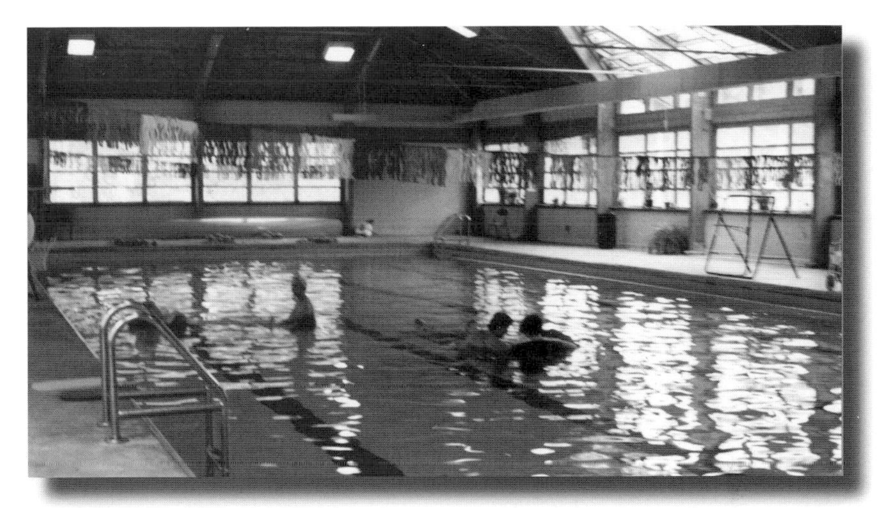

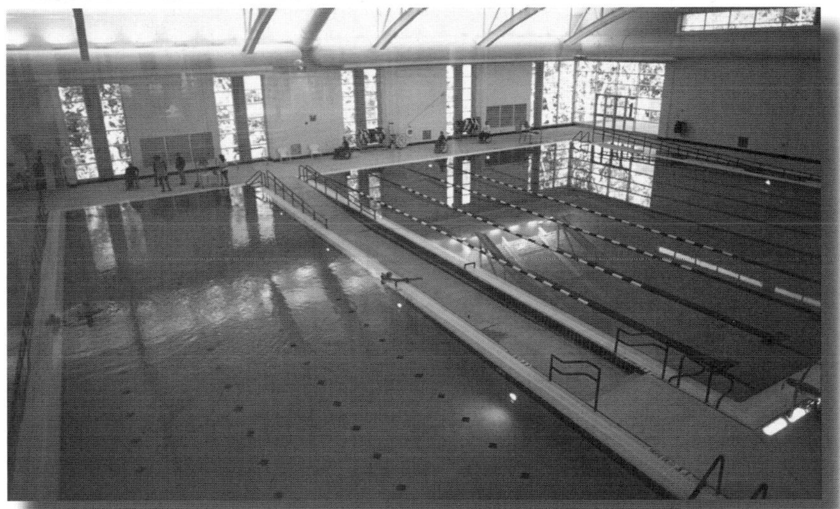

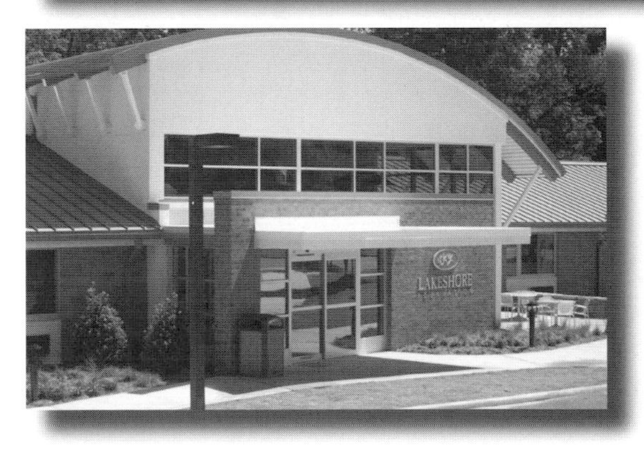

Top: *Wallace Recreation Center has one pool.* **Above:** *Foundation facility has two expansive pools.* **Left:** *Former transitional living dorm is now an athletic dorm.*

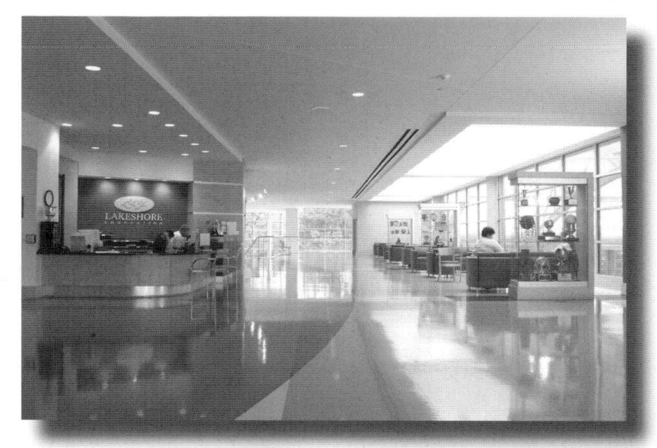

Top: *Foyer.*

Right: *Administrative offices.*

Bottom: *Fitness center.*

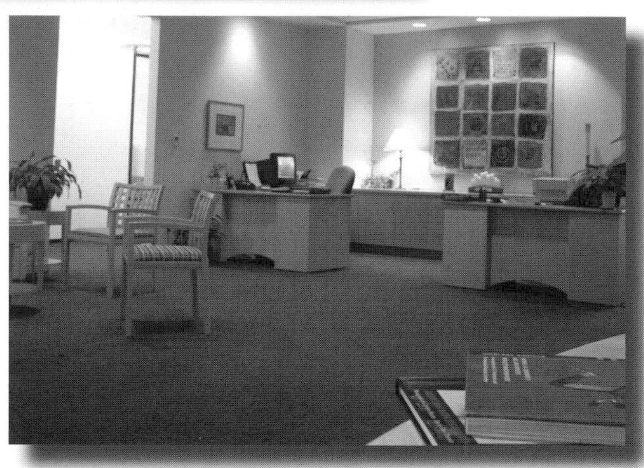

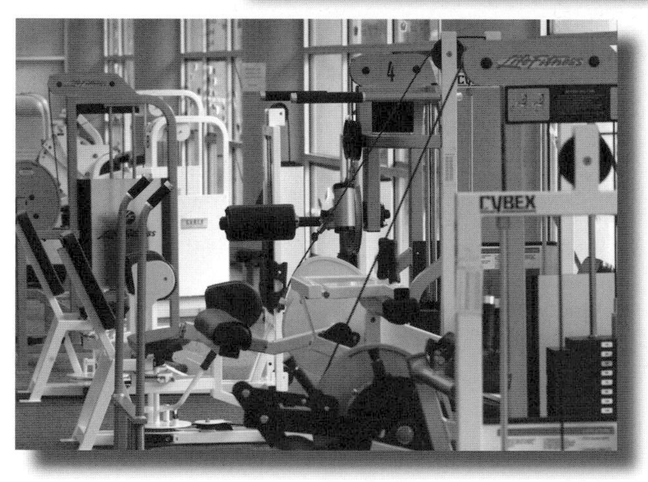

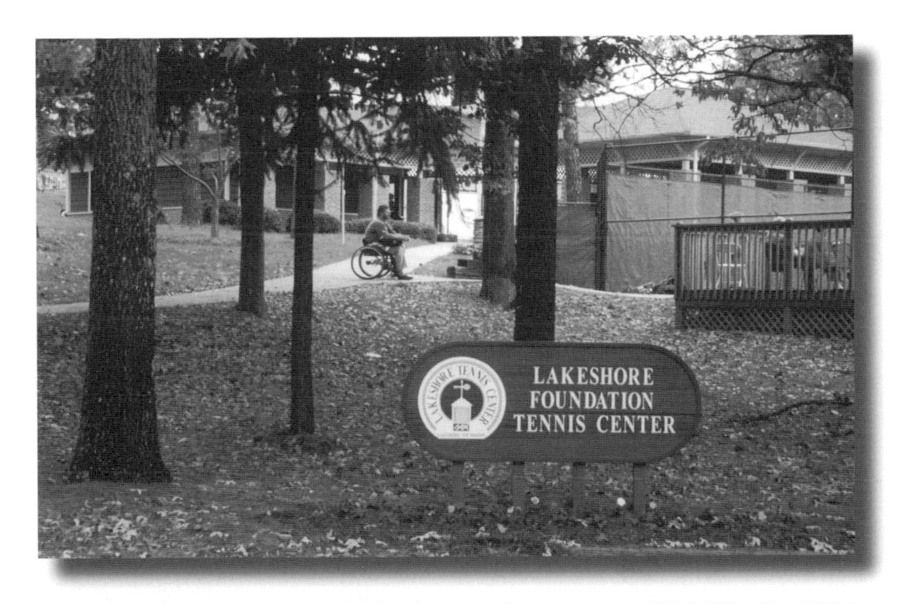

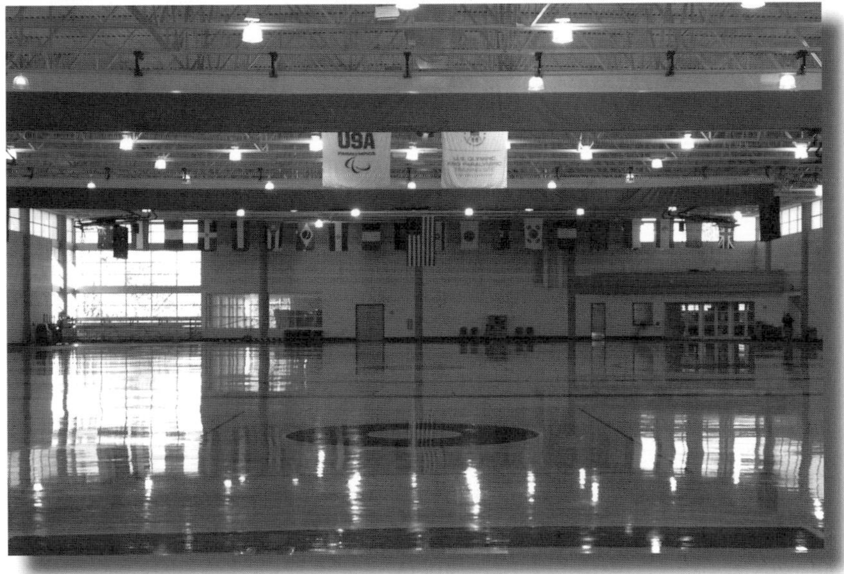

Tennis center and fieldhouse are sites of games and training at recreational, local competition, and world championship levels.

26

The Road to the Olympic Rings

When construction on the new Lakeshore Foundation building was well under way in 2000, Mike Stephens arranged for a new Birmingham area resident to take a tour of the facility, thus setting in motion a journey that three years later would result in the Foundation's being officially designated as a U.S. Olympic and Paralympic training site.

The building tour was for Herman Frazier, who had gained international fame in 1976 Olympic competition in Montreal, Canada. He became a 1976 Olympic gold medalist as a member of the men's 4 x 400 meter relay for the United States. He also scored individually in the Montreal Olympics, winning a bronze medal in the 400-meter dash.

These Olympic triumphs formed a solid base for Frazier's professional career in athletics, as he rose to become senior associate athletic director at his university alma mater, Arizona State University, and then was recruited in 2000 to become athletic director at the University of Alabama at Birmingham (UAB). Along the way, Frazier had become high profile as chairman of the Fiesta Bowl, and, in 1996, by being elected as one of three vice-presidents of the board of directors of the largest and most powerful Olympic organization in the world—the United States Olympic Committee (USOC).

Soon after Frazier moved to Birmingham to accept the UAB position, Mike Stephens became one of those showing him some of the area's positive attractions. For Mike, it was a source of pride to make it possible for Herman Frazier to learn about the long and strong track record that the Lakeshore Foundation had in programs for athletes with physical disabilities.

"It was important that Herman be able to see Birmingham in a positive light," said Mike. "I knew of course that Herman was interested in accomplishments in the athletic arena, and I knew that Lakeshore Foundation had such accomplishments. There were several of us in the Birmingham area who really wanted Herman to see all of Birmingham's positive sides. Birmingham had come a long way since the ugliness of the 1950s and 1960s civil rights conflicts."

Lakeshore Foundation's president, Jeff Underwood, and the staff he supervised conducted the tour that showed to Herman Frazier the almost-completed facilities in the expansive, stunning new Lakeshore Foundation building.

"Jeff Underwood and the other staff members at Lakeshore Foundation had led the way in planning for the new building and in seeing that project through," said Mike. "It was appropriate that they be the ones to show off this almost-completed facility to Herman Frazier. Although I had served as the one to connect Herman with the Lakeshore Foundation, I actually remained back in the Lakeshore administrative area while the building tour was being conducted for Herman."

TO MIKE, THIS building that Herman Frazier was seeing symbolized the dawning of a new era in Mike's own relationship with Lakeshore.

The Lakeshore Foundation building project was a tremendous undertaking. It was by far the biggest single building project on the Lakeshore campus that had taken place in the years that had passed since Mike had established the Lakeshore Foundation, since he had ceased to lead the day-to-day operations of both the Foundation and Lakeshore Hospital, and ultimately since he had ceased to lead the ReLife rehabilitation company that had overseen both the Hospital and the Foundation.

"To me personally, the construction of Lakeshore Foundation's new building was an incredible physical plant that served as a visible bridge to the era when I was functioning in a role solely as a Lakeshore Foundation board member, albeit a very interested and involved board member," said Mike. "I remember thinking on that day when Jeff and other staff members were escorting Herman Frazier through the build-

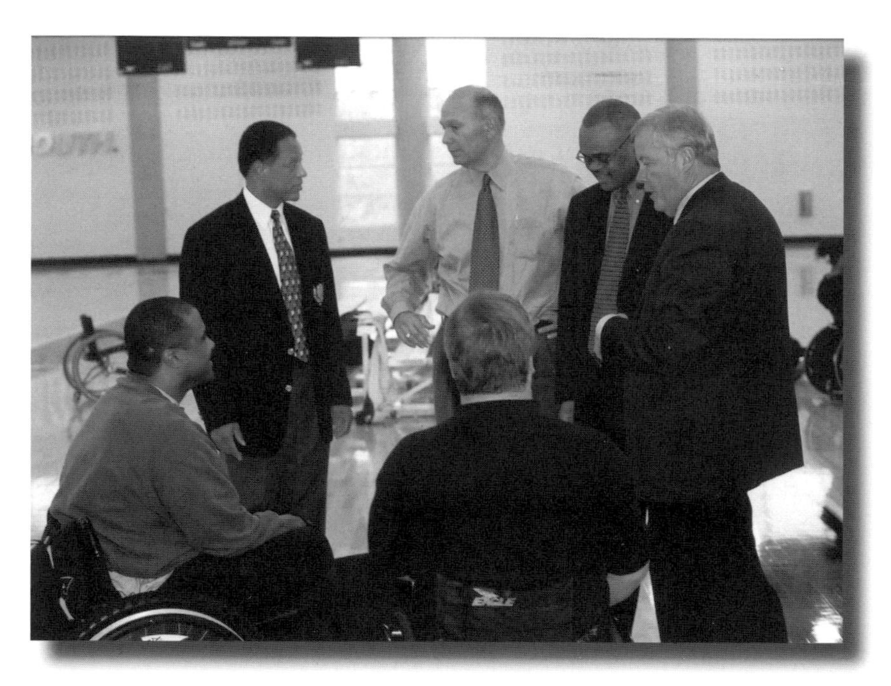

United States Olympic Committee VP Herman Frazier, second from right, standing next to Mike Stephens.

ing, 'To me, this building—a model building—really does serve as a symbol of the beginning of yet another new Lakeshore era—*their* era!' "

When Frazier completed the tour of the Lakeshore Foundation building, he came to Mike and told him what he thought about what he had just seen. "I could see the excitement alive in Herman's eyes and in his words of praise for what he had seen and learned regarding the Lakeshore Foundation," said Mike. Frazier told Mike that he felt Lakeshore had enormous potential to serve athletes on a worldwide stage—possibly to become one among a handful of elite training facilities sanctioned by the USOC.

Herman Frazier's admiration went far beyond the magnificent new building that he was seeing, said Mike.

"What Herman was also seeing—and what other USOC leaders later would see as well—also had to do with Lakeshore's more than two decades of experience exposing the physically disabled to quality sports and recreational activities," said Mike. "If someone really looked into Lakeshore's history, it was apparent that not only were we building physical facilities that no one could surpass worldwide, but in addition, the Lakeshore Foundation had progressive staff members who could provide high-quality support services to athletes. Too, Lakeshore had a history of interacting with medical professionals who had far-reaching reputations in the world of athletics, such as internationally known orthopedic surgeons Dr. Lawence J. 'Larry' Lemak and Dr. James R. 'Jimmy' Andrews.

"If someone just took inventory of the many awards and medals captured by athletes with physical disabilities who had trained at Lakeshore, it was extraordinarily impressive. Lakeshore athletes had been capturing those awards and medals for years with the help of training they received at our first athletic facility, the Wallace Recreation Center. Since we soon would be occupying our new, much more expansive building, it wasn't much of a stretch to envision our further increased capacity as a training site.

"When USOC Vice President Herman Frazier toured Lakeshore Foundation's facilities and really understood what the Foundation was all about, he knew that the Foundation could serve as one of the answers to some of the deep problems the USOC was experiencing in its lack of quality training programs for Paralympic athletes. Herman realized that, if the USOC could incorporate the Lakeshore Foundation into its network of training centers, the Foundation's new building coupled with our deep experience could overnight place the USOC in a much stronger position relevant to what it could do for Paralympians."

LAKESHORE FOUNDATION PRESIDENT Jeff Underwood said there had been discussion for years that it could be a constructive fit for the Lakeshore Foundation to take some role in training Olympic and Paralympic contenders.

Among those who knew Lakeshore well—who understood the contribution Lakeshore already was making in the world of sports and recreation—discussing such future potential for Lakeshore was an understandable topic.

Jeff said that some of the seeds for that thought process had taken root after the 1996 Paralympic Games in Atlanta, when the United States' physically disabled athletes overall had not done so well in competition. There was a feeling that Lakeshore Foundation's long track record in disabled sport might one day contribute to the training of Paralympic hopefuls.

In fact, said Jeff, when planning was under way for Lakeshore Foundation's new building, there was increased hope for a possible future Olympic/Paralympic connection: "One of the goals that our staff expressed to members of our Lakeshore Board of Directors, associated with the construction of our new facilities, was that Lakeshore might be able to achieve a future formal designation as a USOC training center."

After Mike Stephens arranged for Herman Frazier to be taken on a tour of Lakeshore, and Frazier was so impressed, those wheels began to turn more in earnest.

It would be in the year 2000 when Lakeshore submitted a formal proposal to be designated as a training facility sanctioned by the USOC.

In that same year, a national task force conducted a review of how the USOC was implementing and supporting Paralympic sport. One of the members of that task force was the Foundation's President, Jeff Underwood—yet another indication of the growing reputation of the Lakeshore Foundation and the respect that it drew.

IN THE YEARS immediately leading up to the year 2000, when Lakeshore Foundation filed a formal proposal to become a training site for the USOC, several controversies had been swirling around Olympic organizations.

Some of that controversy applied directly to the USOC; some of the discontent applied directly to the Paralympics; other subjects of controversy related to drug use among athletes, and also to Olympic officials charged with taking bribes.

Widely publicized charges of bribery comprised an unfortunate

Olympics focus in the late-1990s, when the International Olympic Committee (IOC) conducted an investigation into charges that, relevant to which city would host the 2002 Winter Olympics, some IOC members had accepted bribes from the bid committee representing Salt Lake City, Utah. As a result of that investigation, four IOC members resigned, six other members were expelled, and reforms were instituted to change the host-city selection process.

On another subject of international Olympic concern, doping among athletes participating in Olympic events had become a pressing issue with the IOC. In 1999, a World Conference on Doping was held in Lausanne, Switzerland, and was attended by representatives from the Olympic community, governments, and various international agencies. As a result of that conference, the World Anti-Doping Agency (WADA) was created. Later, in anticipation of the 2004 Athens Olympic Games, the World Anti Doping Code (WADC) was created, with a goal of "doping-free sport."

And then there was an ongoing swirl of controversy surrounding the level of USOC support provided to athletes with physical disabilities. There were persistent ongoing charges that disabled athletes who trained for and competed in Paralympic events were not receiving nearly the level of support that was accorded their able-bodied counterparts who trained for and competed in Olympic events.

As the 1990s were drawing to a close, the saga of Paralympic sport was mixed.

On the one hand, all around the world, disabled athletes who competed in the Paralympics were steadily finding themselves greeted with more recognition and more inclusiveness. A good example came in some of the provisions in the 1998 amendments to the Ted Stevens Olympic and Amateur Sports Act, which had become law in 1978 and was named for the long-serving senior United States senator from Alaska, a powerful Republican in Congress. Just as Senator Stevens in his 1978 Olympic and Amateur Sports legislation had laid out the legal framework under which the USOC operated, in some of the 1998 amendments he addressed ways the USOC could better serve disabled athletes. Some of the 1998 provisions dealt specifically with athletic eligibility and representation relevant to the Paralympic Games.

However, at the same time that Paralympians seemed to be gaining ground, advocates for disabled athletes said it was not nearly enough ground. In 1999, a disabled-sport-related federal discrimination suit was filed against the USOC and the IOC—grabbing headlines around the world. This suit attracted an especially high level of attention because it was filed on behalf of a disabled individual who actually was an insider with the USOC. His name was Mark E. Shepherd Sr. After having suffered a spinal cord injury in a 1986 auto accident while coming home from his job as a California policeman, Shepherd had become a star in wheelchair basketball—a two-time world champion and a Paralympic medalist. And, at the time the 1999 suit was filed on his behalf, he was manager of the USOC's Disabled Sports Services; in this position, he was a USOC official representing athletic programs and athletes with disabilities. The Mark E. Shepherd Sr. suit claimed that the USOC was discriminating against athletes with disabilities by providing them with separate and inferior services as compared to able-bodied athletes. This alleged short-changing, according to the suit, meant that disabled athletes were receiving less than able-bodied athletes in the way of services, programs, benefits, insurance, medical care, and training. As a result of the alleged short-changing, the suit charged, the USOC and the IOC which supervised it were in violation of several federal laws, including the Americans with Disabilities Act, the Rehabilitation Act, and the Civil Rights Act.

"All in all, the late-1990s had proved to be a difficult time for the Olympics' public image, and Olympic organizations were in search of constructive ways to do a better job and to improve their image by identifying, addressing, and correcting problems," said Mike Stephens. "Where the Paralympics was concerned, these efforts within Olympic organizations of course related to improving services for disabled athletes—including the improvement of training programs.

"Therefore, when the Lakeshore Foundation made application in 2000 to become one of the athlete-training sites for the USOC, we felt the timing of our application was good, particularly in light of the fact that a good word had been put in for Lakeshore by one of the USOC leaders, Herman Frazier."

As Lakeshore Foundation leaders submitted a proposal for Lakeshore to become an official USOC training site, they believed the Foundation had far-reaching resources to train athletes.

In their view, Lakeshore Foundation had an edge in training that would meet the needs of disabled athletes training for the Paralympics; they also felt that the Foundation's resources could serve able-bodied athletes who trained for the Olympics.

They believed that Lakeshore Foundation thus was worthy of earning a training-site designation that would be signified by the famous Olympic symbol known as the "Olympic Rings." The symbol of "The Rings" was proudly displayed by other training facilities that had been officially designated as USOC training sites. That symbol, known to people around the world, consisted of five intertwined rings—in the colors of blue, yellow, black, green, and red—representing the unity of the five inhabited continents.

Shortly after the Lakeshore Foundation submitted its proposal to become a USOC training site, a development took place within the USOC that ultimately would signal good news for this Lakeshore Foundation proposal.

That 2001 development was the creation of the USOC division that was specifically devoted to disabled athletes and to furthering the Paralympics.

Bearing the official name of the United States Paralympic Corporation, this new USOC entity would more generally be referred to as USOC's Paralympic Division, or simply as the U.S. Paralympics.

On March 1, 2001, the USOC announced the individual selected to head this new division—Charlie Huebner. An able-bodied sports administrator whose name already had become well-known in the world of disabled sport, Huebner previously had served as executive director of the United States Association of Blind Athletes. Huebner became the first employee of the U.S. Paralympics.

In an interview for this book, Huebner looked back at what the USOC's purposes had been in establishing a new Paralympic Division: "When the USOC in 2001 created U.S. Paralympics, the focus was very clear. It was to work with the 22 Paralympic sports and Olympic national governing bodies to enhance sport performance for Paralympic athletes, to enhance funding and support for Paralympic athletes, and to enhance revenue and awareness for Paralympic athletes. It was an entirely new division that was created for those purposes."

Several years later, Mike Stephens would look back on the U.S. Paralympics leadership that Charlie Huebner had provided since his appointment and express these sentiments: "Charlie Huebner proved to be a strong advocate, an exceptional person, and a dedicated soul who would do more for U.S. Paralympics and for athletes with physical disabilities than had been done by anyone I had ever known."

AS THE USOC entered the 21st century, it was clear the organization was taking some positive steps—such as the creation of the U.S. Paralympics.

At the same time, the USOC became embroiled in widely publicized internal turmoil that for a period of time created ongoing instability. Amid charges that the USOC had an unworkable governing structure and a leadership that was guilty of severe mismanagement, several USOC officials resigned, including one turnover after another in the top leadership of both the USOC's volunteer board of directors and its paid staff. As conflicts worsened, Congress became involved. On Capitol Hill, hearings about USOC problems were held by the Senate Commerce Committee, chaired by Senator John McCain. The committee appointed a special five-member commission to propose USOC reforms, including the overhauling of the cumbersome USOC infrastructure. Within the Olympics, a task force on governance and ethics was looking at similar issues. And, at the USOC headquarters in Colorado Springs, Colorado, frustrated USOC staff members went into closed-door meetings to air the organization's problems with two U.S. senators who took a special interest in the future of the Olympics and Paralympics—Senator Ben Nighthorse Campbell, Republican from Colorado, and Senator Ted Stevens, Republican from Alaska.

Some of the developments that came to a head in in this difficult period were:

- In May 2002, Sandra Baldwin resigned as president of the USOC Board of Directors—one day after admitting that she had lied about her academic credentials in her official biography.
- In February 2003, Marty Mankamyer resigned as president of the USOC Board of Directors, after she had become a target of increasing criticism by some other USOC leaders, including some vice presidents of the board. She was accused of fanning the fires of conflict within the USOC, and with trying to push Lloyd Ward out of his job as CEO of the USOC by exaggerating charges of ethics violations that had been leveled against him.
- In March 2003, Lloyd Ward resigned as CEO of the USOC, after having been under the heat of months of investigation. Ward had come under scrutiny due to an accusation that he had violated ethics rules by trying to steer some international Olympics business to a company with which his brother was associated. Although official USOC sanctions never were leveled against Ward, and although he contended he was guilty simply of "an error in judgment" rather than overt wrongdoing, he said he had decided to resign willingly in an attempt to shift USOC focus back on the athletes and on Olympic and Paralympic goals.

By the time the USOC turmoil was brought under manageable control, the organization would be operating in the calendar year 2004. By that time, the USOC would have a revised mission statement—a new mission statement that for the first time in USOC history included a written commitment to serve not only Olympic athletes but also Paralympic athletes as well. Too, the USOC would have a drastically restructured infrastructure, which would center around a newly revamped board of directors that would have only 11 members, in contrast to the 123-member board that previously had held the reins.

THERE COULD BE no doubt that the internal turmoil that reigned within the USOC placed some stumbling blocks in the path of the proposal that the Lakeshore Foundation submitted in 2000 to become an official USOC training site. Too, said Charlie Huebner, the review of the Lakeshore Foundation proposal had to move at a measured pace because, after the USOC created the U.S. Paralympics in 2001, there had to be sufficient time to put in place a Paralympics performance plan and to respond to the Foundation's proposal in light of that plan.

As the newly appointed director of the U.S. Paralympics, Charlie Huebner played a key role in reviewing the Lakeshore Foundation proposal. Also reviewing the proposal was James E. "Jim" Scherr, who at the time was chief of sport performance at the USOC—a position that included oversight of USOC training sites.

Huebner recalled a trip he made to Lakeshore during his first six months on the job as director of the U.S. Paralympics. It was Huebner's first on-site visit to the Foundation, and he made the trip along with Jim Scherr. At the time, finishing touches were being put on the Foundation's new building, and programs still were being run out of the Wallace Recreation Center. "Lakeshore was pretty phenomenal. We toured the facilities, met with all the leadership, staff, executives, and board. They outlined their capital campaign and their plans. We were very, very impressed with their leadership, very impressed with their expertise, and with their facilities."

USOC's chief executive officer, Lloyd Ward, paid a later visit to Lakeshore. "He obviously was just as impressed as we were," said Huebner.

However, before Huebner and Scherr could complete a review relevant to the USOC, Huebner said that a Paralympic performance plan had to be put in place. Until that time, said Huebner, "we weren't prepared to respond to the proposal Lakeshore leaders were putting in front of us."

Then there was the other issue—getting the Lakeshore proposal through the unwieldy USOC review process while the USOC was in such upheaval. "It was a very difficult time at the USOC," said Huebner. "My entire staff walked into a hornet's nest. There was no honeymoon [from the time he came to his new U.S. Paralympics job in 2001]."

On the positive side, Huebner said that plans moved along well in getting a new Paralympic plan in place. Too, he said that he and Scherr were able in a timely fashion to get their heads together about what the USOC's requirements were in regard to training centers to meet both Olympic and Paralympic needs.

"Once we defined those training-site needs, Jim Scherr and I strongly believed that it was in the best interest of the U.S. Olympic Committee to designate Lakeshore Foundation as an Olympic and Paralympic training site. And we took that to our (USOC) leadership at the time." He said that he and Scherr made the case for Lakeshore Foundation because of what the Foundation could do not only for Paralympic athletes but also for Olympic athletes.

However, even though Huebner and Scherr took the recommendation to their bosses, it did no good because "our leadership changed," Huebner said—ongoing USOC resignations at high levels meant that he and Scherr soon had new bosses.

Another stumbling block to the Lakeshore proposal was that, at the time, the only way a new USOC training site could be designated was to have the approval of the entire USOC board.

"And, you know, at that time, we had a USOC board that was made up of 123 people," said Huebner. "It was very difficult to get decisions about anything. I don't think [the Lakeshore Foundation proposal] was moving up to the Training Center Committee [of the large USOC board] to a vote."

IN THE MIDST of this convoluted training-site review process, a delegation from Lakeshore Foundation made a trip to discuss its proposal with USOC officials—in meetings held in Salt Lake City, the site of the 2002 Winter Olympic Games.

That Lakeshore delegation consisted of Michael Stephens, the founder of Lakeshore Foundation; William P. "Bill" Acker III, the Foundation's board chairman; and Jeff Underwood, Lakeshore Foundation president.

As a result of those discussions, the USOC made an offer to the Lakeshore Foundation delegation that was so disappointing that the delegation unanimously turned it down.

The offer was this: First, the USOC could not designate Lakeshore Foundation as a full-fledged Olympic/Paralympic training center that could serve both the able-bodied and disabled athletes; instead, the USOC wanted to grant Lakeshore a designation only as a Paralympic facility. Secondly, the USOC could not award the Lakeshore Foundation the right to display the famous symbol of the five interlocking "Olympic rings"; instead, the USOC was proposing that Lakeshore display only the Paralympic logo.

Mike Stephens recalls what came to pass during the fateful trip that he, Bill Acker, and Jeff Underwood made to meet with USOC officials: "After we arrived and had been wined and dined by USOC leaders, we got down to the discussions. Bill and Jeff and I were in my hotel room, and people from USOC were coming in and out discussing their offer—all about becoming just a Paralympic training site and how 'we [the USOC] would love to have you [the Lakeshore Foundation] use the logo of the Paralympics.' "

Mike said that he, Acker, and Underwood were in agreement that they were opposed to that option—they did not believe it served the best interests of the USOC or the Lakeshore Foundation. "Our united message to the USOC was, 'No, we're not going to do this,' " said Mike.

He said the compromise being presented by the USOC was a world apart from the view shared by Acker, Underwood, and himself.

"On our end, we were of the view that Lakeshore Foundation had all the necessary resources to train the able-bodied while at the same time the obvious qualifications to become the first center in the country with special facilities expressly designed to serve the disabled athletes. And our view further was: 'If Lakeshore has the facilities and programs and staff, why shouldn't Lakeshore be granted a full designation, complete with the Rings, just like other USOC training centers?'

"Actually, we felt insulted by such an offer. We felt that such an option was a slam against the wheelchair athletes—a continuation of the same sort of attitude within the USOC that already was drawing criticism."

From the perspective of Mike, who had incurred a severe physical disability when he was 26 years old and had dealt with it ever since, he could strongly relate to the emotions of disabled athletes. Hearing the USOC compromise idea came as a very personal blow to him. His mind swirled with distressing thoughts.

Our people are just as good as the able-bodied people. They are just as good as athletes; they have the same heart. This offer from the USOC is the same as telling our athletes that they don't deserve to have the Rings flying over Lakeshore Foundation.

In the end, Mike Stephens, Jeff Underwood, and Bill Acker made it clear that, rather than accept the offered option, they were willing to walk away.

In Mike's view, there was a certain amount of surprise among some of the USOC representatives that the Lakeshore delegation did not say "yes" to the compromise option: "I got the impression there were some who were kind of astounded at our taking this stand on it—kind of the attitude of 'We are the USOC. Why would you turn us down on something?' "

The final decision about the USOC designation for Lakeshore Foundation had not been made by the time Lakeshore's delegation departed Salt Lake City to return to Birmingham.

But when the decision did come later, it would not be the consolation prize. It would instead be the full designation.

When the designation came in 2003, Jim Scherr had risen to the post of interim, or acting, chief executive officer of the USOC. (He would be granted the CEO position on a permanent basis in 2005.)

"It was Jim Scherr who presented the Lakeshore proposal to the USOC Board of Directors, and they approved it," said Charlie Huebner.

When the Lakeshore proposal was approved, Lakeshore was designated as a USOC training site for both Olympic and Paralympic athletes. The "Olympics Rings" emblem went on display outside the entrance to the Lakeshore Foundation.

"This designation of Lakeshore Foundation as an official USOC training site clearly became one of the major milestones in the history of the Foundation," said Foundation President Jeff Underwood.

IN 2005, SHORTLY after Jim Scherr's title at USOC went from "acting CEO" to fully designated CEO, Scherr spoke, in an interview for this book, about how pleased he had been with the Lakeshore Foundation's performance as a USOC training site.

He said Lakeshore was performing at a very high level in supporting athletes to achieve excellence that could lead to winning medals, that Lakeshore was very proficient in conducting camps that trained athletes from young ages on up, and that Lakeshore had a strong program to promote its programs related to the USOC.

In the eyes of Jim Scherr, the Lakeshore Foundation was living up to the potential he had seen when he first visited the Lakeshore campus: "Lakeshore has one of the finest physical plants of any nature that I've seen, and a staff of dedicated, competent and caring people."

Scherr had a personal reason to have deep respect for what the Lakeshore Foundation had achieved in programs for physically disabled athletes. Although Scherr himself was able-bodied, his father had a physical disability and had become a good athlete despite that disability. "As a boy on a farm, my father got an arm caught in a winch. Although he was left with a withered arm, he became a champion rodeo cowboy in North Dakota and also became a very good baseball player." Through watching his father, Scherr had come to appreciate the positive can-do spirit at Lakeshore. "My father never used his own disability as an excuse. It never held him back in his athletic endeavors. He was a good model for me."

Lakeshore Foundation had become a role model, said Scherr: "Lakeshore is already fulfilling a role model role for both the Paralympic movement and the Olympic movement. Lakeshore has a Paralympic

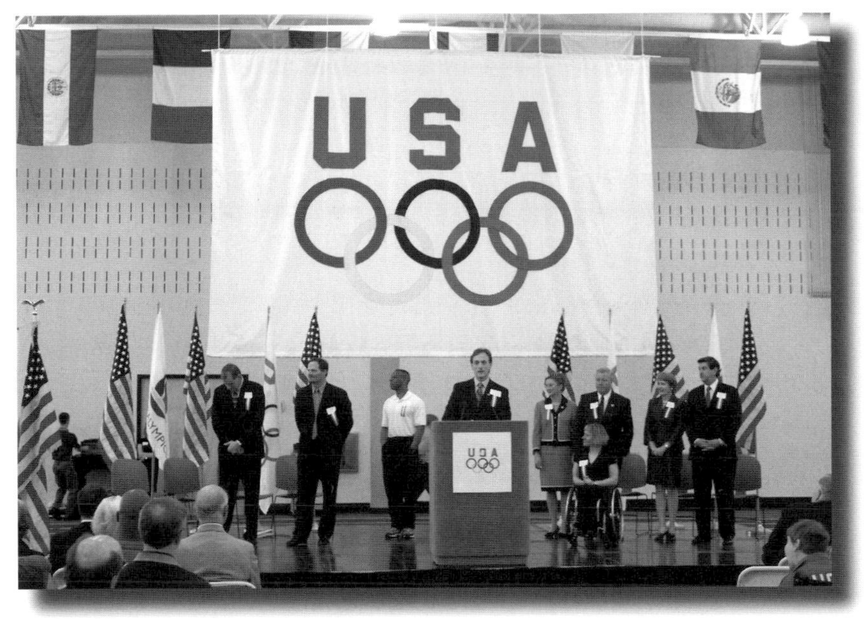

The unveiling of the Olympic rings on the occasion of Lakeshore Foundation being formally designated a USOC training facility. Governor Bob Riley is at far right.

ideal at heart, and also has the Olympic ideal at heart."

In regard to all its training sites, the USOC continually monitored and surveyed the sites' performance, said Scherr. He noted that Lakeshore was doing well in its marks. Even though Lakeshore was still relatively new in its role as a training site, Scherr said that "Lakeshore consistently ranks at the top in the amenities and services it is providing."

In relation to Lakeshore's longtime track record in support of athletes with disabilities, Charlie Huebner said that after Lakeshore was designated as a USOC training site, Lakeshore became "a template for what we're trying to do around the country. . . It's very exciting to say, 'Hey, what is being done at the Lakeshore Foundation in Birmingham is what we should be doing all over the country in the areas of sport programming, in the areas of revenue generation, in the areas of awareness, and in the areas of outreach.' "

CHARLIE HUEBNER GAVE much credit to Lakeshore Foundation's founder, Michael Stephens, and to its president, Jeff Underwood, for the quick and strong partnering success between Lakeshore and the USOC.

With Jeff Underwood, Huebner noted, it was a plus that Jeff had served on a Paralympic Task Force for the USOC and already understood current USOC structure and issues: "Jeff had a very good sense of what needed to be done and how it needed to be done."

As for Michael Stephens, Huebner said as he came to know Mike, it came clear to him that he knew of no one else in the United States who had a more passionate, dedicated commitment to the Paralympic movement. "Mike is brilliant," said Huebner. "He's a mentor, an advisor, a friend, and a leader."

Just as the leaders of the USOC praised Lakeshore Foundation's performance as a USOC training site, so did the athletes who came to Lakeshore as a result of that designation.

Below are some examples—the views of some participants who attended training camps hosted by Lakeshore in 2005:

Attending a Lakeshore developmental camp for able-bodied athletes was 18-year-old Conor Beebe, a wrestler from Western Springs, Illinois. Conor was one of 40 teenage wrestlers from various states who came to Lakeshore to hone their skills in wrestling technique. This camp was part of a network of developmental camps in various sports—camps designed to identify and nurture talent in young athletes who might one day win Olympic medals. Conor Beebe had been wrestling since second grade, and he was about to enter Central Michigan University on a wrestling scholarship. His immediate goal was to become a National Collegiate Athletic Association (NCAA) champion in freestyle and Greco-Roman wrestling. Conor spoke of how impressed he was with the wrestling camp support services provided by professionals at Lakeshore—the strengthening and conditioning, the tips on nutrition, the guidance from the sports psychologist. "The sports psychologist here at Lakeshore helped me out a lot," said Conor. "It helped me to hear him explain how that when I go out on the mat I can clear my mind of everything except what I have to do on the mat." Conor also spoke of how much he liked the idea of being at a facility like Lakeshore that catered both to able-bodied and disabled athletes.

Among athletes with disabilities who came to Lakeshore's training camps to train for Paralympics sport, it was common to hear comments about Lakeshore's specialized facilities and highly trained staff.

"A place especially geared for Paralympians! This is the best!" said 36-year-old Sharon Kelleher of San Jose, California, who was among tennis players who came to Lakeshore for a tennis camp. She had been paralyzed at age 17 in a car accident and had gone on to become a Paralympic athlete who was the top-ranked female in the U.S. in

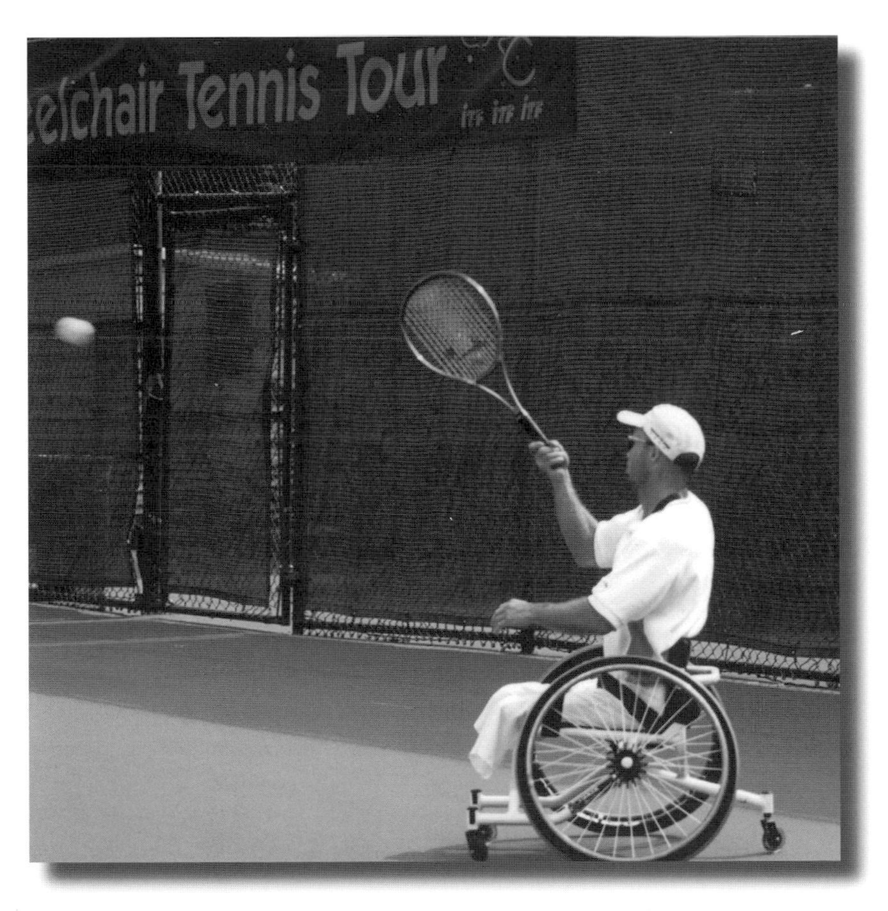

David Hall, serving on Lakeshore's courts.

the women's tennis division. Having had exposure to a wide range of high-quality training facilities, Sharon Kelleher said that Lakeshore was unique in being tailored to the training needs of herself and her Paralympic colleagues, all of whom had some type of physical disability: "Lakeshore is perfect for us!"

Joining in the praise for Lakeshore facilities and staff was Lynn Nelson of Portland, Oregon, who came to Lakeshore for a quad rugby camp. At age 14, Lynn was left with paralysis in parts of both his lower and upper body as a result of a blood clot in his spinal cord. By the time he came to Lakeshore to train in 2005, he already had become a bronze medal winner on Team USA in the Athens 2004 Paralympic Competition—a member of a high-profile team coached by Lakeshore's own staff member Kevin Orr, a team that was featured in the popular feature film *Murderball*. As he took part in Lakeshore's quad rugby camp, Lynn Nelson noted: "The accessibility at Lakeshore is incredible. I know of nowhere else in the world where they have something like this for disabled athletes."

Part VII

The 'People Network' of Lakeshore Foundation

27

The Cornfield

The Lakeshore Spirit: It's akin to what takes place in a cornfield. Centuries ago, as Indian tribes moved northward from Mexico into what is now North America, they brought with them a plant that would become a staple foodsource throughout the world. They understood how each stalk of corn grows and feeds the others until they eventually multiply into a mutually sustainable system.

As Lakeshore Foundation has grown and developed and as the Foundation's people have spread the Lakeshore spirit, Mike says that those individuals "can, in a sense, be compared to those who become part of a highly productive cornfield. It's no secret that at Lakeshore Foundation our 'pollen' is the Lakeshore spirit. That's what we are all about at the Foundation—nurturing others as we are being nurtured, by the sharing and spreading of the Lakeshore spirit.

"If someone is touched by the positive spirit of Lakeshore Foundation, that person can become a seed for further good. The person can share and spread the spirit while working at or being served by Lakeshore Foundation, or the person can use the Lakeshore spirit that has taken root inside him or her to touch individuals in other locations, in other programs, in other settings—thus becoming a seed that helps to grow new 'cornfields' wherever he or she might go."

Lakeshore's focus on teamwork and support allows its staff members to maintain an environment in which those served become part of this inspirational process. "Our staff members realize that tremendous human benefit is derived when clients and their loved ones share their own experiences and encouragement with other clients and their loved ones.

"We realize that a person who has a physical disability might receive his or her greatest help from a teammate on one of our Lakeshore sports teams or from someone he or she meets in our fitness center," Mike notes. "Similarly, we realize that the parent of a disabled child might receive his greatest lesson of the day from another parent who has walked a similar road. Sharing is crucial to helping people."

The mere absence of lab coats or formal uniforms makes a big difference to Lakeshore Foundation's "common ground" environment. Although staff members are well-trained and have valuable experience, they don't emphasize their credentials and degrees to those they serve.

Evidence of this attitude dates back to the beginning of the Foundation's history and is central to its mission and philosophy, Mike said: "Our staff members realize that they are not on one side of an invisible wall of superiority, providing services to clients and their loved ones on the other side. Our staff members are here to work together with the people they serve."

Every individual who comes to Lakeshore Foundation comes to improve and to support the lives of physically disabled people: "No individual is more important or less important than another." Although each person retains his or her own individual identity, there exists a commonality of purpose.

"At Lakeshore we don't see any given individual as being rich or poor, old or young, black or white," Mike emphasizes. "That's one of the beauties of the Lakeshore Foundation. We look beyond your limitations to see your possibilities. We look beyond your missing limb, or your paralysis, or the physical damage you might have incurred from an illness or disease.

"We are not looking at the height of a cornstalk or at the leaves on the stalk. We strip away the leaves and the silk surrounding the ears of corn and look for the essence of the soul that lies at the heart of each ear of corn: the spirit. At Lakeshore Foundation, the glue that holds people together and creates so many success stories has to do with a belief in the human spirit to prevail even when there has been tragedy or loss or disability. We believe that one human being, no matter his or her station in life, has the potential to inspire and motivate another human being."

LAKESHORE FOUNDATION'S LEVEL playing field lets people open themselves to new experiences. Individuals with physical disabilities can learn how to enjoy themselves again. When they can achieve and thrive in the Foundation's nurturing environment, they can feel more and more comfortable doing the same thing in their home communities.

Mike recalls a visit to Lakeshore Foundation by leaders of a well-established rehabilitation center in another part of the country. They were interested in learning some of the secrets to Lakeshore Foundation's success in its sports, recreation, and fitness programs for the physically disabled.

"One of the representatives from this rehabilitation center was discussing the ongoing search for new prostheses and new systems to help extend the functional capabilities of physically disabled individuals," Mike recalls. "Now, I'm all for these new prostheses and new systems, and I know that well-thought-out advances in these areas can help a lot of people. However, I told these visitors who were seeking our Lakeshore Foundation ideas: 'You want to know some of the secrets to what we're doing here at Lakeshore Foundation? Well, we provide an environment in which disabled people are so comfortable, and in which they can see so much of their and others' potential, that they are willing to take off their artificial limbs and put their crutches in the corner if that gives them better access to all the fun and enjoyment that we're having at Lakeshore.' "

WHEN MIKE ESTABLISHED Lakeshore Foundation in the mid-1980s, he had a specific goal in mind: He wanted the Foundation to use sports, recreation, and fitness to help nurture and rebuild the lives and spirits of individuals with physical disabilities. Some of the secrets to that success rested in Lakeshore Foundation's widely hailed programs, in its carefully planned state-of-the-art headquarters building, and in its recruitment and wise use of staff members who have "the right stuff."

However, some of the most touching and lasting secrets to Lakeshore's success rests with the ever-growing "people network" of the Foundation.

"When I refer to Lakeshore Foundation's people network, I'm referring to a wide spectrum of people who in some way are touched by the Foundation and then who go out themselves and positively impact others," Mike says.

The proof, he said, can be seen in the many people whose lives have been positively changed as a result of the Lakeshore Foundation. In the following chapters, some of these people tell their own stories about how they achieved success in confronting the challenges of disability.

28

Joe Ray

Healing Waters

Imagine Lake Martin, near Alexander City, Alabama, in the mid-1980s. Here, a young Joe Ray is learning how to water ski. The catch: Joe is paralyzed from the waist down.

Joe is attending a therapeutic camp located on the lake's balmy shores, Alabama's Camp ASSCA (Special Camp for Children and Adults). Here he meets Phil Martin, who is in charge of Adaptive Aquatics, the water sports program offering services at the camp. Both men will change each others' lives forever.

Joe Ray was 20 years old when, in 1978, he was paralyzed from the waist down by an automobile accident. Through rehabilitation and sheer willpower, Joe soon became a gifted wheelchair athlete. Skilled and fearless, Joe would later become a winning road racer and member of a talented wheelchair basketball team that had to beg for playing space in various Birmingham-area community facilities before ultimately finding a home at Lakeshore's Wallace Recreation Center in the early 1980s.

However, despite his burgeoning athletic career, Joe never expected that he would learn to water-ski, let alone teach others how to enjoy this unique, exhilarating sport.

When Martin suggested that Joe try water-skiing, Joe's usually daredevil, adventurous spirit balked. "Shoot, I can't water-ski," Joe laughed. "I've never water-skied in my life. I can't do that."

But Martin insisted. Soon Joe was water-skiing. From the start, Joe was a natural. He seemingly had been born to fly over the water, swooping in and out of a boat's wake, at a heart-stopping speed.

Hooked on water-skiing, Joe began taking part in Phil's water-skiing program whenever he could. Soon he found himself helping Phil teach other disabled persons how to water-ski. In a short time Joe had gone from being a young man who couldn't imagine himself on water-skis to being a water-skiing instructor.

"At first I had my own selfish reasons for helping Phil to teach other disabled people to water-ski. At the beginning, I did the teaching mainly to have access to Phil's program, so I got in more water-skiing time," Joe remembers.

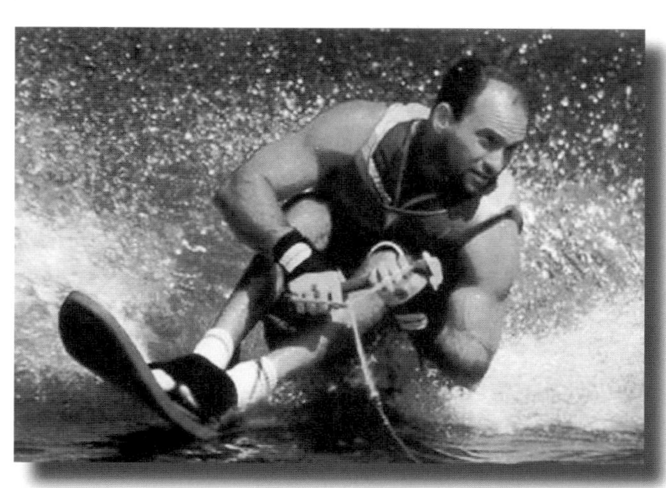

Joe carving up a wake. **BOTTOM:** *Joe at age 51, en route to winning three gold medals at the 2009 Worlds in Vichy, France.*

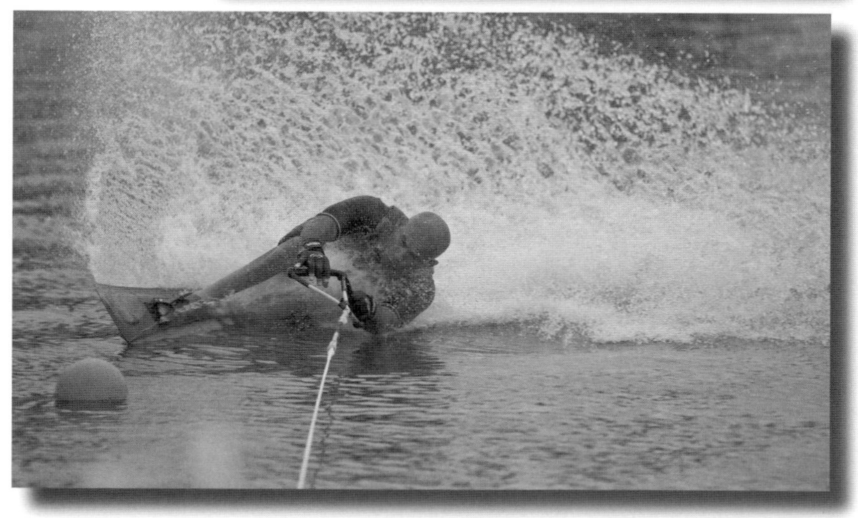

"But then I started figuring out what all this was really about. I found that I was enjoying teaching water-skiing to others who, like me, had disabilities. I enjoyed seeing them get excited about being able to do something they had never done, and had never thought they could do. I thought, 'Wow, this is so cool. I've got to teach some more people!' "

Soon, Joe began skiing competitively . . . and winning.

"As I became more heavily involved in competing, I saw that there weren't really that many disabled individuals who were competing in water-skiing. That inspired me further in my teaching. I thought, 'Hey, I've got to help teach water-skiing to more people with disabilities, so we can get more competitors out there.' "

Inspired by what Phil had accomplished through Adaptive Aquatics, in the late-1980s Joe established a his own water-skiing program, SpudRay Aquatics, named after his own nickname, "Spud."

Then, in 1999, Phil approached Joe and suggested that they merge SpudRay Aquatics with Adaptive Aquatics. Joe became the new executive director of Adaptive Aquatics.

As Joe became more deeply immersed in leading a nonprofit organization to teach disabled people to water-ski, he often found that he was traveling a rocky road.

Running such an endeavor took money. Although Joe used volunteers to provide teaching and lifeguarding support, he had to have equipment—a ski boat, a personal watercraft for his lifeguard, and special equipment for the disabled water-skiers. He had to have funds for marketing, as well as travel expenses associated with his teaching.

Managing such an endeavor required considerable organization and a lot of time, and Joe was also working full-time as a computer programmer and analyst.

By his very nature, Joe had always been determined. Despite his accident, he continued to move forward in life. He was feisty and approached obstacles by fighting back. Joe called attention to architectural barriers in buildings. He stirred up waves by campaigning for more athletic events to be open to athletes with disabilities. This included boldly defying the rules one weekend in Birmingham by maneuvering his wheelchair in the high-profile Vulcan Run race that was open only to able-bodied participants.

However, the spunky approach that had served Joe well throughout his life was put to a test after he became the champion for Adaptive Aquatics. Fundraising was his first challenge. As he began making the rounds to civic clubs and corporations, seeking financial support for his foundation, Joe faced deep insecurities.

Making speeches did not come naturally to Joe. He also felt uncomfortable during some of his one-on-one fundraising appeals to corporate leaders. Joe simply had not been exposed to or coached in the arts of speechmaking and strategic conversation. "My high school senior class had all of 28 people in it. During my early days of public speaking on behalf of Adaptive Aquatics, making those speeches was very hard for me. At first I felt this nervousness of simply not knowing what to say."

There were times when he feared that his unpolished speaking would cause his audience to question whether he really had the ability to run the water-skiing program he was advocating. However, Joe did well enough with his presentations of Adaptive Aquatics' track record that it became easier to speak in front of potential donors. As Joe spoke from the heart about the successes of his students, more organizations invited him to make presentations.

Despite his nervousness at the podium and in one-on-one presentations during those early years, Joe garnered enough fundraising support to keep Adaptive Aquatics afloat. Unfortunately, he was still not able to serve as many disabled clients as he would have wanted. However, he found increasing support from a number of organizations, including Blue Cross and Blue Shield of Alabama, the large health insurance company where Joe was employed for almost 30 years before he began working fulltime at Adaptive Aquatics.

Other obstacles that bothered Joe in those early years included "The Doubters," the naysayers, the people who made it clear they doubted, for one reason or another, that Joe could succeed long-term with Adaptive Aquatics.

"There were some people who obviously felt I could not finish what I had started, that I had bitten off more than I could chew," said Joe. "I had to work hard to get beyond that."

Despite the obstacles, there was that brighter side to the picture that kept Joe pumped: Even as the administrative and fundraising tasks posed perpetual challenges, he found that carrying out the actual mission was fulfilling beyond his wildest dreams. When he was out on the water teaching someone to water-ski, he felt satisfied.

AS JOE WAS managing his small foundation and working his full-time job, he was also winning medals and setting records as a competitive athlete.

Consistent with his determination to excel as an athlete, Joe approached water-skiing with the same fervor that he did his other sports—road racing, track and field, wheelchair basketball, and tennis.

In 2001, he won a national water-skiing championship and an international water-skiing championship, and he set an individual water-skiing world record. During that same year, his Lakeshore Storm wheelchair basketball team won a national championship.

In 2003, he won another national championship, and world championship, and set another world record. In wheelchair basketball, he was a member of another national champion Lakeshore team.

Although Joe continued to play other sports, there was no doubt that water-skiing was his passion.

In Joe's early days of teaching water-skiing, he ran the program out of the backyard of his home on Lay Lake—located just south of Birmingham, near the town of Wilsonville, which for years he had considered his home.

On the one hand, Joe was grateful to have a home located on this beautiful, peaceful lake, a site that could do double duty as the place where he lived and as the place where he taught water-skiing. On the other hand, Joe knew that as long as he ran Adaptive Aquatics out of his small backyard, the compact location was hindering the number of people he could serve and how broadly he could serve them.

"When a disabled individual has a great experience out there on the lake water-skiing—particularly his or her first experience—it's so important that the skier be able to share that experience with friends and loved ones who are watching and cheering from the dock," said Joe. "There is great value in having space for a cheering section."

Unfortunately, there was no space for a cheering section in Joe's back yard at Lay Lake. When the opportunity to relocate and to expand arose, Joe seized it. A choice 2½-acre piece of lakefront property was available for purchase only about a quarter of a mile from Joe's home, still on Lay Lake. The only downside was the price.

AS JOE LOOKED for a way to purchase his dream site, he approached Mike Stephens for help. After hearing Joe's plans for Adaptive Aquatics, Mike agreed to purchase the lakefront property and donate it to the Lakeshore Foundation, which in turn would lease it to Adaptive Aquatics for use as the program's new home base.

Aware of Adaptive Aquatics' impact on disabled people's lives, Mike believed in the program, particularly in Joe's leadership. Mike and Joe first met in 1979, shortly after Joe's accident. Joe had come to Lakeshore's campus to study computer programming. During Joe's time there, he became one of the early residents in Lakeshore's transitional living unit, one of Mike's pet projects.

Mike had not known Joe for very long before he saw how fiery and controversial Joe could be when he was trying to open up new opportunities for the disabled. "While I gave Joe hell for stirring up such disruption in the Vulcan Run with his defiance, at the same time I was in admiration of his reasons and his passion," Mike recalls.

Joe's success as an athlete also impressed Mike. As Joe continued to have a connection with Lakeshore in the 1980s as a star athlete, Mike was pleased to see him and his teammates playing wheelchair basketball in the Wallace Recreation Center—a facility for which Mike had campaigned. Mike watched with pride as the adept basketball players whizzed around the Wallace Recreation Center's sleek basketball court after the team had met so much rejection. Mike enjoyed watching the gutsy, skilled, and versatile Joe Ray who managed to excel in every sport he attempted. Mike understood why Lakeshore Athletic Director Frank Burns gave short-but-lightning-fast Joe the nickname of "Spud," comparing him to the short-but-fast Atlanta Hawks basketball star Spud Webb.

Joe's willingness and ability to become a role model for other disabled individuals, especially children, made an early impression on Mike:

"I saw back in the 1980s that Joe just had that ability to connect with others. I was particularly impressed with the way he inspired Bart Troxell, a young boy who had been injured in a bus accident and who, through Lakeshore, began trying sports. (See Chapter 14: Bart and His Heroes.) That ability to connect and inspire was one of the traits that made Joe so successful with Adaptive Aquatics."

IN SUMMER 2010, construction work was completed on the new Lay Lake home for Adaptive Aquatics. Surrounded on three sides by the lake, the site provided a breathtaking view of the waters beyond.

The location provided a strategically designed starting dock and a separate exit dock, to make it easier to launch and to conclude a water-skiing session. In addition to facilities for water-skiing, Joe noted that there also was a dock for the times when Lakeshore staff brought kayaks to the camp.

In the planning, design, and construction phases, careful attention had been devoted to making the facilities safe amd easy to use.

"Look at the spacious area right next to the boathouse," Joe said, pointing to an expanse of flat deck surface. "If you're standing there, you have access to a clear view of a skier's experience out in the water. That area is what we call our 'Grandstands.' That's where people in our skiers' cheering sections gather, to stand while they watch and cheer on the skiers.

"Now that we have the new facilities in operation here, there's just no way to describe the great atmosphere of interaction and support. These spectators look out and see that the skier is actually skiing, and suddenly from the Grandstands we hear all the cheering and yelling and clapping! It's great for everyone—those of us out on the lake, and the proud observers who are back on land, standing on deck and cheering."

MIKE POINTS OUT one trait in Joe that stood out above all others in his success with Adapative Aquatics, his resolve:

"Joe hasn't just dreamed dreams to help himself. Joe has dreamed dreams to help many other people, and he has been willing to work hard to see that his dreams would bear fruit. I saw an opportunity through Joe to bring the experience of water-skiing into the lives of so many additional disabled individuals.

"The kind of dreaming that Joe has done is realistic dreaming, and it's also an unselfish dreaming. The unselfish dreams of Joe Ray have had a far reach. He continues to function as an outstanding role model."

To many people with severe disabilities, Joe has become an inspirational role model—a high-achieving disabled individual who has lived independently, had a career, enjoyed life, and helped others.

He became particularly influential in the world of paraplegic athletics. At age 51, Joe brought home three gold medals from the 2009 World Disabled Water-Ski Championships in Vichy, France. In 2010 in Indianapolis, Indiana, he was a star at the 21st Disabled Water-Ski National Championship and 2nd Pan-American Championship. Winning event after event, he took home eight gold medals, made the USA Team, and, as a seven-time world-record holder, came close to breaking his own world record.

Despite his success, or perhaps humbled by it, Joe has continued to hold Adaptive Aquatics clinics at Camp ASCCA. After Adaptive Aquatics moved into its new facilities in 2010, the organization began hosting up to 20 water-skiing clinics each year, most of them on Lay Lake. At that point, there were three leading organizations referring clients to Adaptive Aquatics: United Cerebral Palsy, Easter Seals, and Lakeshore Foundation. Because of growing outside interest, Adaptive Aquatics begain to offer sports and recreation programs to injured military personnel, in addition to civilians.

Overall, Lakeshore Foundation is the number one organization with which Adaptive Aquatics now interacts," Joe said in 2010. He said it was very fitting—"for the long-term sustainability of Adaptive Aquatics"—that Lakeshore Foundation had partnered with him to make possible Adaptive Aquatics' new home base.

In 2010, Adaptive Aquatics celebrated its 30th anniversary. As a part of the organization's legacy, first under Phil Martin's leadership and then under Joe Ray's, Adaptive Aquatics had introduced thousands of disabled individuals to water-skiing.

Some of Adaptive Aquatics' water-skiing students had physical challenges that had been dealt by birth defects such as cerebral palsy or spina bifida. Others were dealing with debilitating diseases such as muscular dystrophy or multiple sclerosis. Still others had sustained injuries that had resulted in paralysis or amputations. Among Adaptive Aquatics' water-skiing students were two brothers who were nearly blind.

The students represented a wide range of ages—from the very young to the elderly: "The youngest we have skied was three years old, and the oldest—someone who had polio years ago—was past 80."

Joe grinned as he talked about the joy on the faces of some disabled senior citizens who had an opportunity to water-ski. "This might be the first time some of these elderly men and women have ever water-skied." he said. "It's just as fulfilling for them as it is for a young kid."

Instructors and volunteers who worked in Adaptive Aquatics matched these disabled students with whatever adaptive equipment was necessary to enable them to water-ski. For some students, Adaptive Aquatics might use equipment called "outriggers" on the side of the ski, so the ski would not tip over. For a student with especially severe physical limitations, it might be necessary to use a "sit ski," a larger, wider ski on which the person basically would sit while enjoying a ski ride.

Joe recalls a little girl with severe cerebral palsy: "She couldn't move at all," said Joe. However, with the help of special equipment, she could water-ski.

On the refrigerator at Joe's house in the fall of 2010 was a note

The inimitable Joe Ray, having fun and spreading it to others.

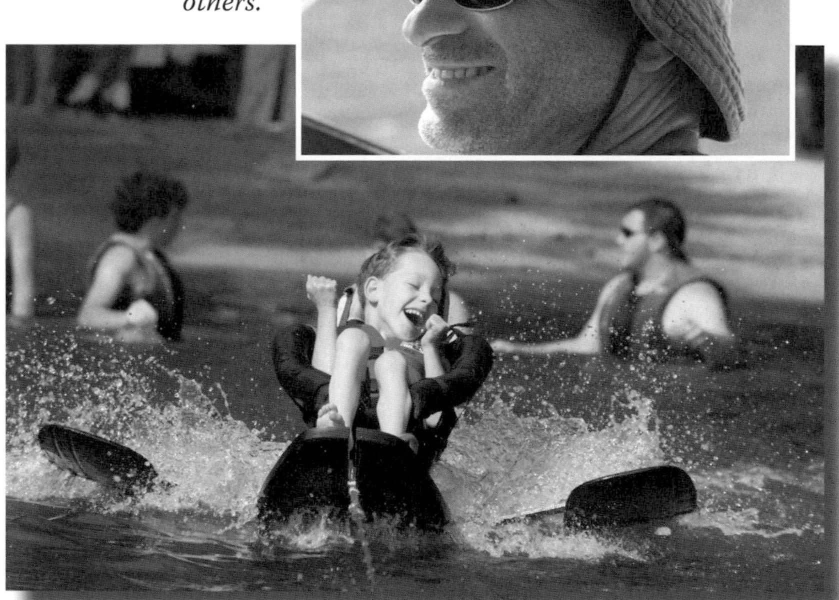

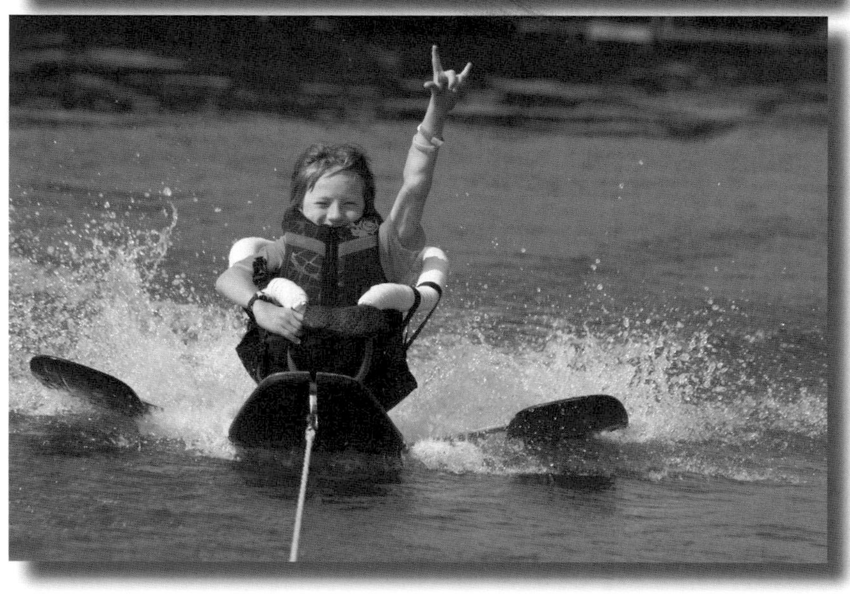

from a child he had introduced to water-skiing. The note contained a cartoon drawing of a young boy on a ski, accompanied by a short but meaningful written message: "Mr. Ray, thank you for letting me ski."

This note is just one example of letters that have come to Joe. He remembers: "As I continued to build the water-skiing program, it soon became apparent to me that I didn't feel as uncomfortable speaking before groups and raising money for the program when I actually talked from the heart about what it was all about—the joy we brought to these water-skiers who had disabilities."

A few weeks after the Adaptive Aquatics new location was ready, an official ribbon-cutting ceremony was held on the grounds. On hand with Joe to cut the ribbon was a teenage boy in a wheelchair. From when he was a child, this boy was a frequent skier at Adaptive Aquatics—one who turned into an accomplished skier. His name is Evan Majewski, and he has cerebral palsy. Evan has become a symbol of success, an inspiration, even for Joe Ray. Joe refers to him as the "poster boy" for Adaptive Aquatics.

The first time Joe ever saw Evan was in a checkout line at Walmart. Since both Joe and Evan were wheeling around Walmart in their wheelchairs, there was an instant feeling of common ground between the two. As Joe made eye contact with Evan, he felt compelled to mention to Evan that he operated a very special water-skiing program. Joe asked the youngster, "Hey, buddy, how would you like to learn how to water-ski?"

Although Evan's mother was wary, she nevertheless took her child to Lay Lake to see what Joe's Adaptive Aquatics was all about. Soon a ski boat was pulling her wonder-stricken water-skiing son over the Lay Lake waters, and a whole new chapter of adventure was launched in the life of Evan Majewski.

"When parents see their child out there water-skiing," Joe says, "usually the child does not seem as fragile as the parents thought he was."

He notes that parents of disabled children as a rule tend to be very protective. Joe describes the reactions of a disabled child and the child's parents the first time the child water-skis: "We let the parents ride in the ski boat, and we do a lot of counseling with these parents, right there in the boat. We also tend to shed a lot of tears. I take a camera and hand it to the parents and tell them, 'Okay, take as many pictures as you want to take!' Then the chain of reactions begins.

"With the kid, the skier, I've seen that little 20-second range of emotions: The child tends to start out like, 'I'm not sure . . .' and then tends to experience a little bit of terror, and then, to be up and skiing with that facial expression that says, 'Oh my God, this is the greatest thing in the world!' From that point, many of these kids are hooked for life on water-skiing. As for the parents sitting there in the boat taking it all in that first time, I've seen their range of emotions as well. The parents tend to go from anxiety, like, 'Is this really safe?' to, when their child is actually skiing, 'Oh, this is awesome!' "

As the years went by, Joe found it increasingly important to convey to disabled individuals that they could achieve in spite of a disability—and often achieve because of a disability.

"I tell people that in a way I feel lucky to have become disabled," he muses. "I think it has driven me. Without my disability, I believe I would be working at some ordinary job, maybe living in a trailer home and going bowling on Thursday nights and not really doing anything that makes a difference in anybody else's life. There's no doubt that what I've been able to do since I became disabled has enriched my life many, many times over."

29

Bob Lujano

Rugby and Religion

In 1979, a 10-year-old boy waits with his grandmother and cousin at a Chicago church to see the newly vested pope, John Paul II. Confined to a wheelchair after a quadruple amputation, Robert "Bob" Lujano has no idea what will happen next: a blessing that will renew his interest in life and lead him to Lakeshore Foundation.

When Bob, a Texan, was taken to see the pope in the fall of 1979, the occasion released him from nine months of hell on earth. A rare blood infection had ravaged Bob's body, resulting in the amputation of both his legs at the thigh-level and the amputation of both his arms just below the elbow.

Despite Bob's severe disability, his paternal grandmother, Hope, knew that it was important to the Catholic boy to see his pope. It was important as well to Hope, who was deeply committed to her faith as well. Hope was her grandson's mainstay; in fact, the reason she was in Chicago was to serve as Bob's caretaker while he went through a rehabilitation program at the Rehabilitation Institute of Chicago.

So Hope Lujano set out to brave the crowds that were gathering for the papal visit, pushing her grandson in his wheelchair while Bob's cousin Gloria Carassco walked alongside them.

First they went to Grant Park, where the pope led the largest Mass ever celebrated up to that time in Chicago. The crowds in the park were as large as 200,000; some estimates were much higher.

Bob's grandmother and cousin decided they could find a better vantage point from which to see the pope if they made their way to a cathedral that would be among his stops. But, even when they arrived at the grounds outside the cathedral they had chosen, the size of the crowds was still daunting.

The threesome was to have some company as they waited.

A police officer with the Chicago Police Department appeared on the scene. His name was Jim Zwit. Spotting the disabled boy and the two women, Zwit appointed himself as their escort.

Bob has never forgotten the kindness shown to them that day.

"Jim Zwit just seemed to take on the attitude of 'Hey, I'm going to hang out with these people and help them,' " Bob recalled. "It was very cold that day, so this police officer brought me a blanket. He would bring me hot chocolate. He would bring me food to eat. When I needed to go to the restroom, he would take me. He was taking care of me as we waited there for those seven hours to see the pope."

When the pope arrived, Zwit knew that only a few in the massive crowd would be lucky enough to get really close to the pope when he stepped foot onto the cathedral grounds. Zwit wanted to make sure that this little boy who had lost his legs and arms would be among those lucky few.

Since he was wearing his uniform and carrying his badge, Zwit crossed the police lines with Bob. He also knew which exit the pope would be taking when he would leave the cathedral and, via a platform, make his way to greet the gathered crowd.

"When I saw the pope, I was awestruck. Why, all of us just lit up like a Christmas tree when we saw the pope," Bob said. "To me he just radiated. He illuminated a certain aura that I've never seen in any other human being—like a holiness aura. I was overcome with joy, just overwhelmed. I remember thinking, 'This is the pope, the person who spearheads the Catholic Church, tracing all the way back to Saint Peter.' "

As the pope made his way to the platform outside the cathedral, Bob was there within touching range. The pope caught sight of Bob and took the child's head in his hands.

"He placed his hands on me and gave me his blessing, in Latin," said Bob. "I remember kissing the pope's ring. He asked Jim about me."

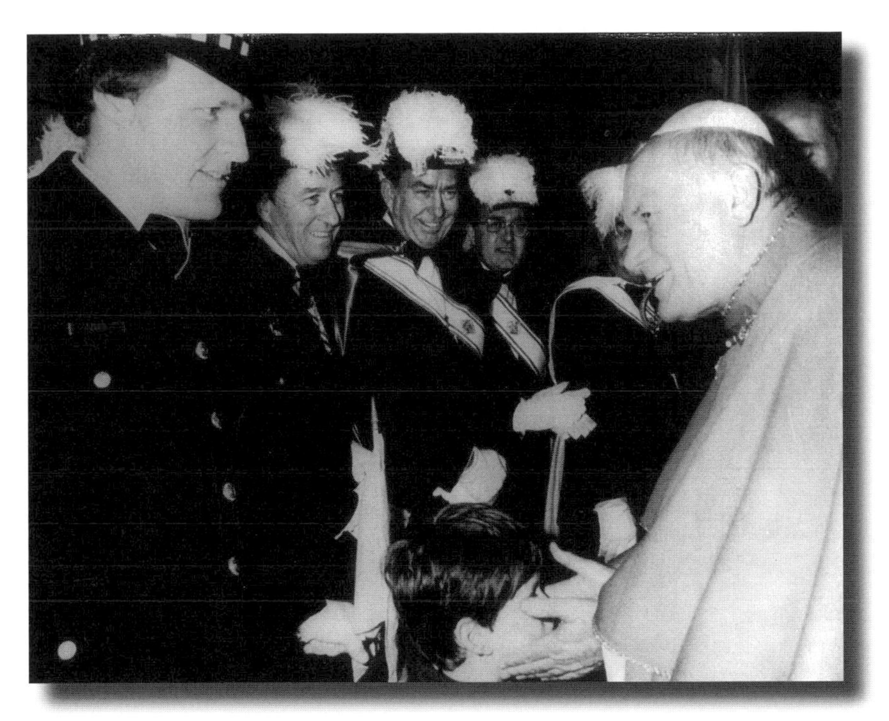

Chicago policeman Jim Zwit escorted the child Bob Lujano to a special moment with Pope John Paul II in 1979.

To Bob, it would seem, from that day forward, that this papal blessing gave him the strength to go on: "Although the pope's blessing was a brief moment in time, it left me with a spark, a motivation. It was like it was God's way of saying to me, 'Hey, everything is going to be okay. You know, don't worry about it.' I just very much felt at that moment that no matter what lay ahead—no matter what surgeries or pain I had to endure—the Lord was going to provide."

Bob started life as a healthy, active child growing up in Irving, Texas. To his family he was known as "Bobby" or by his nickname "Shooter."

Both Bob's dad and his paternal grandfather were big sports fans, and at an early age Bob got turned on to sports. For Bob, the big thing was baseball. His favorite major league baseball player was Pete Rose of the Cincinnati Reds. Bob's T-ball team, the Falcons, had an undefeated season and became the city champions of Irving.

"I played shortstop and second base," Bob remembers. "My dad told me that my job was to stop everything that the opposing team sent my way. And I tried very hard to do that." When Bob executed a particularly good T-ball play—and Bob consistently played well—his dad would praise him and say, "Great, Shooter! Now, that is the way Pete Rose does it!"

Even after Bob's mom and dad separated, there was still a lot of love to go around to the Lujano children. Bob's paternal grandparents, Hope and Bill, joined forces with his dad to help with parenting. Bob and his sister Lisa went to live at the home of their grandparents in Newton, Kansas, a small town about 25 miles north of Wichita.

Bill was a Mexican immigrant who had come to deeply love his adopted country and who won a Purple Heart fighting for the U.S. during World War II. He gained considerable respect in the town of Newton, as he took a leading role in founding a Catholic church there. Consistent with his love for sports, Bill Lujano also founded a fast-pitch softball tournament in Newton.

And then there was Hope, who was an angel in Bob's life. "My Grandmother Hope was the backbone, the heart and soul of the family. She also taught me about embracing our Catholic faith."

A BITTERLY COLD weekend in January 1979 marked the turning point in Bob's life. He was nine and a half years old.

On Saturday night, Bob had enjoyed skating with his friends at the local rink. Later that evening, he returned to his grandparents' house to get a good night's sleep, so he could get up bright and early Sunday morning to perform his role as an altar server at church.

But when it came time for Bob to get out of bed on Sunday morning, something was terribly wrong. Bob had become suddenly and desperately sick, too sick to even move. "I knew that I felt very, very warm," said Bob. "And when my grandparents came in and turned on the light I told them, 'I can't get up!' "

The reason that Bob felt so warm was that he had a dangerously high fever of 104 degrees. He would retain a vague memory of being placed into the car shortly afterward to be rushed to the local hospital there in Newton, and then he would lapse into unconsciousness.

Bob Lujano was on the brink of death. He had contracted a rare, vicious, and fast-moving bacterial infection, *meningococcemia*. The same bacteria that caused meningitis—meningococci—were raging wildly through the blood flowing in his body, clogging up blood vessels, blocking blood circulation.

"My whole body was dark purple, like a big bruise, because the blood was not circulating," said Bob. "At the hospital, they pretty much wrote me off. They actually called in the priest to give me last rites."

In a last-ditch effort to save Bob's life, an ambulance was summoned to transport him from the Newton hospital to a larger hospital in Wichita. The journey was a treacherous one, on roads covered with snow and ice. Along the way, Bob went into cardiac arrest three times.

"My grandmother was in the car that was following the ambulance," said Bob. "Later she told me, 'Bobby, we knew you were going into cardiac arrest because they kept stopping the vehicle and performing CPR on you.' "

Hope also told her grandson of a promise she made to God during that terrifying trip to the Wichita hospital: "Bobby, I promised God that if He would save you, I would dedicate my life to taking care of you."

"When I reached the hospital in Wichita, the doctor knew right away that he had to proceed to amputate both my legs," said Bob.

The powerful meningococci bacteria were carving a rapid path through Bobby's body, setting in play a ruthless process that was destroying his flesh. The specters of gangrene and impending death were hanging over his head

The leg amputations were high, above the knees, only some 8 to 10 inches from Bob's hips.

"In addition to amputating my legs, they also performed a series of blood transfusions to try to clear out the contaminated blood," said Bob. "My blood was so toxic that it was leaking through the walls of my blood vessels and just literally eating my flesh."

In addition to eating away at his legs, the relentless bacteria also were beginning to make inroads with the upper part of Bob's body. Still, doctors held out hope they could save Bob's hands and arms.

But then, a month after his initial illness, that hope went away.

"ONE DAY I was lying there in the hospital, wide awake, when the doctor came in and asked me, 'Bobby, can you move your fingers?' My entire hands were just dark purple, and I could barely wiggle one of my fingers. The doctor shook his head and said, 'That's not enough, Bobby. We're going to have to amputate.' "

On that day, both of Bob's arms were amputated just below the elbow. Young Bob was now a quadruple amputee.

For Bob, losing both his hands and a good portion of both arms in the wake of having lost both his legs created his lowest emotional point since he had became ill.

"That was probably the most depressed I ever felt. After I lost my hands and arms, I just remember crying, sobbing," he said.

Bob would be in the hospital for six months. Including the amputations and skin grafts, he would undergo surgery nine times between January and June 1979—the same year in which he later would meet the pope.

Months after Bob met the pope in Chicago, he was back in school in his own home state of Texas. His dad had remarried and was living in Dallas. In keeping with her promise to God that she would continue to help support her disabled grandson, Hope went to Texas with Bob and remained there for months.

His dad, Robert "Bob" Lujano Sr., played a crucial role in helping Bob to be comfortable with himself, in making him feel at ease as a very young quadruple amputee.

"If people stared and pointed and even laughed at me when they saw I had no arms and no legs, I could see that it did not upset my dad. Actually, my dad would sometimes laugh with them, like it was no big deal," said Bob. "If I had seen my dad getting upset, I would probably have become upset and defensive. So, since my dad didn't get upset, it didn't upset me either."

Resuming life in Texas also opened a new positive chapter in terms of Bob's expanding family. He saw his father's new wife, Edna, not as a stepmother but as a loving, supportive mother in his life. Similarly, when younger brothers Joseph and Julian were born, they were never "half brothers" to Bob; they were brothers.

In his school life, Bob could feel the sting of limitations that came with his disability. Later, he would look back and laugh about some of it. "Whenever anything was going on recreationally at school, in physical education class or whatever, it seemed that I was mainly relegated to playing checkers."

But in the Lujano household, things were different. His dad and new mom created an environment in which Bob was not over-protected, in which he was given leeway and privileges, and in which he also was expected to adhere to certain standards. Bob was not excused from assuming responsibility and achieving because he was disabled.

"It was impressed on me from an early age that I should be independent," Bob emphasizes. "My dad would say, 'You are going to dress yourself. Get yourself ready.' "

Edna Lujano liked an orderly house, and Bob made her proud by keeping his room in order.

"One of the best things that ever happened to me was my dad grounding me for making C's," Bob recalls. "What my dad really wanted was that I make A's. He told me, 'Shooter, just because you are a disabled kid doesn't mean that you can't make A's.' "

Along with the expectations also came the privileges. At the Lujano home Bob wasn't relegated to playing checkers. His parents even allowed him to engage in rough-and-tumble sports: "I remember that a lot of kids would come over to our home in Dallas, and we played football. I would go out there in the grass and roll around and tackle other kids, and they would tackle me. Despite not having arms and legs, I was like, 'Well, I am still going to play, and I am still going to socialize.' "

As he grew into adolescence, Bob developed his own theories about the socializing part. He had a plan: "After I lost my legs and arms, I convinced myself at a young age that I really needed to have a very approachable personality. I could see that people were going to come up to me because of the unusual way I looked and that they were going to stare and maybe even laugh. So I was going to take it and not get defensive about it. And also I was really going to go out of my way to make myself approachable to them—to make myself, you know, fit in, and do all that I could do to be as, I guess, 'normal' as I could be—to be just this regular kid."

WHEN BOB GRADUATED from high school, he first thought he wanted to become a Catholic priest. He enrolled at the University of Dallas, a Catholic university, but, after two years there, Bob believed he could serve God in other ways.

As he changed gears, Bob decided he wanted to become a lawyer and transferred to the University of Texas at Arlington (UTA) to major in pre-law.

Groundbreaking work in collegiate wheelchair sports was underway at UTA, which had a scholarship program for wheelchair athletes. There Bob was introduced to wheelchair basketball.

"I was 20 years old. I thought it was pretty groundbreaking when I learned about wheelchair basketball. Although I wasn't on the wheelchair basketball team at UTA, I would practice with the team."

At that time, Bob wasn't dependent on a wheelchair to move around. He was using prosthetic legs to walk. However, injuries from a car accident resulted in the removal of even more of his left leg. Faced with balance issues, he stopped using his prosthetic legs and began using a wheelchair.

When Bob began applying to law school, he had good grades but not top ones. Viewing law school as no longer a viable option, he began to think that perhaps he could pursue a career in the sports and recreation arena that he had loved so much since childhood.

Bob became seriously interested in pursuing a master's degree in sports management and recreation. Luckily enough, Bob's dad had been transferred to Tennessee; the University of Tennessee offered a master's degree in sports management. So Bob moved to Knoxville. He would be glad he went in that direction.

As a part of completing his degree at the University of Tennessee, Bob interned at a massive operation in Atlanta that facilitated the Atlanta Paralympic Games, which were held a few days after the Centennial Olympic Games during the summer of 1996.

Jack Pursley, a professor at the University of Tennessee, knew the world-famous Georgia native Max Cleland, who wielded considerable influence over the Games. Cleland was a decorated Vietnam hero who had lost both legs and one arm to battle injuries before serving in Georgia state political offices and then holding a high-profile federal post in Washington. Dr. Pursley paved the way for Bob to meet with Cleland.

"When I went to meet with Mr. Cleland, he just rolled out the red carpet for me," Bob recalls. "Since he was a triple amputee and I was a quadruple amputee, of course we had that in common."

After Bob told Max Cleland that he wanted to work with the Atlanta Paralympic Games, Cleland connected Bob with Andrew Fleming, president of the Atlanta 1996 Paralympic Games Organizing Committee (APOG).

The APOG job immediately began to mold Bob's career path. As an APOG "venue director," Bob oversaw the preparedness and maintenance of APOG East, a facility that housed a police department, a military unit, and the headquarters for training and accrediting 12,000 volunteers. Bob performed well, and, after his internship was completed, he was hired to stay on for several additional months.

"I knew after the Paralympic Games that I wanted a career working in disabled sports and recreation, working with disabled people," Bob says.

Enter quad rugby. Atlantan Bill Furbish, who also worked for APOG, first introduced Bob to this spitfire sport. A known wheelchair athlete, Furbish had become a star in water-skiing before founding a quad rugby team in Atlanta: Rolling Thunder.

To be eligible to play quad rugby, a wheelchair athlete must have both upper and lower extremity impairment. The sport is both exciting and grueling. In an incredibly fast-paced environment, players collide their wheelchairs without inhibition. Skilled quad rugby teams compete to score points by carrying a ball similar to a volleyball over the goal line by passing, dribbling, and carrying it down a basketball-sized indoor hardwood court. A combination of football, basketball, and ice hockey, Quad rugby originated in Canada, but did not catch on in the U.S. until the 1980s, when it rapidly gained popularity. Years later it would be hailed by the United States Quad Rugby Association as "the fastest-growing wheelchair sport in the world."

Also known as "wheelchair rugby," quad rugby has been referred to as "murderball," a testament to the sport's fast pace and intensity. Spectators marvel at the skill, agility, and fearlessness of quad rugby players, who, despite having such pervasive disability, play the rough-and-tumble game as though they have no disability at all.

Quad rugby was a sport that suited Bob. He began playing on the Atlanta Rolling Thunder team before going on to play on Lakeshore Foundation's quad rugby team, known as the Demolition. With Demolition, Bob would go on to medal internationally.

"From the time Bill Furbish introduced me to quad rugby in Atlanta, I started playing right away and loved it!" said Bob.

Bob's first visit to Lakeshore was as a member of Rolling Thunder, which was competing against the Demolition at Lakeshore's Wallace Recreation Center. When he first encountered Lakeshore, Bob knew very little about Lakeshore Foundation's programs: "At the beginning, I just knew Lakeshore as a place where I was going to compete in quad rugby."

Bob would quickly learn more about Lakeshore Foundation and its programs. The more he learned, the more impressed he became. When he was told there was a job opening on the Lakeshore Foundation staff, he applied. Until Lakeshore, Bob had been working in other types of jobs, including with a medical products company and a telecommunications company, not in the sports management and recreation field for which he had studied.

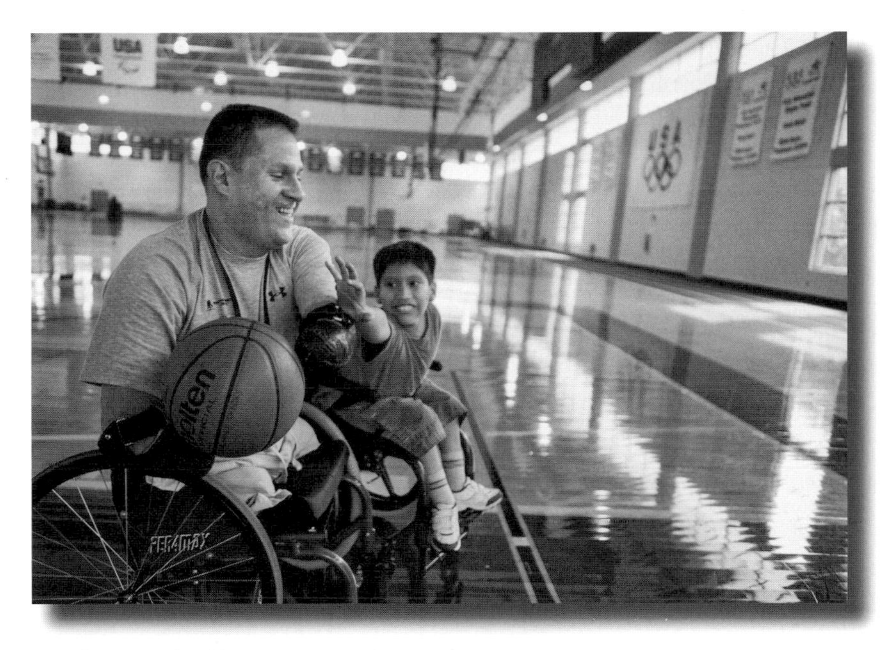

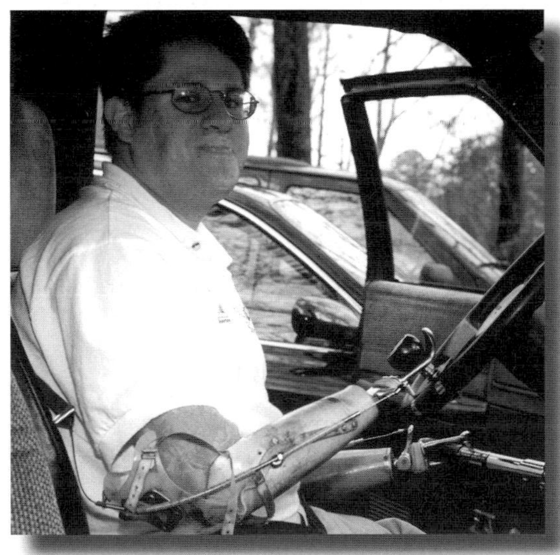

Above, Bob Lujano plays basketball with Renado Jurado on one of Lakeshore's hardwood courts. Left, Bob behind the wheel of his car.

On November 1, 1998, Bob began working at Lakeshore Foundation as a youth coordinator. He was elated.

BOB'S JOB AT Lakeshore Foundation focused on involving children in sports and recreation programs, particularly Lakeshore's after-school programs and Super Sports Saturday. He taught sports skills at the entry level, such as how to use a wheelchair and dribble a basketball at the same time. If kids had the potential and the desire to take part in competitive sports, he could steer them in that direction as well. By identifying sports abilities in kids, he could connect them with coaches at Lakeshore who would then work with them in various types of competitive team or individual sports.

Because of his own physical disability, Bob could identify with the disabled children at Lakeshore. He knew firsthand what a gift it could be for them to be able to participate in sports and recreation.

"Even though a few years had passed since I was a young kid, I knew that in most school systems there were still very limited opportunities for kids with physical disabilities to participate in sports and recreation," Bob said. "In that regard, many school systems had not changed much since when I was a kid relegated to playing checkers during physical education classes."

Bob felt he had found his dream job at Lakeshore Foundation: "To be able to come to Lakeshore and work with youth . . . well, in my opinion I felt that the Lord had directed me there. After I was left with my disability, I could not help but think, 'What purpose do I have? What purpose does the Lord have for a guy with no hands and no legs? What can I do to make a difference in this world?' Well, to me, the Lord said, 'Bob, you can go to Lakeshore Foundation and work with kids. You can help teach them to be independent and show them that, despite what they do not have, they can have a life. Bob, you have a future, you have direction, you have purpose. This is what you are going to do.' "

The more Bob worked at Lakeshore Foundation and saw lives being changed, the more he thought of it as being unique: "To me, Lakeshore is a liberating place. It's a place of freedom."

Bob also saw that Lakeshore was a place where kids could find the motivation to become more independent. It was a place for positive pushing, for encouragement, and for growth.

One child who struck a chord with Bob was Mark Zucker, an 11-year-old with cerebral palsy living in the Birmingham suburb of Mountain Brook. Extremely dependent on his parents, Mark used a motorized wheelchair so that he did not have to exert himself physically. When Mark became involved at Lakeshore Foundation, that began to change. "We got Mark out of that power chair and into a manual chair," Bob recalls.

It wasn't easy. At first the boy had to work just to push his wheelchair a few feet. But the important thing was that Mark was learning, learning to catch a ball and to push his wheelchair. Bob proudly remembers when Mark took ten minutes to maneuver the manual wheelchair the same distance that once had taken him half an hour. Plus, Mark was learning to handle a ball and to push his wheelchair at the same time. He soon joined Lakeshore Foundation's junior wheelchair basketball team.

With his newfound skills, Mark began to be more independent outside of Lakeshore. Bob says, "You know, if you can push your wheelchair up a hill and you can catch a ball, then it also begins to affect you positively in your everyday life independence. That's what happened with Mark. His mother came to me and said, 'You know, Mark no longer wants me to help him brush his teeth, comb his hair, or put on his shirt. He wants to do all that himself.' "

BOB JOINED SOME high achievers at Lakeshore Foundation by taking on the double role of staff member and athlete—standards for both were high.

Lakeshore Foundation had a long track record of winning medals at regional, national, and international levels. Its athletes spent hours working out, practicing with their team, playing in games, and traveling to competitions and meets. Since Lakeshore's teams tended to do well, the teams' schedules included tournaments at higher levels of competition.

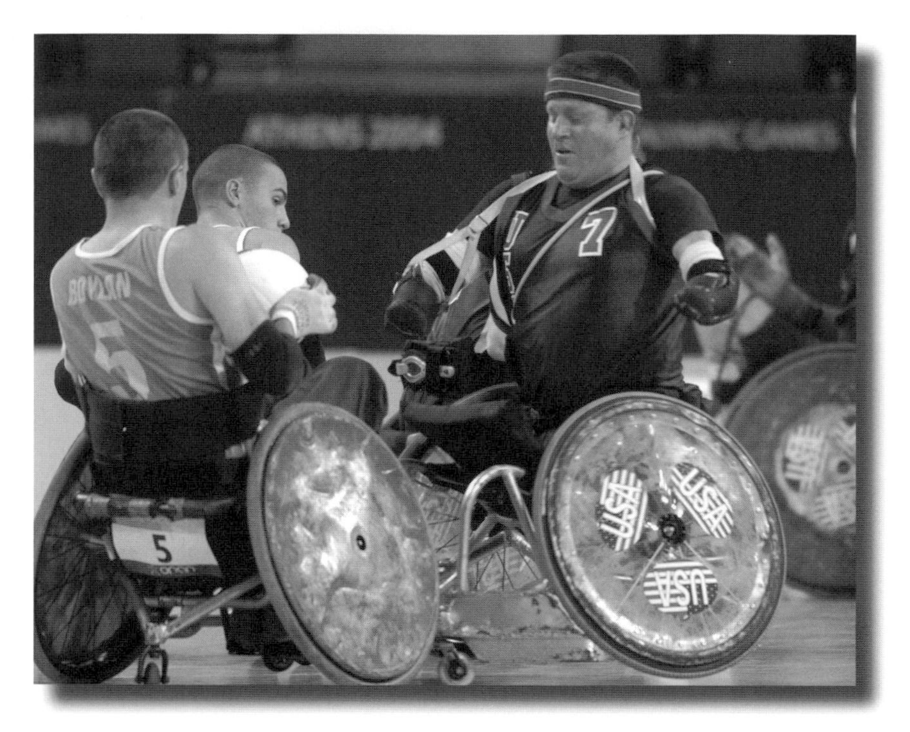

Bob Lujano and other Lakeshore athletes competing in quad rugby.

Such was the case when Bob became a member of the Lakeshore Demolition quad rugby team. This team was well-known as one of the best teams in quad rugby—actually, one of the best quad rugby teams anywhere in the world.

(Demolition's success was due, in part, to its founder and coach, Kevin Orr, who was so successful as Lakeshore's quad rugby coach that he was selected to coach the elite Team USA that competed in the international Paralympics.)

A TOURNAMENT SPONSORED by the United States Quad Rugby Association (USQRA) took Bob Lujano and his Lakeshore Demolition teammates to Chicago in the spring of 2005 for the Heartland Sectional Playoffs. "To go on to nationals, we had to win at the tournament in Chicago," Bob said.

Chicago was a special place for Bob. This visit was especially poignant because Pope John Paul II, who had blessed him at the Chicago cathedral 26 years ago, was gravely ill. As Bob arrived in Chicago, he was painfully aware that that pope who had so touched his life—and the world—lay near death thousands of miles away in Rome. As soon as Bob could, he made his way to the same cathedral as before and went inside to pray for the pope.

Bob had attracted attention since his amputations at age nine. As Bob left the cathedral on this day, a CBS News correspondent approached and asked him some questions. On hearing Bob's story, the reporter said he wanted to share the details with a CBS producer.

"I just went in to say my prayers, and this guy comes up to me and says, 'Hey, who are you? What happened to you?' "Bob remembers with a laugh.

As it turned out, Pope John Paul II died that weekend, on Saturday, April 2. In Chicago, an American city that had especially embraced that pope, the grief was palpable. Bob had his own all-consuming grief. He knew that he had to manage that grief as he moved forward in the quad rugby tournament.

The interview that CBS had requested with Bob, about his connection with the pope, took place in Chicago that weekend. Bob was interviewed by one of CBS's most experienced and popular correspondents, Bob McNamara.

During what continued to play out as an almost surreal weekend for Bob, he went through a kaleidoscope of feelings. In contrast to the deep sadness he was feeling about the pope's death, Bob was happy to be reunited with Chicago family members who gladdened his heart. To top it all off, Bob was reunited with an old friend who had retired from a career with the Chicago Police Department and now was working as a private investigator: Jim Zwit.

This emotional reunion with Jim Zwit, the kind police officer who had taken Bob to see the pope, had been 26 years in the making: "When I saw Jim Zwit, it was on the Saturday night just hours after the pope had died that afternoon, and it was right in the middle of our playing a game at the quad rugby tournament. They had pulled me out of the game to take a short break; and Jim and his son come running over to me. I looked at Jim, so glad to see him, and just all these memories . . . all these memories came back at that moment."

At the end of the weekend, the Lakeshore Demolition won the tournament. The team was headed for the nationals. And the player who was selected to receive the coveted award as the tournament's Most Valuable Player was Bob.

ON THE EVENING of August 3, 2005, *Larry King Live* aired an interview with internationally known quad rugby players.

King interviewed Bob Lujano and four of his teammates. The team was there promoting the recently released documentary titled *Murderball*—a film that months later would be nominated for Best Documentary Feature at the 78th annual Academy Awards. The film, which gave a behind-the-scenes look at quad rugby, traced the rivalry between Team USA, coached by Lakeshore Foundation's Kevin Orr, and Canada's quad rugby team—all leading up to the two teams' competition in the 2004 Paralympic Games in Athens, Greece.

Just the reality that Bob was talented enough at quad rugby to play on such an international stage, and to be one of quad rugby's spokespeople on CNN, spoke to the success of his quad rugby career.

During the popular cable-television program that he hosted on that August 2005 evening, CNN's Larry King asked Bob about the upper and lower extremity disabilities of himself and his team members.

"I'm actually a quadruple amputee," Bob explained. "I did lose both of my arms and legs to a rare blood disease." Bob went on to explain to King and the TV viewers that his fellow Team USA teammates had impairment in their extremities as a result of various causes, including severe spinal injuries.

Later in the interview, King asked about the athletic backgrounds of the Team USA members. Bob said, "I think all of us have one thing in common, in that we all were very much athletes, you know, before our accidents, and very much competitive-natured."

And so it went . . . as Bob was among those to take the lead in a worldwide opportunity to explain to the public about the history and motivation and players behind this game known as quad rugby.

Bob's decision to commit himself to a career in quad rugby put him on the road toward the same rewards and challenges of any other successful athlete. "Quad rugby helped me keep my body in shape, make friends that would last forever, and travel around the world to places I otherwise would never have gone," Bob said. "At the same time, for me and for my teammates, what we would accomplish would be done with a lot of hard work and with tremendous personal sacrifice."

Through the years, Bob and his Lakeshore Demolition teammates shared the gratification of winning many a game. Also, as Bob had a chance to enjoy success as a Team USA member and to participate in Paralympic competition, medals and honors continued to come his way.

Bob won a gold medal at the World Championship Wheelchair Games in New Zealand, a silver medal at the World Games in Sweden, and a bronze medal at the 2004 Paralympic Games competition in Athens that was featured in *Murderball.*

"I still view winning the bronze as being a real honor," Bob explains. "After all, we were playing at the top level in the world—in the equivalent of the international Super Bowl."

The thrill and satisfaction that Bob found through quad rugby created a lasting joy that he didn't take for granted. "I have viewed playing quad rugby as an affirmation. Quad rugby has brought me an opportunity to enjoy a competitive sport I love. And if I did not have my disability . . . and even if my disability were something different in the sense of having a disability that did not affect both upper and lower limbs . . . I could not have played quad rugby."

And Bob Lujano could not imagine what it would have been like not to have had the opportunity to play quad rugby.

In 2008, Bob celebrated a decade of serving as a staff member and athlete at Lakeshore Foundation. During that time, he had seen a tremendous growth and development of the Foundation. In 2001, Lakeshore Foundation opened its new building. In 2003, the Olympic Rings emblem went up at the Foundation's campus, signaling Lakeshore's prestigious designation as a United States Olympic Committee training site for both Olympic and Paralympic athletes.

And, along the way, Bob had seen growth and changes in Lakeshore Foundation programs and a broadening base of those served by the programs. As Lakeshore's membership broadened and diversified, Bob found himself working with members who had incurred physical disability as a result of chronic health problems such as arthritis, diabetes, and heart disease. Along with this expanded membership came an influx of members who were in their middle and senior years—adults who shared Lakeshore's progressive facilities along with children, teens, and young adults.

"At Lakeshore Foundation, I'm now working with kids as young as age three and senior citizens as old as 101," Bob explained in 2010. He said that he enjoyed his interaction with individuals in these diverse age groups who had various physical disabilities.

When it came to Bob's own career as a Lakeshore quad rugby athlete, he had to confront age-related issues: "I turned 41 in the summer of 2010. I have decided it's time to be done with U.S. quad rugby." At the time, he was still in the process of deciding whether he would continue to play a while longer with his home quad rugby team.

Regardless of how much quad rugby he did or did not play in the future, Bob said he already had enjoyed a great ride with the sport. Regardless of how much he played competitive sports in the future, Bob was determined to continue to keep his body strong and in shape by making use of Lakeshore's top-of-the-line workout facilities.

Bob continued to overcome barriers without giving it much thought. If stairs were in his way and it was difficult to get his wheelchair over them, he would get out of his wheelchair and use his strength to slide or roll his body to maneuver the stairs. While other people might marvel at Bob's abilities to do this, Bob didn't marvel. That was just how he lived his life.

Bob did marvel, however, at the opportunities that continued to come his way as a result of his disability. "I give thanks for my life," he concludes. "Actually, I give thanks for my disability. There are many reasons why I thank God for my disability."

30

The Rightmyer Family

Color-Blind

Three young men and a young woman met because they all loved disabled sports. Two were black, two white. At first, they did not seem like family, but Casandra, Master, Brian, and Jessie redefined what it means to be a family and what it means to achieve with every dribble of the basketball, every pass, and every goal.

They are the Rightmyers, and they are family.

As the award-winning film *The Blind Side* was capturing worldwide audiences in 2009, another "blind side" was occuring in the little Alabama town of Deatsville. There, two nurses, Melanie and Joe Rightmyer, were raising their daughter Casandra to be a bright, talented, and athletic young woman despite her confinement to a wheelchair. Born with spina bifida, Casandra was tenacious and fierce, and she enjoyed most of all her participation in the junior wheelchair basketball team at Lakeshore Foundation. In fact, she loved it so much that she often made the hour-and-a-half trip to Birmingham just to play.

There, the Rightmyers met Master Hinkle and Brian Bell. Despite the odds, the Rightmyers would open their home and their hearts to the two young men and, later, Jessie Atwell. Despite the odds, they would become a color-blind family bound by love and trust.

Casandra, Master, Brian, and Jessie came to know one another because each had a physical disability and an interest in sports. Of the four, Casandra was the only one with a disability since birth.

Master was left paralyzed from the waist down at age three after an aneurysm on his spine ruptured following injuries he sustained in a car wreck.

Brian's leg was amputated just above ankle level—a result of an incident involving a train. When he was a few weeks shy of his tenth birthday, Brian slipped while walking between two railroad cars, and a train car rolled over his leg.

Jessie underwent amputations on both his legs, at a level below the knee, after he was stricken with spinal meningitis at age five and complications of the illness attacked his legs.

Master, Brian, and Casandra were the first to meet.

MASTER HAD LIVED far from an easy life. His mother passed away when he was eight years old, five years after he was paralyzed.

"My mother was only 29 years old when she died," he recalls. "She had cancer, and she waited to seek treatment."

Master's dad was not a presence in his life. After his mom died, his grandmother helped take care of him. But, later on, Master's grandmother would also develop cancer. Soon, she was unable to take care of him. By the time the Rightmyers took him in, Master, a high school junior, had been living for a time with his sister, who, residing in a cramped apartment, also had a newborn. It was time for Master to move again.

Running out of housing options, Master was about to leave Birmingham to move in with a relative in north Alabama when the Rightmyers approached him about living with them. Leaving Birmingham meant leaving behind Lakeshore Foundation and his participation in wheelchair basketball, which he had been playing since second grade when an elementary school teacher told him about Lakeshore's sports opportunities. As Master had grown from a young boy into a powerfully built, athletically inclined teenager, playing sports at Lakeshore helped sustain him through deeply painful losses in his life.

Although the Rightmyers lived ninety miles from Birmingham, access to Lakeshore was not an issue in their household. Lakeshore was so important to the Rightmyer family that the Lakeshore commute was made regularly. Casandra made the long trip to attend Lakeshore's wheelchair basketball practices and games. To the Rightmyers it was simple: Why not have one more resident in their household? Why not have one more passenger in their vehicle on those commutes to Lakeshore?

It was 2004 when Master moved into the Rightmyer home.

A FEW MONTHS after Master moved in, the Rightmyers received a telephone call from Brian's mom, saying that Brian needed access to high school studies that were more geared to his goals to attend college and to play collegiate wheelchair basketball. Brian had already spent the summer with the Rightmyers and felt welcome with them. The Rightmyers felt that Brian deserved a shot at his dream of going to college.

So, when Brian, a gifted athlete, returned from playing summer international wheelchair basketball in the United Kingdom, he, too, moved into the Rightmyer home.

UNLIKE MASTER AND Brian, Jessie didn't meet the family through the Lakeshore Foundation.

A resident of a small town not far from Deatsville, Jessie entered the Rightmyers' lives one day when he went to a Health Department clinic to update his immunizations. The Health Department just happened to be where Joe Rightmyer was working as a nurse practitioner.

When Joe saw the teenager walk into the office on two prosthetic legs, he called Jessie's mother and told her about Lakeshore Foundation's athletic opportunities—and asked her if Jessie might be interested.

"I knew the really good things that Lakeshore already had done for our daughter and for Master and Brian," Joe remembers. "I thought Lakeshore might be good for Jessie, too."

Already attracted to athletics, Jessie had been a competitive wrestler at the school he was attending. Soon Jessie was also traveling from south-central Alabama to Birmingham with Casandra, Master, and Brian, and playing wheelchair basketball at Lakeshore.

Unfotunately, Jessie was not excelling in school like he was in athletics. Through the years, school had been a rough road for Jessie. After his long bout with spinal meningitis, its complications, and the leg amputations, Jessie had fallen behind academically. He was frustrated. With one year of high school to go, there was even talk of Jessie dropping out of school and taking the GED test.

"By the time Casandra approached us with the idea of Jessie moving in, Joe and I were empty nesters," Melanie admits. "A few years had gone by since Master and Brian had moved in, and Master, Brian, and Casandra had all moved out to go to college. So here Joe and I were, confronted with the question, 'Can Jessie move in, so that you can help Jessie, too?' I mean, how do you turn away someone who is so thirsty for education, for learning, for independence, as was the case with Jessie? So we let Jessie move in."

Melanie pauses as she describes how she and Joe went about making that decision: "There are times when you are led to do something not because it's the easy thing to do, but because you know it's the right thing to do."

So, in 2009, his senior year, Jessie enrolled at the same high school near the Rightmyer home that had accepted Master and Brian—Holtville High. "The principal at that school was awesome—for Master, Brian, and Jessie," Casandra explains. "Whenever someone new would move into my parents' home, this Holtville High principal was kind of like, 'Oh, so we have another one!' " And then, Casandra said, the principal would make sure the boys got the support they needed.

WHEN CASANDRA WAS growing up as a little girl confined to a wheelchair, she sometimes had trouble fitting in with her peers. "I had a few friends that I found out weren't really my friends," she acknowledges. "They would talk about me behind my back and laugh at me, making fun of me for being in a wheelchair, for being different."

Although Casandra was academically capable, being rejected by her peers damaged her self-esteem. She began picking and choosing her social situations, and her schooling became a combination of public and home schooling.

Casandra had athletic ability, though, and she loved athletics. After she began playing wheelchair basketball at Lakeshore, new opportunities opened up to her. Among her exciting experiences was traveling as a spectator to Athens for the 2004 Paralympics. This was her reward for being selected at Lakeshore Foundation for the Paralympic Academy program sponsored by the United States Olympic Committee's Paralympics Division. The purpose of the program was to demonstrate to gifted young people such as Casandra that athletes with physical disabilities could achieve at very high levels.

The Lakeshore Foundation and the opportunities it provided became so important to the Rightmyers that Joe turned down a dream job in North Carolina to stay in Alabama: "I couldn't take our daughter away from Lakeshore Foundation."

FOR MASTER, THERE were many adjustments to make after he moved in with the Rightmyers. There was the academic adjustment—he had to complete his English assignments, like it or not. There was also a cultural adjustment. He moved from a predominantly African American, urban community to a predominantly white, rural neighborhood.

But Master's greatest adjustment after he moved in with Joe, Melanie, and Casandra was that, for the first time in his life, he had to deal with having people around him who were asking him to share his feelings.

To some folks, all that interest from others might be welcomed as caring attention. But to Master it was uncomfortable—something to which he had to become accustomed before he could embrace it. He would later say that he had experienced so many tragic losses in his young life that he had emotionally walled himself off.

"It was around the time I was eight or nine years old when I reached the lowest point in my life," Master says, recalling the period when he lost his mother to cancer.

"At my mom's funeral, I was eight years old, glancing over at her casket, and looking around like, 'Isn't my mom going to wake up in a second?' And they were like, 'No, she's not.' That's the day I first grasped that things aren't going to be here forever.

"And then I went bouncing around through family members and stuff, before I actually lived with my grandma."

Somewhere along the way, explained Master, he began to isolate himself emotionally. "I guess I really became unwilling to open up to somebody and maybe then lose somebody else."

After Master moved in with the Rightmyers, Melanie, Joe, and Casandra would ask him the kinds of questions that family members often ask one another. When he came home from school, they would ask him how his day went. When he was going out somewhere, they would ask where he was going and when he would return. If he seemed bothered about something, they asked what was wrong.

Later Master laughed as he recalled his adjustment period to all this. "I just wasn't used to somebody bugging me with all those questions," he said. "That was alien to me. I was used to working it out myself."

AFTER INVESTING SO much of herself in helping kids who had physical disabilities, Melanie would find that the tables would turn on her and that she, too, would go through a period of physical disability.

One day she tripped over a dresser drawer, fell, and broke her foot in four places. In the aftermath of her accident, she was also diagnosed with severe osteoporosis. As a result of the accident and the osteoporosis, Melanie had to use a wheelchair for several months.

Out of this experience, Melanie said she gained more insight into the challenges that her daughter faced. Casandra, too, gained something out of the experience. As Casandra began helping out more with household chores to support her ailing mother, she gained an extra measure of independence.

"This occurred when Casandra was a senior in high school, and during that year Casandra was doing a lot of grocery shopping and a lot of laundry around our house," Melanie recalls. "It was the next year when she left home to go off to college and for the first time began living on her own—attending a large out-of-state university hundreds of miles away from Joe and me. Because of all the household duties that Casandra took on after I was injured, I believe she was much more prepared to go out and live on her own than she otherwise would have been."

As Casandra, Master, and Brian made plans to go to college, all three had college athletics as a part of their plans—namely, wheelchair basketball. And all three were helped along with athletic-related scholarship money.

Master was the first to finish high school and head for college. In 2006, he became a student at the University of Alabama's campus in Tuscaloosa, where he played on the men's wheelchair basketball team.

Casandra and Brian both finished high school in 2007. Both had wheelchair basketball scholarships at a university long known for its wheelchair sports programs—the University of Illinois. They began classes at the University of Illinois sprawling Urbana-Champaign campus and began playing wheelchair basketball there.

For Brian, wheelchair basketball would take him places where he otherwise could never have dreamed of going.

He played abroad several times. He became connected to the United States Olympic Committee (USOC) sports, and was placed in tournaments involving USOC-sponsored Team USA. "I had an opportunity to go to England when I was only 16 years old as the youngest in the group of wheelchair basketball players I was playing with there," he said. As time went on, he would play wheelchair basketball in various parts of the United Kingdom as well as in France and Canada.

Wheelchair basketball would be Brian's financial ticket to college, via his University of Illinois athletic scholarship. "My wheelchair basketball scholarship led to my going to a university that is great academically," said Brian. His scholarship covered all of his tuition and other academic needs at an expensive university. With a strong interest in graphic design, Brian chose to major in communications with a minor in advertising.

His journey had begun years before at Lakeshore Foundation, where he was introduced to the world of wheelchair sports. "It was at Lakeshore where I had a place to train, and a place to meet other people in my situation—other people who had a prosthesis or were in a wheelchair," he said. "At Lakeshore, I met amazing people who were working there on the staff—people who helped me and wanted to see

Casandra Rightmyer with Mike Stephens at the 2004 Paralympics in Athens. She is second from left on the championship wheelchair basketball team below.

LAKESH
FOUNDATION
LAKESHORE SHARKS
2003
JUNIOR PREP
WHEELCHAIR BASKETB
NATIONAL
CHAMPION
(18 - 1)

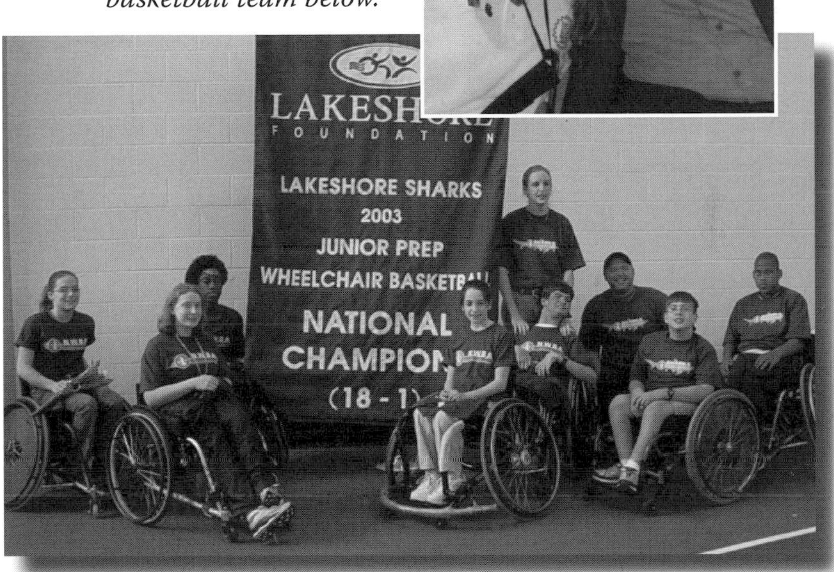

me grow and go out in the world and achieve."

After Brian's journey in wheelchair sports began at Lakeshore, it was the Rightmyer family that helped him get the academic foundation he needed to go on to college:

"I grew up and went to school in a section of Birmingham where the teachers were not that accustomed to working with students who really intended to go on to college. Then I moved in with the Rightmyers and was able to attend Holtville High School."

At Holtville High, Brian found a faculty that worked with him in his studies. He also found faculty and students who expressed interest in his athletic passion—wheelchair basketball. "They were so interested in what wheelchair basketball was all about that they asked Master, Casandra, and me to do wheelchair basketball exhibitions for them, which we did," said Brian. He said on a couple of occasions they asked fellow Lakeshore Foundation basketball players to join them in those exhibitions.

When Casandra went off to college, she already had a history of doing well academically. She continued to do well in her studies at the University of Illinois, making mostly A's in her undergraduate kinesiology major. She had a goal of later earning a master's degree in occupational therapy.

Although academics came naturally to Casandra, she still had her share of struggles as a college coed. As she juggled her busy college life of going to class, playing on the women's wheelchair basketball team—including all those practices and traveling with the team—she often had to stretch herself, and then stretch some more.

She would smile later as she looked back on some of the day-to-day challenges—such as managing her mobility in harsh winter weather to which she, a Southern girl, was not accustomed. There was one snowy, icy morning during her freshman year that she particularly recalled. She was trying to pop the wheels off her wheelchair to load the chair into her vehicle so that she could drive to an early class, but the temperatures were so frigid that the wheels actually froze to the chair.

"I pulled and tugged until finally I was able to pull one of the wheels off the chair. But that other wheel would not budge; that wheel was frozen solid! So I had to lug the chair into my Jeep, with one wheel still frozen onto the chair. But I got it in, and I made it to class."

Other challenges that Casandra faced as a college student—namely her health problems—were far more serious. She suffered from pneumonia, bronchitis, strep throat, swine flu, and kidney infections. At one point she had to take a break from her studies and return home for a semester. But, come the next semester, she returned to the University of Illinois and once again was back to her busy schedule.

JESSIE WAS AT a crossroads in his life when Joe and Melanie Rightmyer considered taking him in with them. His school life had suffered due to his health problems. He had fallen behind in his studies, was a couple of years older than his classmates, and was running out of physical "steam" and psychological motivation.

"Our daughter was so afraid that Jessie was going to become a high school dropout," Joe said. Casandra appealed to her dad and mom, "Can't you take Jessie in, like you took in Master and Brian, and just get Jessie through this last year of high school?"

After Jessie moved in, in May 2009, the Rightmyers went to bat for him in several ways.

They helped in his getting new prosthetic legs that were a better fit. Although he used the prostheses most of the time, the Rightmyers also saw to it that he got a wheelchair to use as backup.

Melanie became Jessie's advocate in convincing the powers-that-be to give Jessie credit for some home schooling that he had had in the past. "Jessie had been so young when he got sick," Casandra explains. "He was so sick—in a coma at the beginning. After that, he had to be home-schooled, and then later on he wasn't even getting credit for his home schooling."

After Melanie intervened, Jessie received credit for his home schooling and enrolled at Holtville High. And, as Joe put it, "Jessie's grades began to come up drastically." The reason? Joe laughs: "Well, in my view Jessie's grades started going up because Jessie's rate of absenteeism in school started going down. After he moved in with us, Melanie and I required that he attend school regularly. If Jessie was feeling a little below par, that was no excuse to miss a day of school."

By that time, playing basketball at Lakeshore had become very important to Jessie, just as it had been to Casandra, Master, and Brian. Even though Jessie was now the only teenager residing in the Rightmyer home, he continued to have the Lakeshore Foundation athletic opportunity. Each week, Joe accompanied Jessie on the commute to Birmingham, so that Jessie could participate in Lakeshore wheelchair basketball.

In Casandra's eyes, it was one of her parents' finest hours when, after having already taken in Master and Brian, they did the same thing for Jessie. "Since they do for others out of Christian love, I think sometimes they don't even really realize what a tremendous positive difference they make in the lives of people they help," she says. "I only hope that I can have the same giving spirit that my parents have."

It was through her dad's caring gesture that Casandra first met Jessie, after her dad invited him to go to Lakeshore with her, Master, and Brian. Casandra was playing on Lakeshore's varsity wheelchair basketball team when Jessie started playing on Lakeshore's junior varsity team.

"In that time frame when I was first getting to know Jessie, I looked upon him almost like a little brother, since he is almost two years younger than I," said Casandra. "When we met, he was 15, and I was 17."

Casandra and Jessie became good friends.

Then, three years later, during the time when Casandra, due to her health problems, was taking a break from her University of Illinois studies to be home in Alabama for a semester, she and Jessie began to see one another in a different light. They started dating, and their relationship converted into a long-distance relationship when Casandra returned to the University of Illinois.

In May 2010, a few weeks before his 20th birthday, Jessie graduated from Holtville High and set his sights on going to a junior college to further catch up academically and then to enter nursing school.

Somewhere along the way Joe had become Jessie's paternal role model. Jessie told Casandra, "I want to do what your dad has done. I want to become a nurse."

Joe and Melanie were proud of Jessie, who had become the first member of his immediate biological family to graduate from high school and head for college.

On July 10, 2010, Casandra and Jessie were married.

The wedding was a big family affair. It took place in the Calhoun Christian Church in Calhoun, Kentucky, where Joe and Melanie had deep family and church roots. It was the church where Joe had served on the church board.

During the five years that Joe and Melanie had known Jessie—now becoming their son-in-law—they had come to know his character.

They liked what they saw. At the wedding, they were happy parents.

"If Joe and I had been the ones picking somebody for our daughter," Melanie remarks, "we would pick somebody like Jessie."

Even after Jessie's high school graduation in May and Casandra and Jessie's wedding in July, the big 2010 events still weren't over for the Rightmyers. In August 2010, Melanie received her master's degree in nursing from the University of Alabama's Capstone College of Nursing. This would serve her well in her job as a cardiovascular health branch director for the Alabama Department of Public Health.

"I received my master's just a few weeks after Casandra and Jessie's wedding, at a time between their return from their honeymoon and before their leaving for Illinois, where both would enroll in fall-semester college classes—Casandra at the University of Illinois and Jessie in a community college nearby," Melanie notes.

FOR MASTER, A combination of Lakeshore Foundation and the Rightmyer family would open doors to lead him to many good things. But, even before those doors started opening, a very young Master was using athletics to bring some fun and uplifting into his troubled life.

Although Master learned to walk as a baby, he would later never remember having walked. Since he was paralyzed at age three after a car accident, the only way of life Master knew was life in a wheelchair. Despite that, Master was always an active child. From a young age, he was drawn like a magnet to athletics—especially to basketball.

"During elementary school, I loved basketball. I just had to play it." Master remembers. When there were adults around, they worried about the little boy zipping about in his wheelchair among all those able-bodied children. "I would grab a ball, and they were like, 'You can't play. You might hurt somebody, might run over somebody!' " But Master just kept playing. When it came to basketball he was determined. "I was like, 'Well, I'm playing ball whether y'all like it or not!' " he said.

It was his love for athletics, especially basketball, that moved an elementary-school teacher to guide second-grader Master toward Lakeshore Foundation's athletic programs.

As Master grew into his teenage years, wheelchair basketball made him into an unofficial mentor for some younger kids. Youngsters saw that being in a wheelchair did not stop Master from achieving athletically. Too, he was a big, powerfully built guy who had a special presence about him. Master would take up time with the younger kids, showing them sports skills and encouraging them.

"Kids can shine when no one else is shining," Master said with a grin. "I like being around the kids."

Wheelchair basketball also helped Master make friends among his peers—especially his basketball teammates. Although Master kept his feelings close, through basketball he could relate to those around him.

And, when he was badly in need of a place to call home, it was the family of his teammate Casandra who rescued him. He would live in the Rightmyer home for more than two years before enrolling in college, on a wheelchair basketball scholarship, at the University of Alabama.

"Without the Rightmyers I probably would not have gone to college," said Master.

And then, at college, it was through yet another wheelchair basketball connection that Master met the girl of his dreams, Anna Kleen.

Anna, a white girl from Minnesota and Master, a black boy from Alabama, found much common ground. They were within a few months of one another in age. Both loved athletics. Both had learned to cope with a physical disability. (Anna had been using a wheelchair since being injured in a car accident as a teenager.)

In June 2010, Master and Anna were married, in the bride's home state of Minnesota.

"The relationship between Master and Anna? That's a good thing!" said Melanie Rightmyer. "They are so, so good for one another."

Melanie was deeply touched at the wedding when Anna's mother came to her and said she felt that Melanie, husband Joe, and daughter Casandra had had an incredibly positive influence on Master's life.

At the wedding, Master asked the Rightmyer family to sit, along with his sister and nephew, in the section reserved for the groom's family members.

"Mr. and Mrs. Rightmyer are family to me," said Master. "Before them, I had never really known the whole mom-and-dad aspect. They became parents to me. I owe them a lot, and they mean a lot to me. It was while I was living with the Rightmyers that I got my first car, had my first college interview, got my first bank account, got my first debit card. It was while I was living with the Rightmyers that I pretty much got what I needed to help me get a life after I lived with the Rightmyers."

Master's new wife, Anna, was very aware of the role the Rightmyers had played in the life of her new husband.

"One night Anna and I went to a movie to see *The Blind Side*," said Master. They sat together watching the story unfold of how the life of Michael "Big Mike" Oher was transformed after Leigh Anne and Sean Tuohy took him into their home.

"Anna punched me and said, 'Hey, that's you!' "

At the center of it all, along the way, was the Lakeshore Foundation. Master saw Lakeshore as a place that made possible athletic opportunities and human connections that helped develop him into an adult.

Although Master had resisted those English essay-writing assignments in high school, he had a natural knack for writing poetry and found poetry as an outlet for his innermost feelings.

He wrote this poem to express what Lakeshore had meant to him:

A SPECIAL PLACE: A TRIBUTE TO LAKESHORE FOUNDATION
By Master Hinkle, 2010

Everyone has a place;
Some go to escape.
When your favorite song just won't do,
And you need to get away.
I, too, have a special place,
A place that I've always loved.
And though it has no arms,
When I'm there I feel so hugged.
Lakeshore is this place,

Blind of status and race.
Where anyone can have a blast,
Because everyone is great.
This place means a lot to me,
It relieves so much stress.
It's the best place in the world to make friends,
And I couldn't imagine being anywhere else.
Since I was a kid,
It's always shown me the way;
That just one smile, or just one hug
Could change the course of a day.
It's the little things in life,
The ones that you don't have to buy.
And the only thing you need
Is the willingness to try.
My special place is one of a kind,
And I hope one day they build more.
But no matter how many are built,
You can never replace a Lakeshore.

31

Exceptional Staff Members

Part 1

The Lakeshore Foundation staff has always been made up of exceptional individuals, some of whom have physical disabilities while others are able-bodied. They all have in common the qualities of talent, resourcefulness, and compassion, plus a dedication to the Lakeshore mission of helping build lives through rehabilitation, sports, and fitness. Here are a few of their stories.

Heather Pennington has always had a sparkle, a contagious enthusiasm for helping others.

A deeply spiritual person, Heather had a desire to carry out a ministry. She came to Lakeshore as a fitness specialist in 1999, two years before the Foundation moved into its new facility. She became a strength and conditioning specialist, receiving national certification and working with Lakeshore athletes—kids and adults, recreational and competitive, and Olympic and Paralympic.

She soon realized that the ministry she desired was taking place at Lakeshore.

Although able-bodied herself, Heather knew firsthand about disability: her uncle was born with cerebral palsy. "My family accepted my uncle like they accepted anyone else," she explains. "He was treated no differently. He worked; he got married; he loved to laugh."

The comfortable way Heather's family interacted with her uncle set a precedent for Heather: "I just never saw anyone with a disability as being any different from me."

Heather later married a man with a physical disability—former firefighter Josh Pennington, who sustained extensive paralysis as a result of a car accident.

During her years at Lakeshore, Heather had an almost magical way of going into a room full of people and connecting with each one.

"New people at first can feel maybe a little helpless, a little bit discouraged," Heather says. "But if they see other physically disabled people at Lakeshore who are being active, living their lives, getting in and out of their cars, getting married, and having children, they see that they, too, can enter that realm."

In 2010, the Penningtons moved near St. Louis, Missouri. There Josh became the program director for a small nonprofit, the Disabled Athletes Sports Association and Heather became a faculty member in the health and fitness sciences department of Lindenwood University.

Heather's students will go into fields such as physical therapy, recreation therapy, exercise physiology, and teaching physical education in public and private schools. "Every one of my students will come across people who have some disability," said Heather.

She passes along the lessons she learned at Lakeshore Foundation. "I want my students to be able to understand that every person was created by God for a unique purpose. It is my goal to impress upon my students how to see a disabled person as just another person."

When Susan Katz first came to Lakeshore Foundation in 2003, she was a young athlete on the USA women's wheelchair basketball team, training for the upcoming 2004 Paralympics in Athens.

"My first feeling when I saw Lakeshore's facilities was, 'At Lakeshore, I'm not an afterthought. This place was made for me.' " She was impressed by the incredible accessibility that existed in Lakeshore Foundation's progressive new building. "It wasn't a building that was built for an Olympic athlete and then adapted for a Paralympic athlete."

Soon after the 2004 Paralympics—where she and her teammates won gold—Susan joined Lakeshore Foundation as a new employee. Armed with her bachelor's degree in communications/journalism from the University of Illinois and her experience producing shows for ESPN, she took a communications job at Lakeshore—spreading the word about Lakeshore Foundation programs through the media.

Through the rapidly expanding forms of social media, Susan especially reached out to parents of disabled kids. She motivated these parents to encourage their children to participate in sports, recreation, and fitness programs, as hers had encouraged her. Born with spina bifida, Susan felt fortunate that, as she grew up in Maryland and California, her mom and dad encouraged her to reach for the same goals as her able-bodied sister, 22 months her junior.

From the time she began playing wheelchair basketball at age 11, followed by wheelchair track and field, Susan's horizons expanded: "It completely changed my life." Her parents encouraged her to participate and to be independent. "During weekend track meets, I had to learn to get all my bags in the airport and travel on my own and take care of myself at a hotel and be responsible for my health and my own care."

After almost four years at Lakeshore, Susan accepted a communications position at the national headquarters of the United States Olympic Committee (USOC), in Colorado Springs. Her job there was to help publicize the Paralympics programs through social media.

What she had learned at Lakeshore Foundation helped tremendously with her job at the USOC. "It was at Lakeshore where I saw programs for physically disabled individuals and saw how people were positively affected. All that experience was so valuable when I went to work at the USOC promoting the Paralympics."

Susan's own athletic activities continued to diversify. After her years of track and field and wheelchair basketball, she moved on to another sports challenge—the triathlon. In her early 30s, Susan still had her eyes on the goal. The Ironman triathlon, she said, "is the hardest thing I've ever done, and the most fun."

CATHY MILLER WORKED in financial and administrative roles at Lakeshore Foundation. She loved her job.

A certified public accountant, Cathy began working at Lakeshore in

1997 and soon became the chief financial officer and, later, the director of administration.

She emphasized that the Foundation's goals made her job fulfilling: "When you are an accountant and thus a 'numbers person,' most of the time you are results/numbers-oriented. But at Lakeshore, although I believe the Foundation does an excellent job in managing finances, a profit motive is not why the Foundation exists. Lakeshore is there to help people attain healthy, active lifestyles."

Cathy is motivated by seeing Lakeshore's clients satisfied.

"Although I am not directly involved in carrying out these programs, I see people coming and going to participate in Lakeshore programs. Periodically I will drop by where some activities are in progress, such as in the fieldhouse, and just watch a little of what's going on." Cathy always feels reenergized when she watches a swimming class, wheelchair basketball game, or personal training in the fitness center.

RONDA JARVIS REMEMBERS a man who had been devastated when a tornado ripped through his Jefferson County home, gravely injuring him and killing his stepchild. Having sustained paralyzed and also grief-stricken over his stepchild's death, he came to Lakeshore unsure of the future and the challenges it would bring, both physical and emotional.

At the time, Ronda was the outreach coordinator at Lakeshore Foundation, a position that allowed her to travel to various communities and spread the word about Lakeshore fitness, recreation, and sports programs. She met this man injured by the tornado. Her goal was "to help him and his family recognize that there was life beyond these traumatic events that had occurred." The man, just one among many Ronda helped bring to Lakeshore over the years, would find new life water-skiing and hunting despite his disability.

Ronda continued to work with individuals like this one and others at Lakeshore Foundation as chief program officer until she was recruited by the Florida-based Wounded Warrior Project in 2008. Her own work with Lima Foxtrot—Lakeshore's rehabilitation program for injured military personnel—drew her to the Wounded Warrior Project.

Her insights stemmed from a deeply personal experience with disability. At age 14, Ronda was diagnosed with a tumor of the spinal cord—*astrocytoma*. Before, she had been an athletic girl growing up in Santa Fe, New Mexico, riding horses and participating in gymnastics, basketball, volleyball, and track.

Although surgery and radiation stopped the tumor, her spinal cord was so damaged that she subsequently used a wheelchair. Wheelchair sports, particularly basketball, would be her saving grace. While earning dual degrees in psychology and social work at the University of Illinois, she also played on a wheelchair basketball team that won five national championships. Later, she would travel to France as a member of a World Cup team that tasted gold-medal victory. She would also win a silver medal with the women's Team USA in the 1992 Paralympics in Spain and a bronze medal at the 1996 Paralympics in Atlanta.

Having had her own positive experiences with athletics in the face of disability, working at Lakeshore was a natural for Ronda. In serving as Lakeshore's chief program officer, one of her greatest joys was interacting with the Foundation's staff. She enjoyed connecting with the incredibly capable, driven staff members.

"At Lakeshore Foundation, it's almost like there's this larger energy that draws people to it. People who are attracted to work at Lakeshore realize that what is being done is much bigger than just getting people back to sports and recreation. What is being done at Lakeshore Foundation is getting people back to life," she concludes.

WHEN JEN REMICK was growing up, she saw a neighbor child, who had cystic fibrosis, as so fragile that she was afraid to play with her.

Later in life, as Jen planned and implemented special events for the Kennedy Krieger Institute in Baltimore, she was introduced to disabilities in a major way. Kennedy Krieger focused on treatment of and research on children and adolescents with developmental disabilities.

"At Kennedy Krieger I saw people with disabilities in a hospital setting, where they were receiving treatment," Jen said. "Then after I came to Lakeshore Foundation, I saw people with disabilities who were active and involved in a setting of sports and recreation programs."

That move to Lakeshore would change her life. Starting first in communications before moving on to coordinating special events, Jen became fast friends with many Lakeshore staff members and clients. She was inspired as she watched their achievements.

Jen loved exposing residents of communities surrounding Lakeshore to special events that could help them better understand their disabled neighbors. For example, one of Jen's favorite events at Lakeshore was "The Amazing Race." As part of that event, modeled after the popular reality television show, able-bodied individuals got a taste of what it was like for disabled individuals to participate in Lakeshore sports and recreation activities.

"For example, during the course of Lakeshore's 'Amazing Race,' an able-bodied individual might play a game in a wheelchair for the first time, or an able-bodied citizen might take on the challenge of having one hand tied behind him, or wearing a blindfold, while trying to climb our climbing wall."

It bothers Jen when an able-bodied person meets a disabled person and asks, "How did you become disabled?" People with disabilities have a "life story" that goes far beyond their disabilities, she emphasizes.

In helping the able-bodied to accept those with disabilities, Jen also saw the fruit of her work with her children. One day her twin daughters, Hailey and Abby, met some severely wounded veterans from Iraq and Afghanistan. Even though they were accustomed to encountering disabled friends at Lakeshore, Jen wondered how the girls would react to seeing severely injured veterans.

When Hailey and Abby walked into a room full of men and women in wheelchairs, with limbs amputated, with visual impairments, they were not taken aback. Instead, Hailey had a question: "Where did all these people get their water bottles?"

It was true. Everyone in the room had a water bottle. Like a typical six-year-old, Hailey was just wondering where she could get a neat water bottle as well. Out of all that room of individuals with disabilities, that's

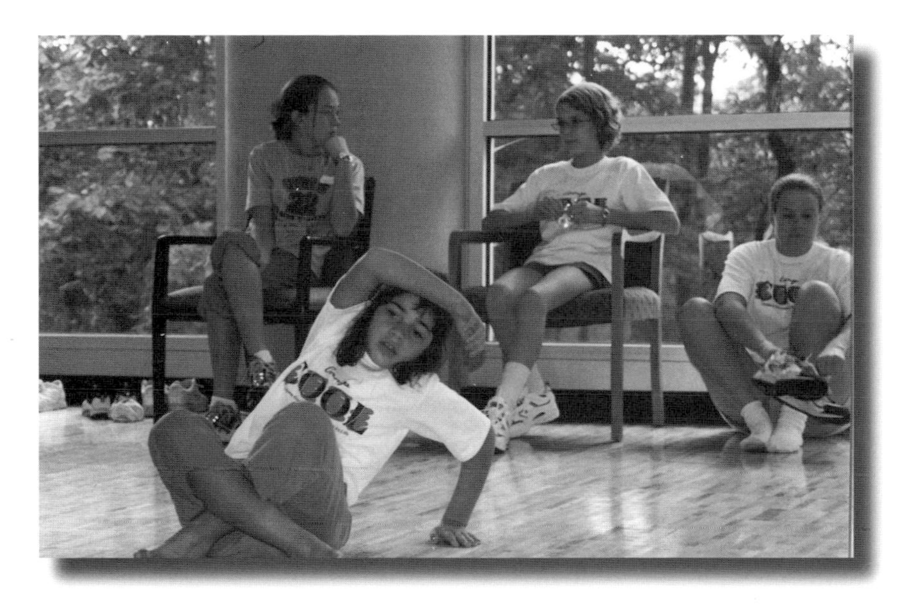

Lakeshore offers programs, like the youth aerobics class pictured, to able-bodied persons as well. It is both a service to the local community and a part of education outreach, bringing those with disabilities and the able-bodied together in settings that help them recognize each other as individuals.

what Hailey saw—just a bunch of folks with water bottles.

"I loved it," said Jen. "It was priceless."

IN 2010, DAMIAN Veazey, a young man who had helped showcase Lakeshore Foundation for five years, discussed some of the ways the foundation was making progress.

A former reporter, sports anchor, news anchor, and television news producer, Damian had come to the Foundation as director of communications after several years of experience in broadcast journalism. It was Damian's job to spread Lakeshore's message to the public.

There were ongoing efforts to inform the public of Lakeshore's state-of-the-art facilities. There were invitations to the community to come to the Foundation to watch sports events, including regional and national tournaments. The Foundation's offerings had grown so rapidly and so extensively that there was a need to balance publicizing well-established programs with showcasing newer ones, particularly the Foundation's disabled veterans initiative.

In addition to traditional media outlets such as newspapers, magazines, radio, and television, Damian began to use social media.

"The possibilities there are huge," Damian remarks. "We have made strides in communicating about Lakeshore Foundation programs through Facebook, Twitter, and YouTube. And we've started our own blog."

Damian and his colleagues also tried to connect healthcare providers with the Foundation's current and future clients. The goal was to inform individuals about Lakeshore through healthcare professionals with whom they already had a trusting relationship. This included reaching out to acute-care hospitals and organizations for individuals with specific conditions, such as cerebral palsy, spina bifida, paralysis, arthritis, or diabetes.

In recent years, Damian had seen increased public understanding of what Lakeshore Foundation does.

In times gone by, one of the main misconceptions about the Foundation was that Lakeshore was a rehabilitation hospital: "But in recent years I have seen considerable indications that we are being successful in knocking down some of that wall. More people understand that Lakeshore Foundation is not a hospital." More people discuss Lakeshore Foundation not in terms of a place of hospital-related therapy, but instead a place where those with physical disabilities could become involved in sports, recreation, and fitness.

When Lakeshore Foundation hired Beth Curry in 2008 as its new chief program officer, the Foundation was gaining someone who already had years of experience working on the Lakeshore campus in the field of rehabilitation.

Before working at the Foundation, Beth had been a staff therapist, supervisor, and administrator from 1984 to 2008 at the HealthSouth

Lakeshore Rehabilitation Hospital. She eventually became the director of clinical services at HealthSouth's Lakeshore facility and a regional HealthSouth therapy director.

Beth said the transition from hospital-based clinical rehabilitation therapy to the Foundation's fitness, sports, and recreation programs for the physically disabled was not a difficult change for her. Her personal interest and involvement in athletics helped. She herself has experience as an avid (able-bodied) tennis player.

When she decided to leave the hospital setting to work for Lakeshore, she felt it was a good point in her life to make the transition. Beth believes that sports and recreation programs have a unique opportunity to expand upon what conventional medical-model therapy can do for an individual who has a physically disabling birth defect, a severe injury that results in lasting disability, or a chronic debilitating illness.

"It doesn't have to be conventional therapy to be therapeutic and healing," Beth said. "Here at the Lakeshore Foundation, our sports and recreation programs can be therapeutic, life-enhancing, and rehabilitative."

On a regular basis after she began her work as Lakeshore Foundation's chief program officer, Beth was seeing disabled individuals become involved in exciting physically stimulating programs that "are enhancing their strengths, their endurance, and their social interactions, as well as their belief in themselves."

PART 2

When it comes to feeling the Lakeshore Foundation spirit, there were some Foundation employees who felt it from two directions: personal and professional.

AIMEE BRUDER BEGAN working at Lakeshore's front desk in 2001. Aimee knew the answers to many questions because she herself had a physical disability. Born with cerebral palsy, Aimee had used a walker until she was 14: "Then I discovered that I could get about much faster in a wheelchair, so I ditched that walker."

A swimmer since childhood, she began winning U.S. Nationals swimming medals at age 17, and, at the international level, she was competing during major Paralympic competitions beginning in 1991. She placed fourth in her very first Paralympic competition in Barcelona in 1991. In the 1996 Atlanta Paralympic Games, she won three bronze medals. Her other medals included silver in Sydney, fourth place in Athens, and bronze in Beijing.

However, even though swimming was her sport, Aimee wasn't afraid to get out of her comfort zone and stretch her wings. She played on the Demolition quad rugby team, had a go at Lakeshore's triathlon, tried out hand cycling, and learned to shoot a gun at Lakeshore's marksmanship range.

"In some of these other activities besides swimming, I might not be the best," Aimee admits. "But I'm going to learn from it."

She donned the required safety gear to take a turn at the climbing wall, a rough-surface, two-story wall equipped with holes and protrusions to grab or step onto. "Although I managed to get only halfway up the wall, I loved doing it!" said Aimee.

Aimee had grown up in Indiana, the only one of four children born into her family with a physical disability. All four siblings were swimmers. Her family didn't coddle her. She grew up in a two-story house that did not even have a ramp until she was in college. That prepared her for a world in which wheelchair access was not widespread.

"I learned at home," she said. "If I wanted to go up and down the steps, I had to figure a way to do that."

After graduating from Eastern Kentucky University with a recreation major with an emphasis on therapeutics, she felt that Lakeshore was her perfect fit.

As Aimee interacted with Lakeshore's members, she shared with them a deep knowledge of what the Foundation has to offer.

"I tell our members, 'Have fun at what you do!' " she says. "I don't just swim to compete. I swim because I enjoy it."

When he was four months shy of his second birthday, Abraham Hausman-Weiss attended his first Super Sports Saturday at Lakeshore Foundation.

As the 20-month-old participated in the scheduled programs, onlookers were amazed as the pint-sized child maneuvered his wheelchair.

"People just couldn't believe this very, very small child was out there maneuvering this big wheelchair," his mom laughs.

Abraham was born with an abnormal mass of fatty tissue restraining his spinal cord. In lay terms, the condition was called "tethered spinal cord." Doctors called it "lipomyelomeningocele." As Abraham grew, the mass grew. Before he had reached his first birthday, Abraham underwent two surgeries that failed to produce the hoped-for results. Abraham would be permanently paralyzed from the waist down.

In 1999, less than two years after Abraham was born, his parents, Natalie and Scott, moved from Cincinnati, Ohio, to Birmingham in order for Scott, a rabbi, to begin working at Temple Emanu-El. Natalie and Scott were still trying to come to terms with the permanency of Abraham's condition. As they settled in Birmingham and learned about Lakeshore's programs for the physically disabled, they wanted their son to become involved.

"The thought of Abraham getting involved in sports and recreation programs at Lakeshore Foundation was exciting to me," Natalie recalls. "And, at first, it was also scary."

Despite Abraham's disability he had many abilities. The boy was strong and quick.

Swimming was the first of his achievements. When Abraham was just two years old, he learned how to swim in the pool at Lakeshore's Recreation Center. In years to come, Abraham would break some records with his swimming.

Independence was another early milestone for Abraham. Kevin Orr encouraged Scott and Natalie to help their son become independent while he was young. Like Abraham, Kevin had dealt with a physical disability since birth, and had used a wheelchair.

"We started early with Abraham's learning how to catheterize himself," Natalie explains. "By the time he was four years old, he could catheterize independently, with adult supervision."

When he grew older, Abraham began participating competitively in Lakeshore track and field activities. Adept at javelin, shot put, discus, and the softball throw, he quickly qualified for nationals. He would later take to tennis and wheelchair basketball. The time would come when Abraham would have a wall full of trophies honors for MVP on the basketball team.

Along the way, Natalie became a staff member at Lakeshore Foundation. In 2004, she took the position of director of development. As Natalie talked to existing and prospective donors about support for Lakeshore Foundation programs, she understood firsthand what the Foundation could do for those with physical disabilities and for their families.

"I so strongly feel that when people hear the name of Lakeshore Foundation, there needs to be an image of all the wonderful Lakeshore possibilities that can await someone who is physically disabled—whether that be a child, a newly injured adult, or whoever.

"We are talking of Lakeshore Foundation's people who are enabling individuals with disabilities to be independent. We're talking of Lakeshore Foundation staff who are helping to make whole the lives of people with physical disabilities. Our son has had so many excellent role models at Lakeshore. It's a success story; Lakeshore has played such a

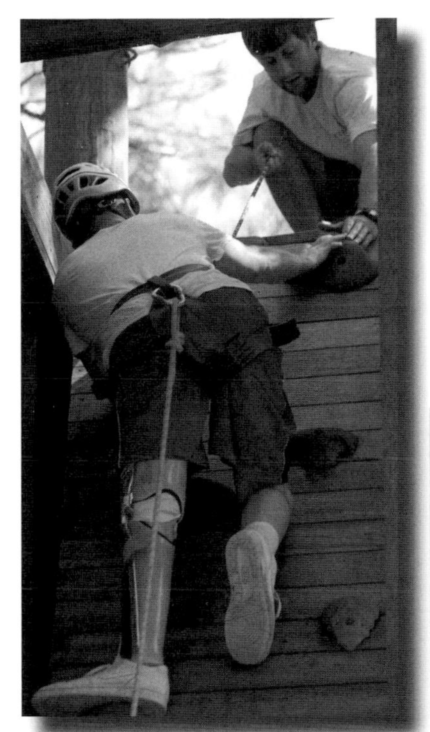

Lakeshore clients participate in archery, climbing, and target shooting, a few of the sports activities which, build confidence and provide fun.

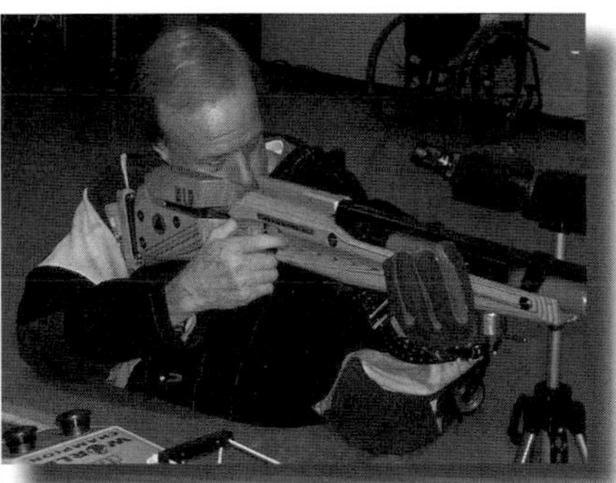

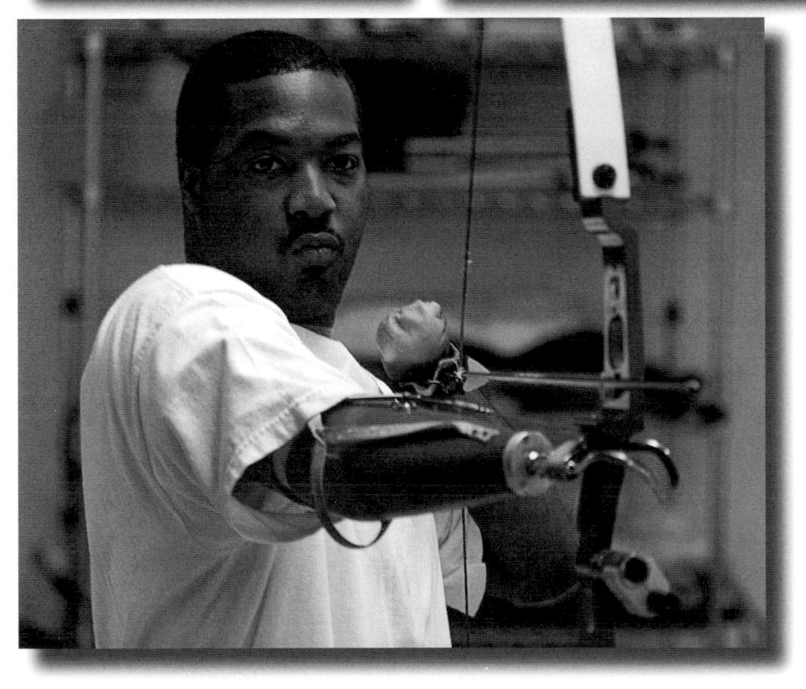

huge, tremendous role in Abraham's life."

Abraham was 13 when he, his parents, and his nine-year-old brother Samuel left Birmingham for Houston, where his dad had been hired as senior rabbi at a large temple. By that time, the Foundation had made an indelible print on Abraham's life. When he had first experienced Lakeshore Foundation's youth sports and recreation programs, Abraham had been a few months shy of two. Now, having just entered his teen years, he had matured into a straight-A junior high school student who took mainstream classes and who was making his plans to go to college. Still athletic and competitive, he had also begun acting in theatrical productions, playing the guitar, and swimming alongside able-bodied swimmers. "All this," said his mom, "is a real testament to the self-confidence our son learned at Lakeshore Foundation."

WHEN AMY BUNN began working at Lakeshore in 1999, neither she nor any of her loved ones was in the market for Lakeshore's programs.

Amy never knew there would come a time when the spirit of Lakeshore would lift her from the depths of depression as she dealt with the most disturbing health crisis she had ever experienced.

Amy had worked previously as an executive assistant at another Birmingham-based company until it was outsourced to Texas. In her mid-50s, she embarked on a second career at Lakeshore as an executive assistant to the president. At Lakeshore, Amy thrived. Lakeshore Foundation became her own mission work; she had already been involved for decades in the mission work of her husband, Lewis, a longtime minister in the Free Methodist denomination.

"From the time I went to work at the Lakeshore Foundation, I really did view my work there not so much as just a job but also as being like a mission," Amy remarks. "I found it so fulfilling to be able to work in a place that did so much good for so many people. It didn't take me long to see that the people who worked at Lakeshore Foundation, combined with the people who came there for services, together made Lakeshore Foundation a very, very special place."

Within weeks after her retirement in 2006, tragedy struck Amy in the form of breast cancer. Months of chemotherapy led her into a hell-hole of acute depression—feelings very foreign to Amy. Even though doctors were aggressively fighting her disease, Amy couldn't make herself believe in a positive outlook.

"Despite the fact I had been very strong in my Christian faith, there came this time in my life when my faith went what I would call 'kablooey,' " Amy admits. "I was really in the doldrums, mainly sitting in my home sobbing and watching television reruns of *Little House on the Prairie*."

Amy's first pivotal spiritual and emotional awakening from this hopelessness came one night. She couldn't sleep. All she could do was think about the ravages of breast cancer and the worst possible outcomes. She went into her husband's home office and began gathering and reading all the breast-cancer literature she could find, both in printed publications and from the Internet. Then she went to bed sobbing. Her husband came to her to offer comfort.

"I said, 'Lewis, I can't read any more of this stuff. Could you just please read it for me? And If there is anything I need to know, tell me.' Lewis was there for me. He took me into his arms and he began praying for me. He prayed and prayed, until around daylight."

Something very freeing happened to Amy by the end of that long night. "It was after that night that I just began to release it. That was the night I began turning it over to God."

And then another miracle came Amy's way—a phone call from Lakeshore Foundation.

The individual who had succeeded Amy when she retired had vacated that position. Amy's services were needed again: "So I agreed to go back to work at Lakeshore Foundation for three months."

Working a steady job proved to be much more physically draining than she could have imagined. She had to push herself. The tips of her fingers were so numb from chemotherapy that she couldn't even pick up a paper clip.

But at Lakeshore, Amy began finding her way back. To build back her strength, she began exercising in the Foundation's fitness center, taking special exercise classes in the pool, and walking on the track. "Why, the results were miraculous!" said Amy. "I would do the swimming, and then I would have the strength to go to the fitness center and work out. I was building my strength."

Amy herself felt the exhilaration that she had seen many Lakeshore clients experience over the years. Although Amy's job still was in administration and not in actual programs, in her own quiet way she became a soft-spoken advocate for Lakeshore Foundation. While Amy had never experienced the despair of physical disabilities such as paralysis or amputations, she had met her own challenges of breast cancer and depression.

"It was after I returned to Lakeshore when I began moving on with my life," she says. "I began living my life with the attitude that my cancer is not going to recur, and that, if the cancer does recur, I'll deal with it."

As Amy told her story, she began smiling about a fact related to a fulfilling passage of time: She had returned to Lakeshore Foundation with the promise to work for three months; instead, when she was interviewed, it had already been three years.

"The way I feel now," she said with a laugh, "I guess I will be at Lakeshore Foundation as long as they will have me."

Young Josh Berenotto was spending a lot of time on the sidelines when he first started to school. Josh had been born with spina bifida and, since he was confined to a wheelchair, his teachers were at a loss as to how he could be active.

Josh's mom recalled the scenario: "Both of Josh's physical education teachers were older ladies, who, bless their hearts, still were of the mindset that, because this child was in a wheelchair, he couldn't do anything. They also were thinking, 'And we certainly don't want him to get hurt!' "

At the same time, both of Josh's parents, Laurie and Tony, were on a mission to find ways to get their child active. "We took Josh camping out in the woods with the Cub Scouts. Maneuvering his wheelchair out in those woods wasn't an easy thing to do, but we went," said Laurie.

Then there was the racing chair. When Josh received services in Shriners-sponsored programs, the Shriners introduced him to his first racing chair. He loved it. After he outgrew it and his parents were looking for a replacement, someone told them about Lakeshore and Kevin Orr, who headed up Lakeshore Foundation's youth programs.

Thus began the Berenotto family's journey to Lakeshore Foundation.

At the time Laurie and Tony Berenotto "discovered" the Foundation, they were living in southeastern Alabama at Fort Rucker, where Tony, an Army pilot, was stationed. When they made their first 3-hours-each-way drive to Lakeshore Foundation in Birmingham, son Josh was not quite seven years old.

Josh began participating in Super Sports Saturday, and the Berenottos felt as though they had discovered a gold mine.

"Josh wasn't on the sidelines anymore," Laurie remembers with a smile.

Time after time, the Berenottos rose before dawn to get Josh to Lakeshore in time for the games. These Fort Rucker-to-Birmingham pilgrimages continued for more than three years. Just as he did with other physically disabled kids who participated in Lakeshore programs, Kevin Orr emphasized to Josh the mastering of independence.

As much as Laurie appreciated Lakeshore, some of Kevin's message came hard for her as the protective mom of a disabled child.

She would never forget the day, early in the family's association with Lakeshore Foundation, when she dropped Josh off at Lakeshore not just for one day of Super Sports Saturday but for an entire week of the Foundation's summer camp for kids with physical disabilities. "I was driving away from Lakeshore thinking, 'I just left my baby with these people I don't really know real well, and he's going to stay there a whole week. Am I crazy?' "

Josh blossomed.

After three years of driving up and down the highway for Josh to participate in activities at Lakeshore, Laurie and Tony decided to move to Birmingham. They reasoned that since Tony was in the military he would be away from the family from time to time with deployments anyhow; so the Berenottos would just make Birmingham—and Lakeshore Foundation—home base for the family.

After the move, Josh escalated his participation in Lakeshore sports. He played wheelchair basketball. He was active in field events—javelin, discus, and shot put. He did weight-lifting. He was on Lakeshore's swim team, and in years to come he would break national records in swimming.

Laurie began volunteering at Lakeshore. She was so good at interacting with clients that she was offered a position at Lakeshore that evolved into a full-time job, becoming an administrative assistant.

Before their move to Birmingham, Laurie and Tony had carefully researched just how Lakeshore Foundation would fit into their family picture.

"We searched the whole country for somewhere else that did programs like Lakeshore," said Laurie. "We couldn't find another one."

32

Snapshots of Clients

When someone comes to Lakeshore Foundation for rehabilitation or fitness, he or she does not become just a client of the Foundation but a member of the family. Here are profiles of four remarkable individuals who did just that, and whose stories illustrate the range of disabilities and the varying ways of overcoming them that are part of the Lakeshore way.

Jess Dixon — New Horizons

Karen and Tom Dixon's baby boy was almost a year old when the couple sat in the office of a neurologist and heard him say, "The best that you can hope for with your son is that he will reach the developmental age of an eight-year-old and live in a group home."

Their son, Jess, had suffered brain damage at birth due to delayed diagnosis of a jaundiced condition. The bilirubin level that caused the jaundice, or yellowing of the skin, resulted in a condition called kernicterus ("kern" for the portion of the brain affected, and "icterus" meaning yellow).

As a result, baby Jess had cerebral-palsy-like symptoms such as floppy, uncontrolled muscle movements. As time went on he would have speech problems, seizures, upper respiratory infections, and other symptoms.

During the first months of Jess's life, his parents were winding their way through a dark and disturbing maze. When Jess was born, the Dixons were living in Florida. They ended up moving to Illinois, where doctors were able to diagnose correctly Jess's condition.

Neither of them expected that 20 years later Jess would be a computer whiz taking college classes and driving himself around town.

That happened to a great extent because of Lakeshore Foundation.

"Lakeshore entered Jess's life when he was six years old after we had moved to Birmingham," Karen recalls. "By that time, Jess had undergone so much therapy in his life that he had come to hate it. He hated doing the same things over and over again. By that time, we had come to know that, despite Jess's physical problems, intellectually he was smart and bright. Jess knew that with all this therapy he was not having fun. We were told about the sports and recreation programs at Lakeshore Foundation, and we thought that would be a fun outlet for Jess."

Through Lakeshore's sports teams, Jess would find the fun he craved. Along with strengthening his physical condition, he also began to communicate more effectively.

"Jess started swimming in Lakeshore's pool. He loved it. He couldn't wait to go." Karen explains. "And with the swimming, we started getting an outcome we had not expected with his speech improvement. At that time, part of Jess's speech problem was that he spoke in a very breathy manner because his respiration was inconsistent. At Lakeshore Foundation, they were teaching him to hold his breath and to do a range of other things. Three months after Jess started swimming at Lakeshore, his speech had begun to improve so dramatically it was unbelievable. Why, Jess had been in speech therapy for four years and he had not made nearly the progress that he made in three months of swimming at Lakeshore Foundation."

Jess also learned how to ride horses, water ski, and dribble a basketball.Although he didn't have the muscle strength to throw the ball into the basket, his sharp mind made him good at reading plays and in playing defense.

Lakeshore athlete Master Hinkle took him under his wing, too. "Oh, Jess grew to love Master!" said Karen. "He decided that he wanted to be strong like Master. They really hit it off."

At Lakeshore, Jess would make close friends. One, a wheelchair basketball teammate, was Jessie Atwell. When Jessie married Casandra Rightmyer, Jess was in the wedding.

Karen says Lakeshore also helped their family: "After we found Lakeshore Foundation, all three of us became a lot less stressed and so much happier."

The journey with Jess and his battle against this rare neurological disorder made Karen reach out in many ways. That journey influenced her to enter a career related to brain research and treatment. In fact, the Dixons moved to Birmingham so that Karen could earn her PhD in biochemistry and molecular genetics at UAB. After receiving her degree, she took both a faculty position in UAB's neurobiology department and a program-development position at UAB's Civitan International Research Center. Then, in 2000, Karen cofounded a group called PICK—Parents of Infants and Children with Kernicterus.

In many senses of the word, Lakeshore Foundation experiences introduced the Dixon family to new possibilities that in turn paved the way for additional new horizons—for Jess, and also for his mom and dad.

After experiencing one adventure after another at Lakeshore, Jess and his dad climbed into his dad's Ford-150 truck and took off on a father-and-son adventure soon after Jess's graduation from high school. They drove all the way to Alaska and British Columbia and back—thousands of miles, just the two of them!

BOBBY LEMAY—STRENGTHENING

On December 1, 2001, Dr. Bobby LeMay went deer-hunting at his farm in Bibb County, just south of his Birmingham home. The longtime Birmingham ears, nose, and throat specialist and his three sons had enjoyed many hours of hunting deer, turkey, and quail there. But, in recent years, hunting had no longer brought LeMay the enjoyment that it had in years past.

"Since I had retired from my medical practice in 1996, I had become interested in several other hobbies, including photography. I had just gotten tired of hunting," LeMay said. Before he headed out to the woods to hunt on that December day, he had already decided it would be his last time. As fate would have it, it was on that hunting trip when 68-year-old LeMay would fall more than 12 feet, leaving him paralyzed for life.

"At around 2 o'clock in the afternoon on that day, I climbed up in a deer stand that had not been used in a couple of years," he recalled. He was alone when he climbed into the stand.

LeMay had been in the deer stand less than an hour when the stand collapsed. "Immediately when I hit the ground I felt this feeling of burning fire from my waist down my legs. And I couldn't move my legs." He knew that he had likely sustained paralysis.

He lay on the ground for more than two hours before anyone found him. Soon a helicopter transported him to UAB for surgery. Although his spine was not severed, he had fractured his neck and severely damaged his spine. Unable to walk and with limited movement in his arms and shoulders, he was forced to use a wheelchair. He also suffered from autonomic dysreflexia, a condition in which, as a result of damage to nerves near the spinal cord, blood pressure rises to dangerous levels.

It was a friend of LeMay's, Mike Stephens, who encouraged LeMay to go to Lakeshore Foundation. LeMay's wife, Amanda, also encouraged him to go to Lakeshore.

LeMay lived for more than nine years after his accident. On repeated occasions he would say that his decision to go to the Foundation proved to be a positive turning point, a milestone, in his rehabilitation. One of the keys to LeMay's improvement was his use of the Foundation's fitness programs, particularly the aquatic program. "The instructor taught me how to accomplish 50 to 75 percent more in the water," he explained. Lending him support and companionship as he exercised in Lakeshore's pool was Amanda, who was an accomplished swimmer and former lifeguard.

LeMay became so inspired by what he learned at Lakeshore Foundation that he hired a personal trainer and outfitted his home and vacation house with gym equipment.

As a physician, LeMay was well aware of the importance for the physically disabled to keep their muscles and joints moving. Without activity, he said, "people can just shrivel up and become emotionally introverted and just physically deteriorate."

After he started doing regular workouts, he became noticeably stronger. Without Lakeshore Foundation, he said, he felt his muscles would have contracted. "I probably would have even had difficulty feeding myself."

LeMay emphasized that, beyond the physically strengthening benefits he discovered at the Lakeshore Foundation, he also found considerable emotional strengthening. He said that through his visits to Lakeshore Foundation he found himself regaining some of his natural positive outlook that had sustained severe blows as a result of his accident.

"To see the things that disabled people are able to accomplish at Lakeshore Foundation is really inspiring to watch," he said. "You can go all day without smiling. And then you get to Lakeshore and you work out alongside these people, and you suddenly find yourself smiling and laughing and joking. You know that something is happening. They start teaching you what you can do to help yourself. At Lakeshore Foundation, you get to where you can smile a lot."

Isaac Godwin —Enlightenment

What should have led to marriage ended with a funeral. The couple, young and in love, drove down the road with their future before them: a wedding, a home, and a baby on the way. Instead, that future was ripped from them, leaving one dead and the other barely alive.

Isaac Godwin was 16. Struck by tragedy, this rebellious teen would become more than just a man in the years to come. He would become a force to be reckoned with.

AS A TEEN, Isaac was a good-looking, standout athlete in Marshall County, where he had grown up. From the time he became a starter on the varsity football team at Guntersville High School, he displayed the talents of a star—a punter, linebacker, and tight end. He dreamed of playing professionally.

Isaac's grades in high school were average; his priority was sports and, later, his girlfriend, Anna Currie. When they were 16, Anna became pregnant. Instead of breaking up, they continued dating, planning a future together, picking a name for their unborn baby girl: Emma Kyle.

Everything changed on May 19, 2004. It was the day after Anna's birthday. On the list of Isaac and Anna's plans was to drive to a local store to buy a birthday present for Anna's twin sister.

The last memory Isaac had of that day was of the two of them getting into his Ford Explorer to head to the store. En route, they were in a one-car accident. Anna and the unborn baby were killed. Isaac was critically injured and airlifted to a hospital in the nearby city of Huntsville. There were no witnesses to the accident, and it could not be determined who was driving; Isaac can't remember.

Initially, Isaac's life hung in the balance. Six days after the accident, he began to regain consciousness. His condition improved. From Huntsville he was transferred to undergo a period of rehabilitation at Shepherd Center in Atlanta, Georgia.

The accident left the 17-year-old with permanent paralysis that confined him to a wheelchair. It also left him to deal with the painful loss of Anna and their baby.

"Anna and I could talk; we got along and we never argued. And she was pretty," Isaac said in a 2005 interview. "I miss Anna. I loved her, and I wanted to spend the rest of my life with her. There is not a day that goes by that I don't think about what could have been."

After Isaac finished his stint at Shepherd Center, he returned home. When the football season began a few months later, Isaac could be found sitting in his wheelchair on the sidelines on Friday nights, longingly watching his high school football team play their opponents. "If my team was getting beaten, it was tough for me, not being able to go out there on the field and help them," he said.

For Isaac, the challenges had gone from making the "big play" in a football game all the way to just managing the taken-for-granted tasks of everyday life. "This meant coming to grips even with something like taking a shower . . . just having to learn a different way of life."

During the autumn of 2004, Isaac began playing sports again, mainly wheelchair basketball at Lakeshore. He graduated high school and enrolled at Snead State Community College, located in the town of Boaz near Guntersville. On the surface, it seemed that Isaac was gradually adjusting; that would prove not to be the case.

After playing wheelchair basketball a few months at Lakeshore, Isaac began to feel frustration rather than accomplishment. Accustomed to his success as an able-bodied athlete, he thought he was not doing well. His dad, Doug, said, "After he was injured, Isaac kept judging his athletic ability based on where he had been athletically before he was injured."

College posed some problems to Isaac as well. After a brief period, he dropped out of community college. Isaac knew he might find college courses to be a major challenge. Doctors explained that he had sustained a slight brain injury in the accident that could cause delays with information processing and retention. He was told that to stand a realistic chance of making it in college he might need to use a tape recorder to help him in class—to record everything that went on and then study it later.

But, at the time he dropped out of Snead State Community College, Isaac didn't blame a brain injury. To him, the issue had to do with where his priorities were at the time: "I wasn't ready to go to college. If you are not ready, you just are not ready. First you've got to get ready."

By this time, Isaac's grief and frustrations already had begun fueling a rebellious streak. "I was wild for a while," Isaac admitted. "I went through a period when I just wanted to do what I wanted to do."

He tried college again, this time at the University of Alabama, but, despite playing on the school's inaugural wheelchair basketball team, he left after just one semester. He had one health problem after another—including a spider bite and two dangerous staph infections. He moved back into his parents' home in Marshall County and went to work at a popular Guntersville general store called Mike's Merchandise.

In the meantime, Isaac began abusing drugs.

"I was down in the dumps, and I was not where I needed to be mentally and spiritually," he acknowledged.

During this wild period, Isaac wrecked family cars three times.

"Isaac totaled three vehicles," said his mom. "And I mean totaled—to the point you would look at these vehicles and wonder how anyone got out of them alive." Miraculously, no one was ever seriously hurt.

Isaac later would be candid about his own fault regarding the wrecks. "I never had a wreck when I was sober," he said. "I was either drinking or taking pills. When I had a wreck and I was the only one in the vehicle, I didn't think much about that. But then when I had a wreck with a passenger riding with me, I thought, 'I could have really hurt someone.' "

That wreck marked a turning point. Liz took the lead in the Godwin household in terms of putting her foot down that Isaac was barred from driving. For months, he did not.

Liz said that, in a time to come, after Isaac pulled himself out of his hole he would tell her: "Mama, until I hit the bottom, I wasn't going to do it . . . And I would have hit the bottom a whole lot sooner if you and Daddy had not kept picking me up."

FOUR YEARS AFTER his paralyzing accident, Isaac enrolled again in Snead State Community College and stuck with it. He soon transferred to Jacksonville State, where his sister had already earned her bachelor's and master's degrees. There, for the first time since he had been injured, Isaac began to create an independent, productive life for himself.

In an interview in early 2011, Isaac was entering his senior year at Jacksonville State, majoring in communications with a concentration in public relations. Semester after semester, he had set a goal for himself to make the Dean's List. In the last semester of 2010 he reached that goal.

He said the drinking, abusing pills, and driving recklessly were in the past.

At that time, there was no serious love interest in his life. He said he was interested in that for the future, "But I wouldn't want to get serious and get married and not be finishing my college degree and look back later and say, 'Hey, I wish I had first stayed in school,' " he said. "I just want to get things done academically first."

What changed?

"I guess I just finally realized I couldn't keep using my 'stuff' as a crutch and dumping it on other people. I matured to the point that I realized my own decisions were going to make things better or they were going to make things worse."

He said he finally reached the point that it bothered him to know he was disappointing so many people. He began to think about how his community saw him: "I knew that I already had gotten to the point I was ruining my reputation with a lot of people. I thought, 'I can do a lot better than this. I don't want to be remembered as somebody who just went off the deep end.' "

BRYAN KIRKLAND — FAST AND FURIOUS

Motorcycles race across the Georgia landscape, scaling hillsides and jumping over barriers. A young man feels exhiliration as the machine beneath him pulses like his heartbeat. He feels it hum and thrusts the throttle to high gear, but suddenly he's falling in a riot of limbs and metal.

Bryan Kirkland would become paralyzed after a motocross accident in his early twenties, but he would not let the accident rule his life. He would power through it.

GROWING UP STRONG and healthy, Bryan was a high-achieving teenage athlete in his hometown of Leeds, Alabama, a few miles northeast of Birmingham. During his years at Leeds High School, Bryan lettered in both football and basketball. He was tapped for "all-state" football honors and took "player-of-the-year" honors in basketball. He accepted a basketball scholarship from Jefferson State Community College but was disappointed when the program was later discontinued.

Rather than end his athletic career, Bryan simply moved on to the next best thing: motocross racing, a high-speed, high-stakes sport involving racing motorcycles at break-neck speeds over rough terrain. The thrill of it was what attracted Bryan to this dangerous but exciting activity. Nothing had ever gone wrong before.

"But that Sunday at the Georgia racetrack, I guess it just wasn't my moment," he recalls. "I took a head dive, into a dirt embankment—broke my neck, crushed my fifth vertebra, and bruised my spinal cord. The accident happened at the top of the hill, and I slid on down to the bottom of the hill, lying face down on the ground. I was never knocked out, and I remember the whole wreck. I also remember that feeling in my body. My whole body was tingling. I couldn't move my arms. I couldn't move anything."

The 1992 accident left Bryan a quadriplegic, his legs paralyzed, and with limited function in his arms and hands.

"The way the doctor described things to my parents that day, it was like I would end up as a vegetable," Bryan remembers. "What the doctor said was that I was going to have to be taken care of by other people for the rest of my life, including having someone to dress and feed me."

Bryan ultimately would decide to approach his disability like he approached racing: fast and furious.

However, in the weeks that followed the accident, Bryan would be reduced to a shadow of his former self. The body of this strapping 6'5" young man, weighing around 210 pounds at the time of his injury, would deteriorate dramatically.

"I got down to around 125 pounds. I was a skeleton," he explains. "My whole body was in shock, and I had a lot of issues, including with blood pressure. From day one, it was a battle."

Immediately after the accident, Bryan was stabilized enough at a Georgia health facility to be transferred to St. Vincent's Hospital in Birmingham. When well enough, he went to UAB's Spain Rehabilitation Center.

"I was learning a new lifestyle. I remember waking up each day in rehab and thinking, 'Well, what am I going to do today?' I was learning the simple things in life, just getting dressed, tying my shoes."

Soon, he decided to transfer to Lakeshore Hospital, where he lived in the transitional living unit. He discovered a new lifestyle there that held some promise, and a new outlook on life.

"At Lakeshore, it wasn't like being in a hospital. There when I would wake up and say, 'Well, what are we doing today?' . . . we might be going fishing.

"I was beginning for the first time to feel just a little more comfortable about being out in public, in a wheelchair. I mean, I didn't want to continue to keep to myself and be such a private person and stay away from people—like I had been doing since my accident. Before the accident, I always had been outgoing and enjoyed other people and enjoyed having fun. Staying to myself just wasn't me."

Despite his former athletic prowess, Bryan stayed on the sidelines for a while. Soon, though, he and a friend at Lakeshore were tossing a basketball back and forth. It was Bryan's first real physical activity as an athlete using a wheelchair.

"I was just in the infant stage after my injury of practicing some motor skills," he said.

Little did he know that he would become a founding member of Lakeshore Foundation's Demolition quad rugby team.

BRYAN ALSO HAD to face new hardships in his relationship with his girlfriend, Shai, who had witnessed his accident at the motocross track. Despite the stress of Bryan's new life, the two stayed together through thick and thin and later married—but not without a serious discussion about what their future would be like.

"After I got home from rehab, I went through a stage when everything was hitting me. I was thinking, 'Well, I won't be able to do this and this and this again.' For me, it was a brief, short time of depression.

"I got to thinking that I didn't want Shai to have to go through what I was going through. I just felt like I wasn't good enough for her. I told Shai, 'It's not that I don't love you. It's just that there is no need for you to have to go through this. I was actually trying to run Shai off."

Bryan chuckled: "Well, Shai just looked at me and told me that I wasn't getting rid of her. She made it clear that she wasn't going anywhere."

With all the cards on the table, Bryan and Shai dated for four years until Bryan felt he was fully independent and ready for the new trials—and new joys—marriage would bring.

After rehab, he moved in his aunt's house, where alterations were made to render the house wheelchair-accessible.

"I lived there for almost two years, and then I moved out on my own—got my own apartment and did it in my own," Bryan explains. "I wanted to prove it to myself and to prove it to everybody else that I didn't have to have anybody taking care of me."

In the wake of his injuries Bryan had to regain not only his independence but also his self esteem:

"I can remember, during the first couple of years or so after my accident, I felt like people were looking at me in my wheelchair and thinking, 'Well, wonder what's wrong with that guy?' I would go into a restaurant and be nervous, feeling that everybody was looking at me. Here I was this big guy who had been knocked on his can, knocked down hard! The pride was hurt, the ego was gone, the confidence was gone. It was like, 'Oh, man!'

"It was just the rebuilding—the whole process," he said. "Just getting it back."

HELP WOULD COME in the form of Home Depot, Bryan's employer. As a sales associate, he would be sponsored by the company as a Paralympic athlete. Home Depot even allowed him to work part time while still being paid for a full-time position. The extra time let Bryan train

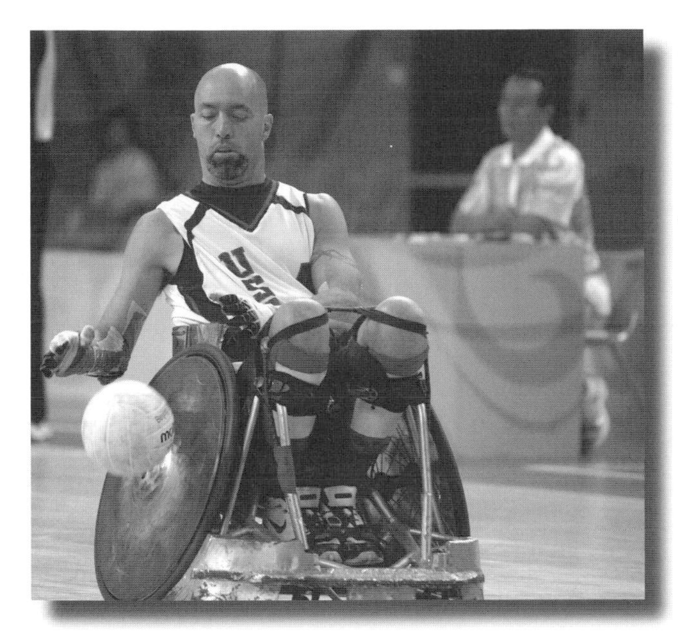

Bryan Kirkland shows his "murderball" form on the quad rugby court.

at Lakeshore without added financial stress.

By the mid-1990s, Bryan was competing competitively in wheelchair racing and quad rugby. In 1998, at the World Championships in England, he set a world record in 100-meter wheelchair racing and won gold, silver, and bronze medals. In 2000, he was on the winning quad rugby team in the international Paralympic competition in Sydney, Australia. In 2004, at the Paralympics in Athens, Greece, he was a member of the bronze-winning American quad rugby team—a team that also was featured in the much-hailed movie *Murderball.*

In 2006, at the World Championship quad rugby competition in New Zealand, he took home the gold. "That was a special thrill, playing in front of thousands of people and being televised nationwide in New Zealand," Bryan recalls.

In 2008 in Beijing, China—marking his third time in international Paralympic quad rugby competition—Bryan's team came took home yet another gold medal.

In addition to wheelchair sports, Bryan took on other interests, like racing little remote-controlled cars. "These are fast ones!" Bryan says, referring to his prized miniature vehicles. “They do like 50 or 60 miles per hour.”

As he went from track to track to race his remote-controlled cars, Bryan found himself in places not accessible by wheelchair. “But I would go to these tracks anyhow, and I would just push my chair up a hill, whatever I had to do,” he notes.

At one particular track, where Bryan was a member, the powers-that-be decided to make Bryan’s visits to that track easier and more enjoyable.

“They built a driver’s stand with a ramp,” Brian explains, a grin on his face. “It was great! I told the folks at the racetrack that they did not have to do that for me—that they did not have to roll out the red carpet for me. But I certainly appreciated it.”

Bryan was touched. It pleased him to know that this wheelchair-accessible driver’s stand would over time not only help him but also other participants in wheelchairs who came to the track: “It’s neat to see people become more aware and more willing to accommodate.”

ALL GOOD THINGS come to an end, though. At age 38, Bryan decided to retire from international sports.

“It wasn’t a physical thing. My body could still play,” said Bryan. “I just wanted to do some other things, including to have more time to spend with my family.”

Bryan had felt the sting of the recession, which had triggered cutbacks by Home Depot—resulting in Bryan losing his athletic sponsorship. However, he said that that was not the driving factor in his decision to retire from international competition:

“I didn’t want to become that athlete who stays in there too long. It’s better to be missed than people be saying, ‘Thank God he’s finally gone.’ ”

Even though there would be no more World Championships or Paralympics, he would still be involved in athletics.

“I’ve said I will continue to compete as long as I am competing at locations that are within the United States,” he explains. “For instances, I’ll still be entering some road races. And I’m thinking about doing some marathons. I still am competitive and I still enjoy being a part of competitions."

On November 30, 2011, it was announced that Bryan was among eight new inductees into the Alabama Sports Hall of Fame.

Lakeshore Foundation had become a deeply important part of Bryan's life. He felt a connection to the entire Lakeshore campus, where he had learned to live again.

"For those of us who participate in Lakeshore Foundation's programs, it's not like we are a cult up there on the hill with an attitude of, 'This is just for us, and you can't come up here.' Lakeshore is all about getting involved, whether you have a disability or not.

"For me, I've never looked upon Lakeshore Foundation like 'This is my sanctuary.' Instead, I've looked upon Lakeshore Foundation as 'This is where I come to train. This is where I come to see people, to communicate. It's not just *my* place, you know; it's *our* place.' "

33

Battle on the Homefront

By its nature, war kills. Many more who are not killed outright are maimed. Ironically, recent advances in battlefield medical response and evacuation have saved the lives of many soldiers in Iraq and Aghanistan who in previous wars would have died before they could be treated. These survivors of catastrophic injuries need the same comprehensive rehabilitation and fitness as the traditional Lakeshore clients. Recognizing this need, the Lakeshore Foundation has welcomed U.S. military veterans into its programs for the past several years and continues to develop services for the long-term care of the men and women injured in service. The profile below is an inspiring example.

Noah Galloway—A Warrior's Fight

Late at night, a soldier drives an armored vehicle across a deserted road in Iraq. But he knows it's not deserted; it's littered with roadside bombs, landmines, and other booby traps. He and his comrades scan the road with night-vision goggles, hoping to outwit their attackers. Suddenly, a flash of light, a rush of noise—then silence. In the aftermath, Noah Galloway lies in a ditch, his leg trapped beneath the seat, his arm dangling by threads of muscle tissue. His battle is just beginning.

Noah came from a family with a strong military background. Following the September 11th terrorist attacks, he enlisted in the Army, saying, "I've got to join the military." After Noah trained as an infantry soldier, he joined the first wave of American military that invaded Iraq in 2003. From the beginning of his deployment, young Noah was in the heat of battle. Time and again he dodged missiles, Molotov cocktails, and gunfire. All this danger just whetted his appetite. He reenlisted for five more years.

In September 2005 Noah was deployed to Iraq for the second time. He was there only three months when, in December 2005, he sustained massive injuries that would change the rest of his life.

Noah was a member of a platoon involved in heavy combat southwest of Baghdad. "We lost a lot of guys," he admits sadly. As the battle waged on, members of the platoon became separated. Hours later, Noah joined a convoy of three armored Humvees embarking on a nighttime mission to locate platoon members who were still unaccounted for.

"I want to drive the lead vehicle," Noah volunteered, climbing into the driver's seat of the lead Humvee with a lieutenant and a gunner riding beside him.

"We couldn't use our headlights, because they could give away our position," Noah recalls. "Roadside bombs have been notorious with this war." They used night-vision goggles to scan the road.

Around 11 P.M., a thin, invisible tripwire changed everything.

"When my front tires rolled over the tripwire, it detonated a bomb," Noah explains. "When the bomb hit our door, it threw our vehicle into the air, flying. There was a canal running adjacent to the road, and we landed in the water."

The lieutenant who was in the Humvee with Noah climbed out. The gunner, not severely injured but temporarily dazed, lay on the ground. As the lieutenant frantically looked around for Noah, he took the risk of using his flashlight to alert the rest of the convoy to the current position of the bombed-out Humvee. Even as he waved the flashlight, the lieutenant knew that the light could alert enemy soldiers who had planted the bomb and perhaps trigger a secondary attack. Spotting a helmet on the ground, the lieutenant picked it up and saw it was filled with blood. He knew it was Noah's blood.

"The lieutenant climbed a steep embankment to get to me in the

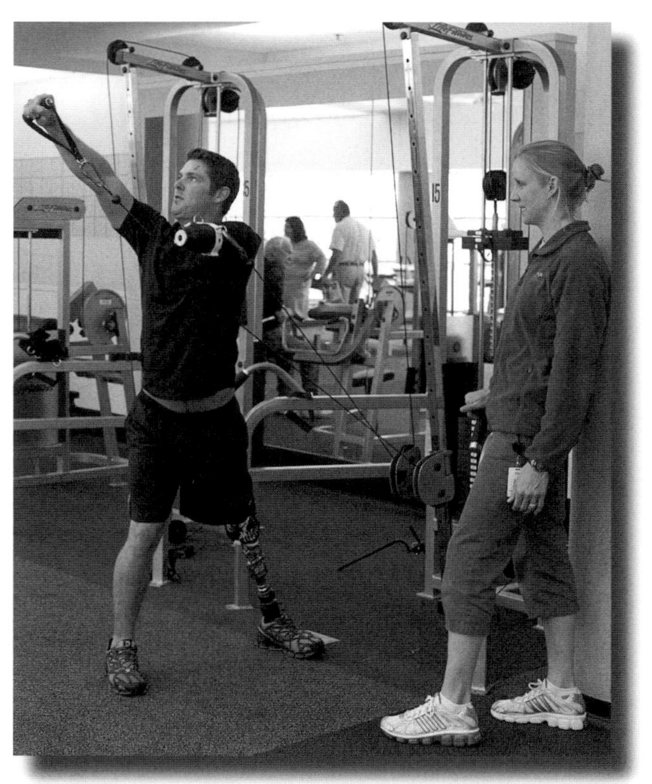

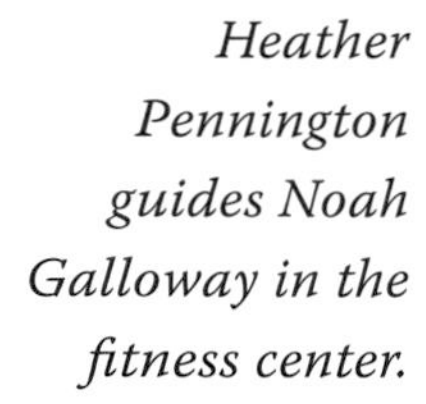

Heather Pennington guides Noah Galloway in the fitness center.

canal," recalled Noah. "When he found me, he said the water was up to my chest. There was a huge hole in the side of my jaw, and he said I wasn't making a sound. The lieutenant said that all he could do was just sit there, hold on to me, and pray."

It took several comrades to pry him out of the heavily damaged Humvee. Reinforcements arrived, and a team of soldiers went to work. "My left leg was caught under the seat . . . in a Humvee there is no real 'under the seat,' it's just seat, and then there's just metal. So it was blown out, and my leg was caught under there," said Noah. "And I had an arm that was hanging on by . . . just, like, a few ligaments, just some muscle fibers . . . just barely hanging on."

Then it was a race against time to get him in the hands of field medics. "There was this other lieutenant that I'd never met, who was yelling at a guy in the backseat to keep me breathing, because he could hear me choking on my blood."

NOAH LOST AN arm and a leg. "I had always been somebody who had been in shape, been healthy. I cared about my image, about how I looked," he admits. "I thought all that was just thrown away. I thought, 'What will I do?' "

He was also facing a divorce. His marriage, already strained by the birth of a premature baby, faced another setback with his injuries. The divorce was finalized soon after he returned to the States. Regardless, Noah soon regained some of his natural spunk and determination. He made rapid progress in his rehabilitation and learned how to use artificial limbs. Inspired by his own father, who lost an arm at age 18, Noah kept moving forward. A new love interest also entered Noah's life—a young woman who had been one of his first girlfriends, in middle school.

So it was that he felt motivated to get involved in some kind of sport.

"I had to adjust to my new body, and I figured, 'If I can get back in shape, I'll feel more comfortable, I'll start accomplishing a lot, and I'll feel a lot better.' I started thinking, 'Why not start competing in different sports?' "

In a stroke of good luck, a family friend told Noah's mother about Lakeshore Foundation. After a phone conversation with Lakeshore's Ronda Jarvis, Noah went to to check things out. He wasted no time in taking advantage of Lakeshore's programs. Using a special prosthetic leg, he started running. Through Adaptive Aquatics, he learned to water ski. Then, shortly after he started coming to Lakeshore, he was asked to be the spokesperson for the Foundation's new veterans' rehabilitation program.

Just as he had wanted to fight for his country in Iraq, Noah knew that he wanted to do the job Ronda described—a job that would help Lakeshore help others in the military who, like Noah, had had their lives altered due to severe injuries.

Speaking in a mid-2007 interview shortly after he took on this spokesman job, Noah explained why he felt comfortable in the role for which he had been recruited.

"It honestly feels like this is where I am supposed to be. It's like everything that has happened in my entire life has designed this person that was supposed to lose his arm and his leg and be in the position that I'm in right now."

The programs that Noah had been asked to help introduce became Lakeshore Foundation's priority in the early 2000s. To be collectively branded as "Lima Foxtrot," Lakeshore's military-oriented programs had been inspired by the massive numbers of severe injuries sustained by members of the United States' armed forces in Iraq and Afghanistan. However, Lakeshore's programs were designed for injured members of the armed forces no matter how they may have incurred disability.

Through these programs, the Lakeshore Foundation introduced injured military personnel to opportunities ranging from wheelchair sports in the Foundation's gym to water sports on Lay Lake and Lake Martin.

Carefully planned and professionally staffed Lakeshore camps were held to teach the injured military. Some camps would be aimed toward those with a wide range of injuries. Others would be specialty camps—aimed at specific groups such as the visually impaired and those who had sustained traumatic brain injury. Camps would go by names such as Operation Down Home and Operation Night Vision.

Not long after Lakeshore Foundation launched the Lima Foxtrot initiative, it would build a group of cottages for use as lodging for visiting members of the armed services and their families. These cottages would be dedicated on Veterans' Day 2010. The whole idea behind the cottages was to provide a holistic, family-oriented approach to rehabilitation and rejuvenation.

When Noah spoke with Alabama governor Bob Riley about Lima Foxtrot, he said, "I would love to be back in Iraq with the men I was working with, and I can't. But I can be here for those who are injured. And I will walk to the ends of the earth or talk till I'm blue in the face to get it done."

Lakeshore's programs for the military also needed to be launched with a view towards the future and long-term care. To serve the United States' military, these programs needed to continue long after the wars in Iraq and Afghanistan. In short, said Noah, the programs should have lasting power and should serve as a symbol that injured military personnel are not forgotten.

"Although people don't do it intentionally," said Noah, "they do tend to forget what happened to the guy who lost his arm or his leg."

As Noah prepared to take part in Lakeshore Foundation camps for injured military personnel, he said he viewed those camps as "a window of opportunity" for those who had sustained life-changing injuries: "Through Lakeshore's programs, they can be shown what they're capable of doing,"

Noah believes it's one thing to tell a soldier with a debilitating injury that he still could play basketball, or water ski, or run, or hunt and fish. But he said it was still another thing—something much more convincing and motivational—to show that soldier even higher goals.

"If you're coming to the Lakeshore Foundation, you're not coming to some hospital place to go through rehabilitation. The Lakeshore Foundation is much bigger than that. When you come to the Lakeshore Foundation, you're coming to a place that can show you how to enjoy life."

By mid-2011, Lakeshore had served some 1,200 injured service members and their loved ones. Participants had come from 37 states, Germany, and Puerto Rico with a wide range of physical disabilities.

"These Lakeshore Foundation programs are exposing military personnel with disabilities to quality-of-life opportunities after injury—helping to get their lives going again," said Mandy Goff, the Foundation's associate director of athletics and recreation and Lima Foxtrot Coordinator. Through the programs, participants are able to become involved in activities that they never dreamed of doing "either because they thought they could not do it, or because they had not been exposed to it."

Once the veterans return home, they can say, 'Hey, I think I'll go back to school,' or "I'm going to work on my relationship with my family.' "

All of this happened because of the sacrifice soldiers, like Noah, made for their country. The battle on the homefront had just begun at Lakeshore Foundation.

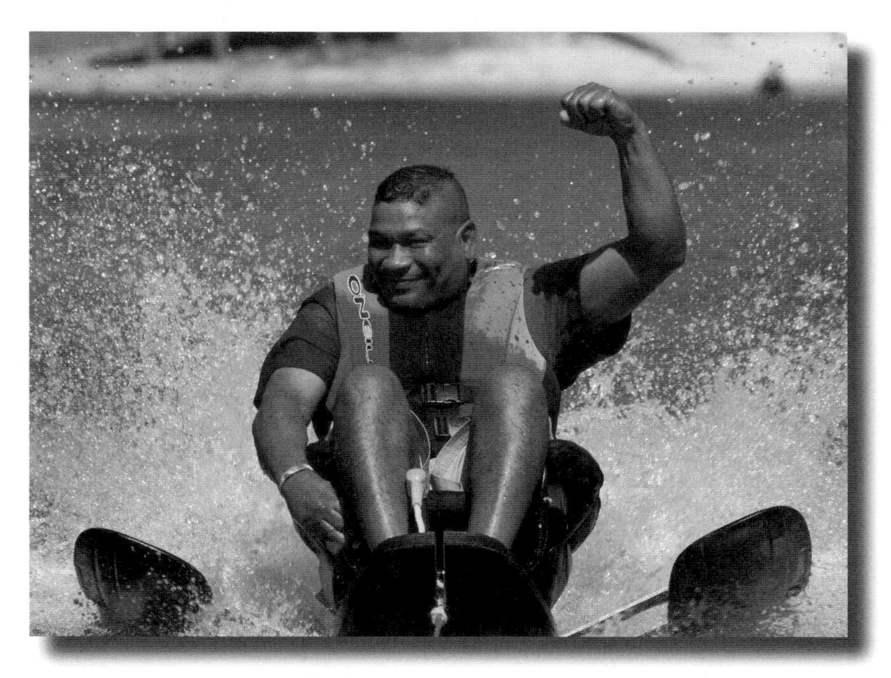

Above: *"Booyah!" A wounded soldier, coming back.*
Below: *A soldier sorts out his prosthetic legs before scuba diving.*

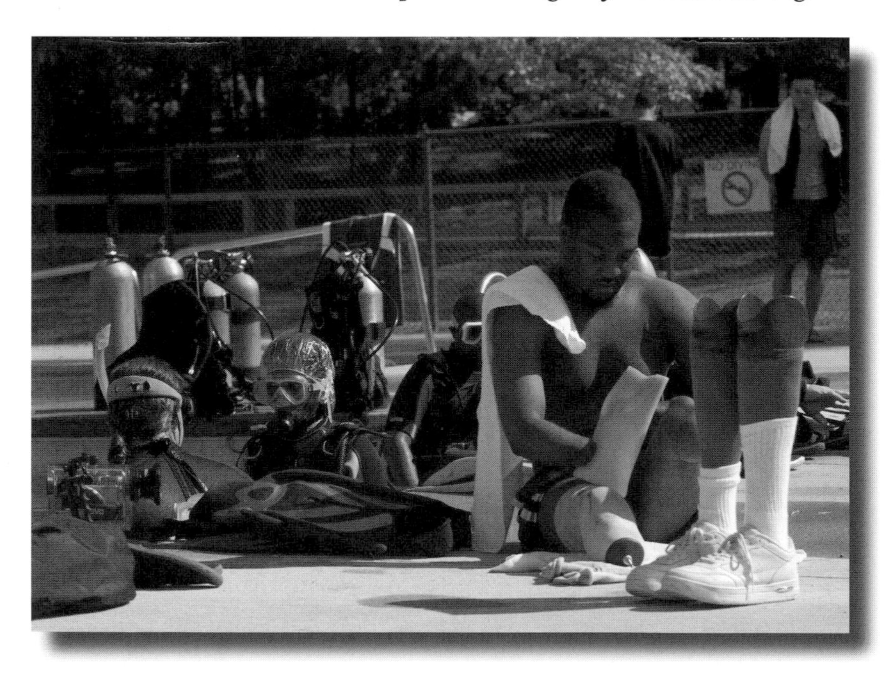

Epilogue

A Message from Brandon

"shot six times . . . n i ask mi self were i go from then 2 now. n i say God seen da best and me, wen everone eles around me, can only see da worst n me, but i still say u can only live for today nt 2morrow. we r liven n the lasts day of ur life . . . so choose tem wildless!!!!! man u when believe how this maid me a stronger person!!! so anything is possble!!! N the faith of the lord. yes. but am nt perfect either. I still go threw trails n tribulations, but love da ones who hate u!!!! luv yall!!! qouta frm brandon"

Looking in the Mirror

Michael E. Stephens

On the facing page is a text message I received on my phone from Brandon Alexander. I had just met Brandon, his mother, uncle, and grandmother in the front of the Lakeshore Foundation Building. It was Brandon's first day at Lakeshore, and he was to start his programs that would give him back as much movement as possible after being left a quadriplegic from the six bullets he encountered on the streets of Birmingham.

The effort it took for Brandon to write the message with severely limited hands reflects his determination. Such desire, supported by the Spirit of Lakeshore, will ensure his success.

No, not a success walking again as Brandon desires, but a success that many never experience in life: true inner strength! This is what will be needed to overcome the many obstacles he will face in his future. Based on the more than 40 years that I have been associated with rehabilitation, I can assure Brandon that, with strong commitment and hard work, he may attain the ultimate success sought by most humans: sincere happiness through the "peace with self" brought by inner strength. I have seen it happen with so many individuals who have physical limitations.

One such individual is the one I face in the mirror each morning—one radiating joy from within. And, yes, my joy from within has only come in recent years. For those of my distant past who doubt it, as they remember my "street fighter" attitude, simply ask for a testimony from those who are close to me now. At long last, my spiritual self has sifted through the assets and ashes brought by an excess of successes and tragedies.

Following some health crises of my own in recent years—including accidents that resulted in serious injuries, and a close brush with death—I am healthy now. Nevertheless, I am in a wheelchair, an experience from which I have gleaned much insight.

THE QUESTION IN most people's minds is how I ever managed to walk again, and to continue walking for decades, following a 1970 swimming-pool accident in which I suffered a spinal cord injury at the base of my neck. The cord was bruised and not cut, which left me temporarily paralyzed, with residual weakness in the torso and legs. Many of the medical personnel who served in my recovery felt I was able to walk again by sheer determination.

Indeed, I was determined! Just as many are after an injury or illness leaves them without what was normal to them before. Prior to my accident, so much of my life had been based on the physical being, and to lose the physical from the shoulders down was devastating! My life up to 1970 had depended on what I could do physically, and that was what I felt made me worthy of acceptance by others. More important, after I became executive director of Lakeshore Hospital in the mid-1970s, I truly believed that success for the Lakeshore rehabilitation campus had to come with me on my feet!

And on my feet was not an easy feat. Over the years, the lack of strength in my body caused a number of falls and other embarrassing moments. Still, I felt I had to look at those in my path eye to eye, to stand to intimidate, and to give the impression that I had escaped the "wheels by my hips" and could move on! However, it was always obvious that I couldn't stop looking over my shoulder at those struggling behind me.

From the mid-1970s on into the early years of the 21st century, so many associated with rehabilitation advised me to use a wheelchair so my quality of life would improve, and I now find they were right. But in the 1970s and 1980s we didn't have laws like the Americans with Disabilities Act that improved accessibility. My work for Lakeshore required stepping up and down a great number of curbs and climbing many stairs in large cities such as Washington, London, New York, and San Francisco. There were times during those challenging, politically charged years when I felt I was doing much more than confronting curbs and steps; I felt that I indeed was "jumping through hoops."

Now, from a wheelchair, I see things that I previously missed in my journey of life from the time I was injured going forward. Most important: It is the responsibility of the occupant of the wheelchair to "make it disappear." Most start their new lives in a wheelchair by feeling inhibited, and that is reinforced by those they encounter; because the average able-bodied person is at a loss as to how to interact with a person in the wheelchair. The wheelchair person needs to break through the barrier by strongly presenting his or her personality, so that all will see the individual and be distracted from the wheelchair.

Here's a most positive revelation: The protocol in assisting one with a disability is not to offer, but wait to be asked. At the same time, when I have been quizzed by friends as to whether it offends me when people rush to open doors or to take my wheelchair and place it in my car, I always respond with a delighted "No." It actually restores my faith in society to observe such kindness in an era when we hear so much about how uncaring Americans have become.

Although conducting many of my activities in a wheelchair has brought some positive things into my life, I will continue to exercise and strive to walk once again to the extent that I can. Yet it is apparent that I will always have to depend on a wheelchair to some degree, and I am very comfortable with that.

MY CLOSE CALL with death and my subsequent recovery revealed great insights of self. That illness isolated me from the mainstream and turned off the spotlight that had been shining on me. The situation placed me in a position in which I felt that I was unable to "earn" others' love. Those who remained around me gave their unconditional love and support; and I learned that, indeed, love is a gift. Their love allowed me to love the person I am and to find a spiritual place in this world.

While always following God's lead, I had continued to live my life mainly in a physical sense and now found that I was missing the part that made life beautiful: I didn't feel the fulfillment of the true spiritual. In the race of my career, the battles I had encountered, and "coasting" after the mid-1990s sale of the ReLife rehabilitation company I had founded, I somehow had escaped the Spirit that others had found at Lakeshore.

So much importance is placed, by society, on the physical that we lose sight of the individuals we are destined to be.

In what seems to be a cruel fate, those who are stripped of physical wholeness (stripped of some movement or some function of the body) often are motivated to look closer at the mind and, in the process, discover the true spiritual self.

It is said that the body is God's holy temple, and that belief guides us to serve and reward the body. But if you ask one to point to his or her temple, a person likely will place a finger to the head—the mind.

So, who we really are is simply residing in the mind, not in the heart nor in the loins. The more one fights that and tries to be something else, the less successful he or she will be in life.

Prior to my 1970 accident, my career of choice was sales. Although I worked hard to be successful, I found myself falling short—not materially but in self-fulfillment. However, it was only after I lay paralyzed in a hospital bed that I confronted that I was not truly happy with my career. I began to think there had to be a choice of life's work that was more "me."

Following my accident, I reflected deeply on the career I had at the time and realized that what I mainly enjoyed about my sales job was my interaction with hospital administrators in providing them with legal publications. I found their profession to be very challenging. These hospital administrators were in charge of a business that operated around the clock, seven days a week; they interacted with all educational levels; and, in the process, they were responsible for an enterprise that was dealing with our most precious commodity, human life. I could not think of a more exciting challenge.

So, upon the completion of my rehabilitation, the new direction of my career would be in healthcare administration. Part of the requirements for receiving my master's degree in health administration was to serve a one-year residency, and I did so with one of the nation's fastest-growing, most progressive private healthcare systems, based in my home city of Birmingham, Alabama. That system allowed me to experience a wide range of healthcare management, and I found that my talent was in building and developing systems and approaches, not in managing ongoing operations.

Although I sought out healthcare administration, I never specifically sought out the rehabilitation component. It sought me out, and I am glad.

After spending almost a quarter of a century in the rehabilitation industry, I knew in the mid-1990s that it was time for my career to transition when ReLife was sold.

A lot of water had gone under the bridge since I was first introduced to the rehabilitation field as a patient. A decade and a half after my injury occurred, while I was leading Lakeshore's parent company, I was proud I had the opportunity to establish the Lakeshore Foundation that would be devoted to sports, recreation, and fitness programs for those with physical disabilities. A few years down the road, while I was at the helm of the multistate ReLife rehabilitation company, I was proud that Lakeshore Hospital was ReLife's flagship hospital, and that both the hospital and ReLife created what became the phenomenal growth of the Lakeshore Foundation.

When I changed the direction of my career in the mid-1990s, it was with a feeling that I had no more to build or develop. By that time, Lakeshore Foundation was, as it is today, in the hands of one who possesses great talents in managing ongoing operations, Jeff Underwood.

I thus had ended that phase of my career, content in knowing that I had found my true career—that I had placed myself in a profession where I could have ultimate success and also where the results could positively touch the lives of many.

HAD IT NOT been for my life-changing accident in 1970, would I ever have found my true career, my true self, my true peace? Of course, I can't answer that. But before 1970, I felt no direction.

While I worked with Anita Smith on this book, time and again I found myself speaking aloud this goal: It is my hope that through the pages of this book many readers—able-bodied as well as those with physical limitations—will learn lessons that will help them discover who they really are and assist them in overcoming any adversity.

In these pages I have shared some of the soul-searching I did in my journey in the hope it will serve as an inspiration to others, both disabled and able-bodied, to do some soul-searching of their own—to find their true selves, their true missions in life.

Trust that in the mystery of the brain resides our destiny and spirit, and, if we can escape its clutter of impressions, we may find our places in society. We have heard such advice before: Those approaching it from platforms of religious belief might call it "God's Plan." Naturalists might call it "getting in tune with nature." Others might simply call it "your fate."

Regardless of terminology, when one is on the right path toward finding and living true self, he or she can sense that the direction is correct and, along the way, can feel a periodic reassuring pull, nudge, or push. Unfortunately, such is not the reality of life for many; with so many choices to pick from, all too many take the wrong paths.

Although it might seem a harsh observance, some of the most successful Lakeshore Foundation "graduates" likely have been focused because they have been dealt limited choices. Limited choices combined with a nurturing environment (Lakeshore) led to successes.

Most served by Lakeshore have had so many choices taken away from them due to disease, illness, or accident. At the same time, at Lakeshore they find themselves in an environment where they are not distracted and can focus on inner self. Those who really succeed tend to be the more independent ones who realize that Lakeshore is an entity that functions to support them in their journey—not to take care of them, but to support them.

ONE DAY IN our early discussions about this book, its author, an experienced medical reporter, posed a probing question to me: "Why has the Lakeshore rehabilitation campus survived while so many entities on similar paths have failed?"

I believe the following can afford some context and answers: A strong base was laid in the 1970s and 1980s for the building and developing of Lakeshore—a durable base that allowed for the evolving superstructure we see today. The guidance and support of those who, since that early period, have taken part in Lakeshore's development, and who have been served by Lakeshore's development, also have fostered Lakeshore's future. The continuing successes of those who work at Lakeshore and are served by Lakeshore—and the lessons derived from the failures as well—continue to perpetuate the Spirit found there. Simply, Lakeshore's respected reputation is the result of a continuing desire of all involved to follow Lakeshore's core culture.

It always has been the Lakeshore goal that no one's dream of spirit would be ignored when he or she traveled along Lakeshore's path. That has applied even to those who have traveled many paths and who shared only a brief time on the Lakeshore path. Lakeshore's development has been influenced by the dreams of many; Lakeshore's spirit has been developed and expanded by the contributions of many. That includes even a number who felt they were not successful. I am grateful to ALL who have made a constructive contribution.

AS I LOOK back on my years with Lakeshore, the road is marked with many milestones. In looking forward, the road is endless. In the distance, there are many challenges. Those challenges also stand as opportunities.

One mission is for Lakeshore Foundation to continue and also broaden its service to our men and women from the military who are returning from service, often from war, with devastating injuries.

The task at hand is to harness the power of recreation, sports, and fitness to help those who, while wearing the uniform of an American military branch of service, have sustained debilitating injuries, often compounded by the aftermath of post traumatic stress disorder. In this mission, Lakeshore Foundation is tackling what I feel is likely the most powerful ongoing challenge that has ever existed in the history of the rehabilitation industry's service to mankind. That challenge is to support injured military personnel in their reintroduction into their home environments, to help them to again interface successfully with their families and with society.

Another Lakeshore Foundation challenge is to use recreation, sports, and fitness to address some of the gaps and pitfalls that are created in today's world. It is a modern world in which a combination of longevity, a more crowded and complicated civilization, and, yes, even the marvels of modern medicine have set the stage for more individuals to survive to confront the ravages of disease, illness, accidents, violence, and resulting disability.

Because of the leadership that Lakeshore Foundation has taken in what some refer to as "disabled sport," the Foundation continues to have a major role to play in pushing for the Paralympian athlete to receive equal accolades to that of the Olympian. Part of that mission is to demonstrate to powerful sports oversight bodies such as the National Collegiate Athletic Association (NCAA) why they should take bigger steps forward in recognizing and supporting competitive sports that embrace those with physical disabilities.

And, all along the way, Lakeshore Foundation retains the charge to continue to provide an environment where "my people" (both staff and clients) may pursue their dreams and not feel they are in the way of others.

I THANK MY God for using me as his crusader for the implementation of Lakeshore's mission. To see the international rehabilitation paradigm completely change for the positive during the course of my career has been fulfilling. Further, to see the dramatic impact that Lakeshore

Foundation has made and continues to make on that rehabilitation paradigm and on human life is both humbling and a source of great pride for me.

Gaining steam in the 1970s, healthcare in America experienced a great growth. During that time, healthcare became a large, profitable business; and rehabilitation services were sucked into the vacuum of growth.

That growth period in many ways became very controversial. However, the changes during that period were good for those in need of rehabilitation; and the Lakeshore rehabilitation campus was at the pinnacle of the changing environment for the severely physically disabled.

Many factors came together for the "perfect storm" to make Lakeshore succeed and continue to succeed. First there was the excellent timing of its development. Then there were the impacts of Lakeshore's comprehensive master plan, its gradual access to a sustainable funding base, and its location on a campus that had, and continues to have, so much potential. Too, of utmost relevance has been the leadership over the years of an outstanding board of directors, without whose support the Lakeshore success would not have come to pass.

Perhaps on an ongoing basis the most important factor laying the groundwork for Lakeshore success, and sustaining that success, has been its staff.

In the early days of Lakeshore's 1970s and 1980s development, a very diverse group of individuals, core leaders, and staff members came together, unbound by a traditional past. These individuals were attracted to staff an environment where they could see that their caring and hard work would have immediate results.

Lakeshore from the beginning was blessed with staff members who had strong personalities. I must say, a diverse group of individuals is an understatement! Those personalities, combined with the sometimes seemingly "stranger than life" situations and challenges they faced, actually led to a number of comical situations—many of which at the time did not appear comical.

In fact, the fast-paced and, I must say, unique environment on the

Lakeshore campus was so ripe with color and action that Lakeshore management and activities became the subject of a cartoon strip that ReLife executive Steve Bates created. A sampling of Steve's "real-life" cartoon characters: (1) Dr. George Traugh, our outspoken medical director, who was well known for his work in rehabilitation research and who had become high profile while serving as Governor George C. Wallace's rehabilitation physician. (2) Dr. Frank McArthur, our bright, rebellious young doctor in charge of acute medical services. (3) Rosie Durham, who, as a Lakeshore administrator, became the first top female hospital administrator in the Birmingham area, ultimately rising successfully through management positions at both Lakeshore and the hospital system operated by the University of Alabama at Birmingham. And, (4) Yours Truly. Although this Lakeshore-inspired cartoon strip never made it to syndication on the comic pages, publication-agency representatives found it interesting enough that Steve's concept went through several stages of consideration in Atlanta and New York.

I include this little anecdote to point out that Lakeshore certainly is not your run-of-the-mill place today, and that it didn't start out that way. The creative, devoted staff members who gathered at Lakeshore in the early years were each respected for his or her expertise and dedication. As a group, they were given a work environment where all would be heard and where most were challenged by other members of the team.

One truly grows in uncomfortable situations; and the bright, diverse staff from Lakeshore's early days certainly provided those situations. Feeding this atmosphere charged with frequent discomfort were the rapid growth of the campus and the resulting opportunities that presented themselves in ways in which all had to think on their feet. The staff's conflicts, challenging resolutions, and ultimate cooperation created a synergy that benefited Lakeshore and its clients.

THAT SAME DYNAMIC, changing environment continues to exist today at the Lakeshore Foundation.

As an example, I want to comment on a pivotal process—a strategic planning process—that unfolded at Lakeshore Foundation in late 2011.

This strategic planning, to create Lakeshore Foundation's latest long-range plan, involved joint meetings of Lakeshore's board, management, and staff. Candor, at times uncomfortable candor, was used by all as they gave their perspectives of how to best serve the Lakeshore Foundation family in the future. Each participant had his or her own view in terms of how to serve—often through additional equipment, space, and services. But, even with the great assets Lakeshore Foundation has today, it was of course impossible to approve all requests, presentations, and plans. As always, choices had to be made, often difficult choices. And, fortunately, as in Lakeshore's past, synergy prevailed.

The course taken by the planning process molded the team into a stronger organization. The candor used by all throughout the process led to transparency that relieved the fears and anxieties of most who experienced these concerns. I believe that the exercise will lead to more effective communication for all involved with Lakeshore.

With the new Strategic Plan now in the hands of Lakeshore Foundation's current team, I have faith that the plan will continue to fuel a sophisticated culture that will take growth and challenges in stride and continue to generate good things.

As this process went forward, it was always clear that, as in the past, there was no way to discuss one part of Lakeshore's development without discussing the other parts. There is always that overlapping, that mutual feeding—of one program to another, of one group of staff members and clients to another, of one goal to another.

For example, both the new research efforts the Foundation is launching and the continued provision of services to disabled veterans will enhance another longstanding Lakeshore Foundation focus—the training of Paralympians. Still very much a part of the Lakeshore Strategic Plan, these unique Paralympic athletes represent what the soaring human spirit can do when it is supported properly. They serve as pride and inspiration for all with physical limitations. They reflect that they are citizens of successful countries that have their priorities and foundations in place.

THE LATEST LAKESHORE Foundation long-range plan that has emerged includes the embarking on a unique approach to rehabilitation research.

In recognition of the fact that Lakeshore Foundation has achieved outcomes not found elsewhere in the world, data will be analyzed and tested to validate successful outcomes of those served by the Foundation.

In a structure designed to serve this research, Lakeshore Foundation has endowed a Chair for Rehabilitation Research (which recruited the best in his field of research, Dr. James Rimmer) at the School of

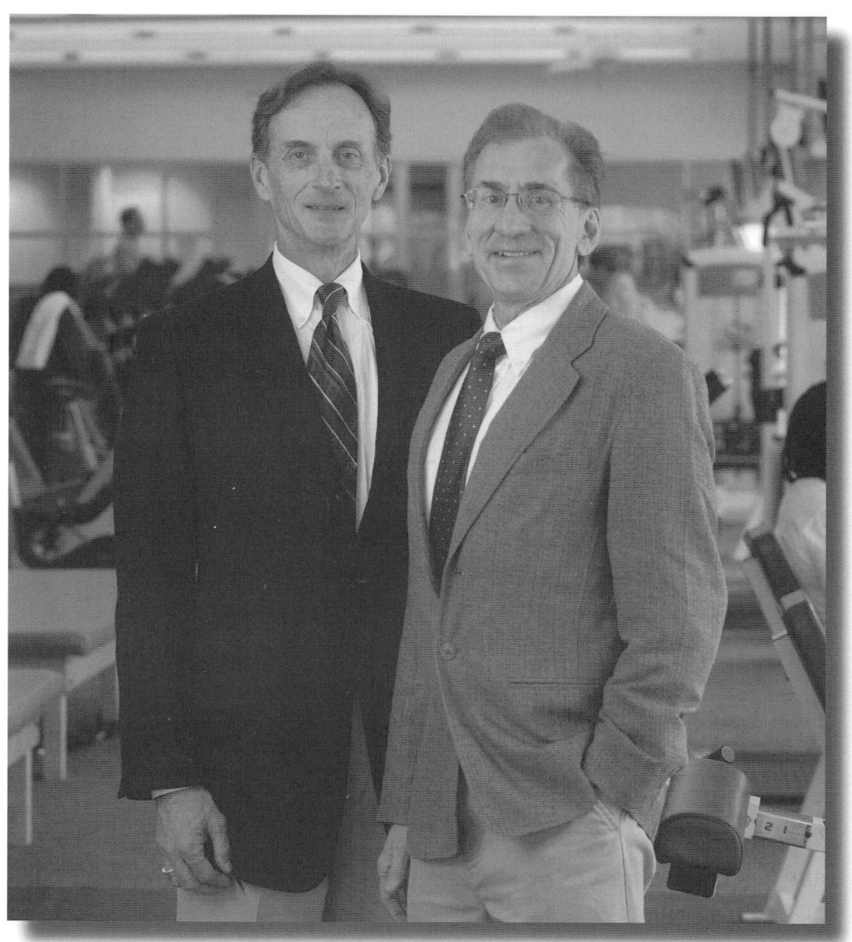

Lakeshore Foundation President Jeff Underwood and Dr. James Rimmer, the Foundation's rehabilitation research medical director.

Health Professions at the University of Alabama at Birmingham (UAB), with the leadership of its dean, Dr. Harold K. Jones. As a crucial part of this Lakeshore Foundation teaming with UAB, the initiative calls for the professor who is appointed to the Chair at UAB to serve also as rehabilitation research medical director at Lakeshore Foundation.

Goals driving the initiative call for outcomes and protocols to be published for use throughout the world. These outcomes and protocols all relate to the good that can be accomplished for those with physical disabilities by putting to use programs of sports, recreation, and fitness and the social structures they provide.

This is an initiative that will bring out the best of all worlds from the cooperation of many. We will be engaging Lakeshore Foundation staff in cooperation with those who represent UAB entities—including, among others, Spain Rehabilitation Center, the School of Engineering, and, in the School of Health Professions, the departments of Physical Therapy, Occupational Therapy, and Nutrition Sciences.

Through this endeavor it is our hope that the resources found in the Lakeshore Foundation's staff and clients will make lasting contributions to the ever-evolving betterment of lives for the physically disabled.

Lakeshore has reached a new plateau with its plan for the future. Building a path for the progress of mankind is never smooth; so many obstacles are encountered. And the greatest challenge is passing the well-traveled paths that cross your own.

But, as I look back at Lakeshore's path over the decades, I see a path that has become both smoother and wider because of the number of those who through the years have chosen to take this path and have traveled it well.

And, like all well-beaten paths in societies, it has become a roadway for the greater number that will follow.

Jeff Underwood's leadership as Lakeshore Foundation's president is solid and what Lakeshore needs at this time.

As I indicated previously in this Epilogue, I have always believed that my own management strength has been mainly to build and develop, while Jeff's strength is managing operations with political skills.

It is strange how fate has always shaped Lakeshore's future, and Jeff's bout with life-threatening cancer is yet another example. That life-altering experience impacted Jeff in ways that I feel will strengthen and aid him as he leads Lakeshore Foundation into the future.

It is my belief that, as a result of his battle with cancer, Jeff now has a stronger inner strength and is revealing more of his good qualities because of the increased confidence he has in himself.

I AM EXCITED about Lakeshore's future. The topflight team is in place with plan in hand. Looking forward now, I can always see the road disappearing in the distance. I often wonder what challenges are ahead after those at Lakeshore accomplish this current plan. Regardless of the challenges, I know they can handle them; for they know it is their responsibility to foster the Spirit that brought the successes of today.

The confidence of my belief comes partly from an inspiring message to which I was exposed during the time the cornerstone of my career with Lakeshore was being laid, in the spring of 1976.

During my visit then to the renowned New Jersey-based Kessler Institute for Rehabilitation, I was given a book, *The Knife Is Not Enough*, written by the Institute's founder, Dr. Henry H. Kessler. An orthopedic surgeon, Dr. Kessler was a pioneer in physical rehabilitation, putting his theories to use both in the United States and in other parts of the world.

On the first page of the Introduction of his book appeared words from Dr. Kessler that were so powerful they continually guided me in the proper direction—leading me to the Spirit still found at Lakeshore today.

These are some of Dr. Kessler's words that touched me so deeply: "The rehabilitation idea has taught me that there is a miraculous biological safety factor in every human being. Resources that lie dormant can be called upon to remold a personality physically and mentally. I have learned also that there is a safety factor for civilization. It is that powerful fraternity of men and women who believe that 'the object of all help is to make help superfluous.' "

Looking back at what has been built at Lakeshore, I can say those words of Dr. Kessler could well serve as a keystone.

During a 1970s period when I was being interviewed by Anita Smith, then the medical reporter for the *Birmingham News*, she talked to me about "human interest" stories. As it applied to Lakeshore, Anita told me that stories about Lakeshore should include personal insights about me to engage the reader with a "human interest."

Similarly, during recent times when Anita has been gathering information for this book, one day she told Jeff Underwood that a part of the book would be devoted to telling of the personal journey taken by Lakeshore Foundation's founder—me. Jeff expressed his delight to Anita, telling her that he thought it wise and relevant to include details of my journey in the book, explaining, "People are always wanting details about Mike Stephens."

While I agreed to share details of my personal journey, I know that Lakeshore is and always has been the core story and that I have served Lakeshore simply as an instrument.

I chose to share my life with the reader in the body of this book and my thoughts in this Epilogue for two reasons:

First, to show from whence I came to overcome obstacles to benefit my chosen part of mankind and lead it to a better good. (All readers may do so, in their own ways, by always serving something greater than themselves.)

The second reason was to reveal the truth of where my heart was and is. My journey has made me a man with a terse, rough exterior. I needed the exterior mostly to survive (as in "street fighter mentality"), to clear my path quickly and not to be distracted along its way. I never wanted to expose my soft underbelly and reveal the emotional wounds of some of the experiences shared in this book which I suffered silently. As a result, many have judged me by my cover, and sadly that is something that one carries to the grave. But it was a sacrifice I gladly made!

I SHUDDER TO think of how I will remember in the future those many additional people, and things as well, that are worthy of inclusion in

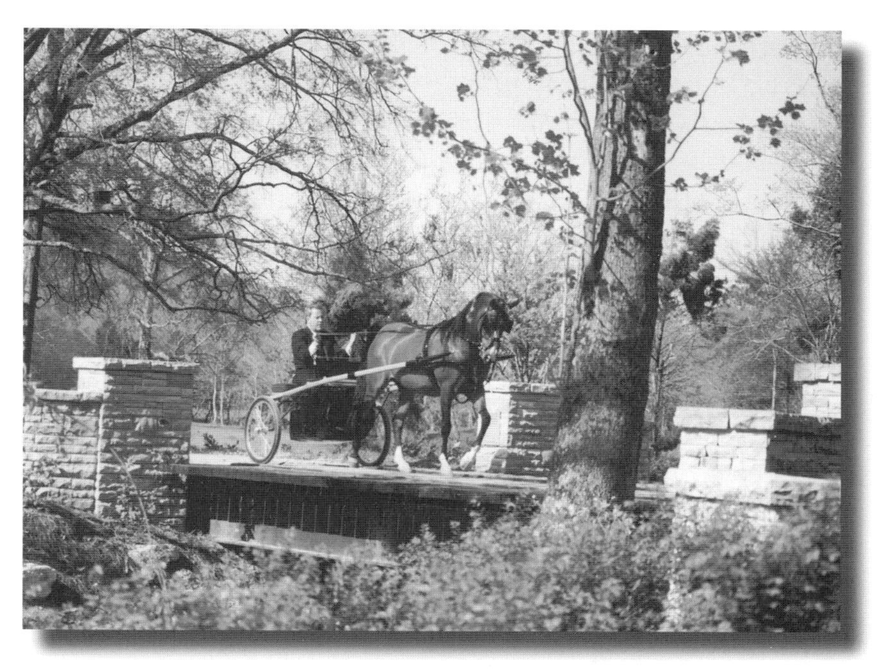

Mike Stephens, getting some fresh air while doing a little cart driving training—and, in the Lakeshore way, simultaneously building his core strength through horsemanship—on a nice morning at his farm south of Birmingham.

this book. Some of those individuals and things that are included stand to represent many others, for there are so many that added a portion of the Lakeshore Spirit.

Over time, those who have been and/or will be touched by the Lakeshore Spirit in one way or another will be noticed (and sometimes envied) by members of our society, because of the desire of others to experience this Spirit. Once touched by this Spirit, one carries the positive feelings for life.

For example, a lady who worked very successfully for Lakeshore beginning in the 1990s, in areas of fitness, coaching, and management, was unknown to me when I started working on this book. She, Allison Morrow, has since brought her experience and her portion of Spirit to provide what was needed for my inner peace.

Early in my rehabilitation following my 1970 injury, I acquired inner strength. However, my journey for inner peace was long and hard. In the 1970s, I felt it was my call of fate not to have inner peace. If I had felt inner peace during that period, I seriously doubt that I could have led Lakeshore to the successes that came to pass.

During my more recent adversities, Allison provided for me what the Lakeshore family provided for those you have read about in this book. Although I had always been aware of the Spirit, until Allison, I had never been touched by it.

My own search for contentment is now complete, and I am pleased to think of how the Lakeshore Spirit will go on to serve the future without me.

The ending of my journey means the end of this book. It is an honor to be included in having built something that will help mankind as long as the Lakeshore Spirit prevails.

At the same time, I am truly sorry for those who passed our way when we were not strong enough to support them.

I love you, Millie Ragland, and I feel your presence with each visit to Lakeshore.